Forensic and Legal Dentistry

Klaus Rötzscher
Editor

Forensic and Legal Dentistry

Springer

Editor
Klaus Rötzscher, Dr. med. Dr. med. dent.
German Academy of Forensic
Odontostomatology (AKFOS)
Speyer
Germany

ISBN 978-3-319-34605-2 ISBN 978-3-319-01330-5 (eBook)
DOI 10.1007/978-3-319-01330-5
Springer Cham Heidelberg New York Dordrecht London

Printed on acid-free paper

Springer is part of Springer Science+Business Media (www.springer.com)

Preface

The need for legal knowledge in the contractual relationship between dentist and patient and knowledge of the legal procedure in civil and criminal law, particularly in the dental field, is increasing. This legal knowledge will help both to minimize personal insecurity and assess the personal position realistically and to interpret medical facts as an expert witness; this is imperative for all parties because of the increasing number of liability cases.

Age estimation and the identification of living/dead persons, together with forensic medicine, the courts, and the police, may improve the recording of dental findings and their documentation.

The review of bite and tooth marks, which has not been properly regarded in German specialist literature so far and which has often not been recognized in daily practice, is supposed to help to disclose the estimated number of unreported cases of maltreatment (particularly, cruelty to children) and, in homicides, to convict a criminal or to exonerate an innocent person.

The medical history of the patient's survey and the survey of the clinical findings by means of various diagnostic measures are part of the treatment contract. The patient's education (including education about the diagnosis, treatment, alternative options, the value and impact of the forecast, the risks, resulting costs, and also non-treatment) only lead to a treatment if the patient consents. Therefore, the dental, oral, and maxillofacial surgery supports the regular development, preservation, and rehabilitation of the stomatognathic system.

On 29 October 1976, during the 102nd annual meeting of the German Society for Dental, Oral and Maxillofacial Surgery in the Mozart Hall of Stuttgart, under the auspices of Professor Werner Hahn, the Working Group (now the German Academy of Forensic Odontostomatology) was established. Extensive legal treatises on the relationship between dentist and patient from the legal perspective already exist, as well as judiciary collections in medical and dental law, which provide insight to court decisions in various instances.

This book is addressed to doctors and dentists, forensic scientists, lawyers, investigative and identification authorities, criminologists, prosecutors, insurance agents, and the students of those disciplines.

In the legal section, the reader shall be informed about the risks of dental treatment and the relationship with the patient, which may extend to liability risks. The legal relationships from the perspective of the dentist (from practice to the practice) are discussed, along with the medical connections on the basis of the treatment, which might cause legal complications imposed by civil and penal law. The insight into relevant legal questions shall help to reduce existing uncertainties and to enable to an assessment of the situation that is more realistic.

Finally, I present my highest appreciation and thanks to all coauthors, and to Mrs. Christina Neitsch (script control) and Mr. Siegmar Klose (IT assistant) for their participation in enabling this book to be published.

Speyer, Germany Klaus Rötzscher, Dr. med. Dr. med. dent.

Contents

Contributors

Herman Bernitz, BChD, MSc, Dip Odont, PhD (Pret) Department of Oral Pathology and Oral Biology, School of Dentistry, University of Pretoria, Pretoria, South Africa

Charles Georget, DDS University of Nancy, Nancy, France

Joseph P. Graskemper, DDS, JD, DABMM Stony Brook School of Dental Medicine, Stony Brook, NY, USA

Claus Grundmann, Dr. med. Dr. med. dent. Municipal Medical-Superviser, Duisburg (North-Rhine-Westphalia), Germany

James Hardy, OStJ, BDS (Lon), MSc, MGDSRCS (Eng), MGDSRCS (Ed), LDSRCS (Eng), Dip F Od, Dip FHID Criminology Department, Portsmouth University, Portsmouth, UK

Oscar Heit, Prof. Dr. Faculty of Science and Technology, University Autonomous of Entre Ríos, Paraná, Entre Ríos, Argentina

Ian R. Hill, OBE, MA, MD, PhD, MRCPath, FFFLM, MRAeS, LDS International Organisation for Forensic Odontostomatology – IOFOS, London, UK

Jean-Marc Hutt, Dr. med. dent. (Strasbourg), Dr. for. sciences (Nancy), Association Française d´Identification Odontologique (AFIO) Private Practitioner, Strasbourg, France

Bernhard Knell, Dr. med. dent. Forensic Odontostomatology, Institute of Forensic Medicine, University of Zurich, Zurich, Switzerland

Forensic Dentistry, Center for Dental Medicine, University of Zurich, Zurich, Switzerland

Russell Lain, Dr. Department of Oral Surgery and Diagnostic Imaging, Sydney Dental Hospital, Surry Hills, NSW, Australia

Dieter Leopold, Univ.-Prof. (em) Dr. med. Institute of Legal Medicine, Leipzig, Germany

Hannu Mäkelä, DDS, PhD LtCol res Finnish Air Force MC, Muurame, Finnland

William O'Reilly, Ass. Prof. Department of Oral Health, School of Health Sciences, University of Newcastle, Ourimbah, NSW, Australia

Wolfgang Pilz, Univ.- Prof. (em) Dr. med. dent. Department of Preservative and Pediatric Stomatology, Academy Carl Gustav Carus, Dresden, Germany

Klaus Rötzscher, Dr. med. Dr. med. dent. German Academy of Forensic Odontostomatology (AKFOS), Speyer, Germany

Peter Sahelangi, Dr. DFM Department of Forensic and Medico- Legal Faculty of Medicine, Hasanuddin University, Makassar, Indonesia

Günter Seifert, Dr. med. dent. Orthodontist, Berchtesgaden, Germany

Rolf Singer, Univ.-Prof. (em) Dr. med. Dr. med. dent. Department of Oral and Craniomandibular Surgery, Clinicum Ludwigshafen/Rhein, Ludwigshafen/Rhein, Germany

Tore Solheim, Prof. (em) Dr. odont. Institute of Oral Biology, Pathology and Forensic Odontology, University Oslo, Oslo, Norway

Jane Taylor, Ass. Prof. Department of Oral Health, School of Health Sciences, University of Newcastle, Ourimbah, NSW, Australia

Eddy de Valck, DDS Forensic Odontologist, DVI Team Belgium, Beigem, Belgium

Yvo Vermylen, Master of Law Department of Dentistry, Katholicke University Leuven, Leuven, Belgium

Puisqu' on ne peut être universel et savoir tout
ce qui peut se savoir sur tout, il faut savoir peu de tout.
Car il est bien plus beau de savoir quelque chose de tout
que de savoir tout d'une chose.

[Since you cannot be universal and cannot know everything,
you should know a little about everything.
It is probably better to know a little of everything
than knowing everything about one thing.]

*(Blaise Pascal, *19.6.1623 in Clermont-Ferrand, Auvergne – † 19.8.1662 in Paris;*
Pensées sur l esprit XXXVII, in: Pensées, Pensée 42 (49).
Bibliotheque de la Pléiade, ed. Galimard, Paris, 1954, pp 1098–1099)

Abbreviations

AAFS	American Academy of Forensic Sciences
ADA	American Dental Association
AFG	Study Group for Basic Research
AFIO	Association Française d'Identification Odontologique
AG	District Court
AG	Study Group
AGB	Terms and Conditions
AGBG	Law Governing the Right of the General Terms and Conditions
AHA	American Heart Association
AK	Working Group
AKFOS	German Academy of Forensic Odontostomatology
AMG	Drug Law
AOZ (Appro-Z)	Licensing Regulations for Dentists
ArztR	Medical Law (magazine)
ASFO	American Society of Forensic Odontology
AsylVfG	Asylum Procedure Act
AuslG	Aliens Act
AZ.	Reference Number
BAFO	British Association for Forensic Odontology
BAG	Federal Labour Court
BÄK	Federal Chamber of Physicians
BDZ (BdZ)	Federal Association of German Dentists (BegleitG) Support Law
BegleitG	Support Law
Bema	Rating Scale Funds for Physicians' Services
Bema-Z	Rating Scale Funds for Dental Services
BfArM	Federal Institute for Drugs and Medical Devices
BfS	Federal Office for Radiation Protection
BGA	Federal Health Office (now Federal Institute for Drugs and Medical Devices)
BGB	Civil Code
BGE	Federal Court Decisions
BGBl	Federal Law Gazette
BGH	Federal Supreme Court
BGHZ	Federal Supreme Court in Civil Affairs: Decisions
BKA	Federal Crime Office

BMG	Federal Ministry of Health
BMV-Z	Federal Contract for Dentists
BO	Professional Regulation for Physicians
BO-Z	Professional Code for Dentists
BSG	Federal Social Court
BSGE	Federal Social Court: Decisions
BuGO-Z	see GOZ
BverfG	Federal Constitutional Court
BVerfGE	Federal Constitutional Court: Decisions
BVerwG	Federal Administrative Court
BVerwGE	Federal Administrative Court: Decisions
Bw	Bundeswehr (Armed Forces)
BZÄK	Federal Dental Association
BZK	District Dental Association Surgery
Chir	Surgery
DBG	The Federal Court of Germany
DGAI	German Society for Anaesthesiology and Intensive Care
DGI	German Society for Implantology
DGKFo	German Society of Orthodontics
DGP	German Society of Periodontology
DGRM	German Society of Legal Medicine
DGZ	German Society for Conservative Dentistry
DGZMK	German Society for Dental, Oral and Maxillofacial Surgery
DGZPW	German Society for Prosthodontics and Materials
DHZB	German Heart Centre Berlin
DVI	Disaster Victim Identification
DZW	The Dentist Week (magazine)
DZZ	German Dental Journal (organ DGZMK)
EC	European Community
EK	Spare Cash
EK-V	Spare Cash Contract
EU	European Union
EWG	European Economic Community
FBI	Federal Bureau of Crime Investigation (USA)
FDI	Fédération Dentaire International
FKO	Functional Orthopedics
FO	Forensic Odontology
FOCH	The Swiss Group of Forensic Odontology
FOS	Forensic Odontostomatology
FVDZ	Free Association of German Dentists
GBI	Law Gazette
GDzh	Directorate of Health Canton Zurich
GesG	Health Act
GewO	Trade Regulation
GG	Basic Law
GKK	Statutory Health Fund
GKV	Statutory Health Insurance
GOÄ	Schedule of Fees for Doctors

GOZ	Schedule of Fees for Dentists
GZHeilk	Law on the Exercise of Dentistry (see ZHG)
IADR	International Association for Dental Research
IANC	International Anatomical Nomenclature Committee
ICAO	International Civil Aviation Organization
ICD-DA	International Code of Diseases of Dentistry and Stomatology
ICD-0	International Classification of Diseases for Oncology
ICPO	International Criminal Police Organization (see Interpol)
ICRP	International Commission on Radiological Protection
IDKO	Identification Commission
IDKO BKA	Identification Commission at the Federal Bureau of Crime Investigation
IDZ	Institute of German Dentists Interpol International Criminal Police Organization
Interpol	International Criminal Police Organization
IOFOS	International Organization for Forensic Odontostomatology
ISO	International Organization for Standardization
JGG	Youth Courts Act
KatS-Kalender	Disaster Safety Calendar
KCH	Jaw Surgery
KfO	Orthodontics
Kons	Conservative Dentistry
KPol	Criminal Police
KZBV	Regional Dental Authorities
KZRL	Regional Dental Authorities: Guidelines
KZV	Regional Dental Association
LBA	Civil Aeronautics Board
LBG	Provincial Court (for the Medical Profession)
LG	Regional Court
LKÄ	Country State Criminal Police Offices
LSG	State Social Court
LZK	Country Dentists' Chamber
MBO-Z	Pattern Proper for Professional Dental Doctors (see BO-Z, MuBerO-Z, and MuBO-Z)
MedBG	Federal Law on Medicine
MedBV	Regulation on Medicine
MedR	Medical Law (journal)
MedSach	The Medical Examiners (magazine)
Mitt	Messages
MPG	Medical Devices Act
NL	Newsletter
MuBerO-Z	Career Pattern for Dentists (see MBO-Z)
MuBO-Z	Career Pattern for Dentists (see MBO-Z and MuBerO-Z)
NAR	Standard Committee of Radiology in the German Standards
Newsletter	Organ of the German Academy of Forensic Odontostomatology (magazine)
NJW	New Law Weekly (magazine)

NVwZ	New Journal of Administrative Law
OLG	Higher Regional Court
OR	Obligations
OVG	Higher Administrative Court (Supreme Administrative Court)
PAR	Periodontology
PHG	Product Liability Law
PKV	Private Health Insurance
Polvo	Police Regulation
PStG	Personal Status Law
RiStBV	Guidelines for Criminal and Administrative Penalties
RVO	Insurance Code
SG	Social Court
SGb	The Social Proceedings (magazine)
SGG	Social Code Act
SGRM	Swiss Society of Legal Medicine
SNOMED	Systematic Medical Nomenclature
SSFOS	Scandinavian Society of Forensic Odontostomatology
SSO	Swiss Dental Association
StGB	Criminal Code, Swiss Criminal Code
StPO	Code of Criminal Procedure
StrSchV	Radiation Protection Ordinance
StVO	Road Traffic Act
Urt.	Judgment Ruling
VerfG	Constitutional Court
VersR	Insurance Law (journal)
Vfg	Ordinance
VG (VerwG)	Administrative Court
VGH	Administrative Court
VO	Regulation
VSFZ	Association of Swiss Forensic Dentists in the Swiss Society of Legal Medicine
WHO	World Health Organization
Zschr	Journal
ZA	Dentist
ZAE	Dentists
ZAH	Dental Assistant
ZÄK (ZK)	Dental Chamber
ZHG	Dentistry Act
ZHKG	Act on the Exercise of Dentistry (see GZHeilk)
ZM	Dental Communications (magazine)
ZMF	Qualified Dental Assistant
ZMK	Dental, Oral and Maxillofacial Surgery
ZO-Z	Licensing Regulations—Dentists
ZPO	Code of Civil Procedure
ZVEG	Judicial Remuneration and Compensation Act (Law on the Compensation of Witnesses and Experts)

Introduction

In the training regulations of university courses for dentistry, there is no single reference to the field of forensic dentistry or forensic odonto-stomatology.

As a chairman of the commission on dental research, I became aware that dentists often are engaged in various fields of criminology, and I was amazed that in many countries, forensic dentistry is fully integrated to the curriculum of dental universities.

In Scandinavia, Gösta Gustafson, Gunnar Johanson, Søren Keiser-Nielsen, and Tore Solheim have been very successful in embedding forensic dentistry. In Germany, Klaus Rötzscher pointed out years ago that dentists work as research assistants in institutes of legal medicine.

It was a special pleasure for me to welcome these colleagues to the interdisciplinary working group for forensic odonto-stomatology of the German Society for Dental, Oral and Maxillofacial Surgery (founded in 1976), and the German Society of Legal Medicine.

Thanks to their energetic work and knowledge, forensic dentistry was established in the Federal Republic of Germany. This book was composed to bring together the main areas of forensic odonto-stomatology as a separate field within the forensic sciences, such as supporting identification of unknown human remains.

Therefore, I owe special thanks to Klaus Rötzscher and hope his book will find entry to dental and forensic training literature and will become an integral part of the library of every dentist.

Univ.- Prof. Dr. med. Dr. med. dent. Werner Hahn
Kiel, Germany, 2000
(† 2011)

Part I

History

1 History of Forensic and Legal Dentistry

Klaus Rötzscher

1.1 Introduction

The different terms of dentistry, dental medicine, odontology, and stomatology, imply different practical and scientific–theoretic functions. According to our requirements, modern dentistry stands for the normal development, conservation, or rehabilitation of the orofacial system. The orofacial system includes the functional system of teeth, masticatory apparatus, jaws and temporomandibular joints, masseter and facial muscles, glands, soft tissues, membranes, and their support by blood, lymph, and nerves.

A dentist is therefore not just an odontologist, but has to think and treat in terms of odontology and orthodontics. Forensic odontostomatology as a special modification of dentistry is an independent scientific branch within the forensic sciences that deliberately puts its research and methods into the service of the administration of justice (Rötzscher 1991/1).

Forensic odontostomatology is supposed to collect all of the results of odontological research to serve criminal prosecution and legal procedure. It is therefore regarded as an independent branch of science, originating from the requirements of a civilized nation's system of law and administration of justice.

K. Rötzscher, Dr. med. Dr. med. dent.
German Academy of Forensic Odontostomatology (AKFOS),
Wimphelingstraße 7, 67346 Speyer, Germany
e-mail: roetzscher.klaus.dr@t-online.de

Some aspects of forensic odontostomatology are (Keiser-Nielsen 1968):

1. Forensically assessing scientific disputes
2. Establishing certain principles that, being generally approved as correct, are supposed to serve as a standard for correct odontological practice
3. Identification of unknown bodies (dead or alive) in certain cases
4. Supporting the investigation and prosecution of crimes
5. Imparting certain juridical knowledge solely leading to an effective cooperation between dentists and the administration of justice

It is often believed that only those few odontostomatologists who serve as expert witnesses need to have some knowledge in this field. However, one must not forget that every dentist is obliged by the code of criminal procedure to be an expert witness should the situation arise. In addition, knowledge of forensic odontostomatology is advisable to avoid possible compensation claims.

1.2 Early History, Part 1

Forensic odontostomatology still lacks a systematics in teaching as well as in research and even in its practical performance. As also seen through a historical survey presented in this chapter, it seems necessary to build up forensic odontostomatology all over the world. At the same time, the forensic odontostomatologist, the forensic pathologist, the police, and the

K. Rötzscher (ed.), *Forensic and Legal Dentistry*,
DOI 10.1007/978-3-319-01330-5_1, © Springer International Publishing Switzerland 2014

public prosecutor should be given an understanding of this scientific branch. The evolution of forensic odontostomatology undisputedly depends on the development of medicine, odontology, and jurisprudence. It is a part of human cultural history. In the primitive societies of prehistoric times, affliction, the urge to help, and the community feeling of kinship marked the beginning of the art of healing. Despite their artistic work in Western Europe >20,000 years ago, cavemen and bone engravers did not record anything relating to odontology (Rötzscher 1991/2).

The hieroglyphs and pictographs of the smaller or larger slave-holding states of the Old Orient (Middle East) show, through the use of the mouth and teeth in their writing system, how much importance was given to these. The most important evidence from Old Egypt is the EDWIN-SMITH-PAPYRUS from the seventeenth century BC. In this document a dislocation of the jaw and its correct reposition are depicted. Findings of dental prostheses and tooth support are attributed to the marvels of antique metal technology and not to human medicine. There was no knowledge about forensic medicine (Breasted 1922).

Little is known about oral hygiene in Mesopotamia. There is more information on the importance of good teeth in the CODEX HAMMURABI, which was written shortly after 2000 BC for Babylonia and Assyria:

§ 200: *If anyone knocks out anyone's teeth, then his teeth shall be knocked out likewise.*

§ 201: *If he has knocked out the teeth of a freed man, then he shall pay 1/2 mine of silver.*

At least after the publication of the CODEX HAMMURABI, no surgery could be performed in Mesopotamia (Mishulin 1948).

1.2.1 Early History, Part 2

China had a culture as noteworthy as Egypt's or Mesopotamia's, which, in its turn, influenced India and Arabia. It is true that there have been books on odontology, but they have not been published (Mildner 1964). From the books on history, law, religious cults, and devotional writing in ancient Israel, one cannot expect anything serious concerning medicine or odontology in particular. And if a man smite the eye of his servant, or the eye of his maid, that it perish, he shall let him go free for his eye's sake (Mironow 1961) (Exodus 21, 24).

And if he smite out his manservant's tooth or his maidservant's tooth, he shall let him go free for his tooth sake (Exodus 21: 26–27). Jewish law, as well as Babylonian law, ranked the value of the tooth straight after the eye (Eye for eye, tooth for tooth, hand for hand, foot for foot (Exodus 21, 24 and Talmud fifth century AD)). The replaced tooth in the Talmud is treated as a cosmetic intervention under "female ornaments." The artificial tooth was made by a craftsman and had therefore nothing to do with medicine (Nobel 1909). The first denture was found in a tomb near Saida in Phoenicia, two right incisors tied together with a gold thread and fixed to the dental neck of the neighboring teeth by means of a loop of gold wire (Renan 1864). Even for ancient Greece, where there was no subdivision into different branches of medicine, it can be proven that there were no medics specializing in odontology.

The therapies of Hippocrates, Archigenes, Celsus, and Galenus were most remarkable. The first Roman laws, written down ca 450 BC, mention gold threads to tie teeth together. The law of the Twelve Slabs (302 ab urbe condita) stated: *Do not throw any gold onto the stakes where dead bodies are burnt, but you may burn the deceased with the gold that keeps his teeth together without violating the law.*

Ancient Roman medicine was part of religion and magic. The first medics were slaves, people set free, or adventurers. Aeneas had soldiers and officers skilled in the art of healing, which they performed only occasionally, because they were mainly trained to fight. Roman law subsumed injuries of the teeth to injuries in general. In ancient Greece and Rome, there are no traces of expert witnesses, although in both societies the law developed in a rather complicated way and both societies had a high standard of medical knowledge. The fall of the Greek and Roman empires led to a decline in culture and affected a step backward in medicine and at the same time in odontology (Geist-Jacobi 1905).

Until the beginning of the Christian calendar, there had been no odontology on its own. In theory and practice, it had always been part of general medicine, which was preferably performed by priests or medical men who had come from the priest's caste.

The Teutonic tribes of the Franks, Alemanns, Goths, Vandals, etc., who were looked down upon as barbarians, were the first to *legally* introduce medical experts. This was done to stop the custom of blood feuds, and thus they assigned a certain responsibility to the community. However, in medicine they did not yet have the necessary qualifications to meet the expectations. We do not know anything of dental treatment in Celto-Germanic history (Rötzscher 1991/3).

The laws of the Teutonic tribes were codified at the same time when these tribes entered Roman territory: first the Visigoths under Eurich (466–456) and then the BurgLindians under Gundobad (474–516), who was the most important legal expert among the Germanic princes. In the sixth century, these tribes were followed by the different tribes of the Franks (Schmidt 1953).

In the first half of the seventh century, a «law» of the Langobards and the Alemanns, the so-called Pactus Alamannorum, came into existence, which was, 100 years later, rewritten as the Lex Alamannorum. Both allow insight into how medical expertise was treated at those times. In the eighth century, the Langobards and the Franks rewrote some laws. At the same time, the Bavarians, the Saxons, Thuringians, and Frisians recorded their own laws. Whereas the legal recordings were basically completed in the eighth century, the Anglo-Saxons did not finish recording laws until the eleventh century, only succeeded by the Northern Germanic tribes (eleventh to thirteenth centuries) (Brittain 1966).

The Nordic laws of the Icelandic and Scandinavian peoples, although latest to be recorded, have retained a certain naturalness. The recordings of the Germanic tribes fell into oblivion; they were hardly known on the continent in the tenth century. New recordings of laws were very rare.

1.3 Middle Age

From the eleventh century, the towns gained their own jurisdiction, and Germanic law was codified again. The presentation of evidence was being improved; sworn surgeons now became forensic doctors. The range of laws extended from facial injuries and bone injuries to castration, paralyses, and chest injuries. The doctor and medical expert remained outside the court. At the beginning, the proof of the truth did not trust medical testimony very much. This medical testimony was mentioned for the first time at the end of the sixth century. The surgeon had to swear – *in ferramenta* – on his surgical instruments. The beginnings of a systematic forensic medicine can be found in the big trade centers of Northern Italy (Rötzscher 1991/4).

The Italian statute law and the first German recordings of law took place at the same time. Johann von Schwarzenberg's Bambergensis (1507) and the first German criminal law meant the ingenious fusion of both sources.

In the thirteenth century, the Chinese Si-wan-hu published the first book on forensic medicine, which was called the first systematic book at all on forensic medicine by MIRONOW (1961). In France, forensic medicine was initially influenced by Roman law and the doctrines of Hippocrates and Aristotle. Later Franco-Germanic and church law became more influential. The year 1278 records sworn-in surgeons around King Philip the Bold and in several cities (e.g., Rouen). Trial by ordeal and torture were the custom of these days, the doctors were there to interrupt the torture, not to stop it. Freiburg/Br. (Germany) had city surgeons beginning from the year 1403; they had to teach forensic medicine as well.

1.4 Renaissance (Fourteenth to Sixteenth Century)

The first known and most precious document of forensic medicine dates back to 1544. It is the report of the exhumation of Francisco Pizzaro, the discoverer of Peru (Avendano de Lima 1960). Its main issue was the final identification of the body. In 1570, King Philip II created the Court of Justice of Senior Surgeons (Tribunal del Protomedicato), whose advice on civil and criminal law was often sought by the administration.

In the fourteenth century, odontostomatology remained within surgery, whereas the extraction of teeth became the job of "tooth breakers," *dentatores*, barbers, and village quacks. The last two were not untrained in medicine, and the expression tooth breaker was not meant derogatively (Rötzscher 1992/1).

Guy de Choliac (died in 1370), who is often called the first author of the French surgery, mentioned, in his book *Great Surgery* (1365), the *dentista* as a name of a profession, because these people gradually took over odontotherapy.

Any information on odontotherapy was only found in the Latin books of the surgeons. Latin could not be read by the barbers or village quacks. Superstition, alchemy, and astrology were in the minds of the *dentatores* and also of the surgeons. It would be a mistake to overlook the importance of the monasteries for the progress of medicine. Pope Honchus III (1216–1227) had stopped all of the clergy from exercising their art of healing. As a result of the change in the scholastic teaching, the national languages were also used in teaching. Paracelsus had started to do the same, and, at the end of the fifteenth century, all medical books and pamphlets were published in any language but Latin. However, because odontotherapy was still part of surgery, independent publications in this field were very rare.

1.5 New History

The year 1700 marked the birthdate of the odontology as a scientific field in two respects: first, Louis XIV, King of France, issued an edict on May 11, 1699 that created the profession of *chirurgiens-dentistes* as a subdivision of surgeons. Second, Pierre Fauchard, a surgeon (1678–1761) in Paris, published a book on odontology that remained the leading textbook for a long time. The *chirurgiens-dentistes* were trained at the College Desarcon, and they were examined by professors of surgery. Only in 1766 were new rules set that prescribed that the future *chirurgiens-dentistes* had to go through a 2- to 3-year apprenticeship with an expert dentist or surgeon. The regulations also became tighter, and those who held a title without justification were punished. The French Revolution of 1789 gave everybody freedom of trade, which was abolished again in 1803 (Dérobert 1941). Prussia had stopped the freedom of trade in all medical professions on February 12, 1665.

Despite of all of these advances in dental medicine in France, there was no similar development in Germany. *Dr. Eysenbarth* (died in 1727) was a medical doctor with many privileges in Magdeburg, who would cure all his patients after his own fashion (as German folklore sings even today). In Bavaria, there was a similar doctor roving around until 1772 with the highest approval. In 1748, the Collegium Medico-Chiruigicum was founded in Saxony under August II, and, only 3 years later, he opened the first surgical hospital, which even employed a teacher of odontology. A new edict of September 29, 1785 allowed medical practice under a special oath, but there was no special formula for dentists. The edict of December 23, 1869 abolished the swearing in (Jefimow 1950).

A court circular of 1828 conceded "first-class surgeons" the right to prescribe internal medicaments. A ministerial edict of 1825 even stated that every surgeon was, at the same time, a dentist, because odontology was an integral part of surgery. This edict clearly showed the position of the dentists in the nineteenth century. Only those who did not qualify as first-class surgeons had to take a special examination, which remained in effect even after the medico-surgical schools were closed, thus leaving two different approbations even until today. When the German *Zentralverein* was founded in 1859, there were new hopes for the dentists. In 1869, the Northern German Union passed a law concerning the requirements of dentists that later on became law in the new German nation. At the same time, the Union proclaimed the freedom of professions (Rötzscher 1994/2).

In England, dentistry was the barber's job. The guild of the barber-surgeons received their first privileges only in 1462. There were two classes, the surgeons and the barbers. The title of dentist only appears at the end of the eighteenth century. There is no further knowledge of the first odontologists. In 1868, Berdmore published the handbook on odontology in England. In comparison with its French contemporaries, it was only insignificant. The year 1858 saw the founding of the Odontological Society of Britain. A short time later, the Institute of Dentists was founded, which was followed by the London School of Dentistry in 1859. In the same year, the first examination took place. In 1878, the registration of dentists became mandatory and the unregistered ones have been controlled since 1921.

Belgium passed its first laws concerning dentistry in 1818, by introducing examinations by a provincial commission. New laws only followed in 1880. In 1815, Sweden introduced a kind of examination in front of a medical supervisory authority. In 1860, Svenska Tandläkaresellskapet was founded, and, in 1885, an outpatient clinic was created to house a medical school. There was no difference in the practice of dentistry in the United States. Before 1840, there was no regular teaching even for the general medicine. Hyden and Harris, who founded the Baltimore College of Dental Surgery in 1839, were the fathers of American odontology. The years 1760–1770 can be regarded as the birth of dentistry in Russia, when the German OBEL was one of the first dentists who was granted the right to open a surgery of his own after an examination at the Medical College of St. Petersburg. According to a law of 1810, these foreign specialists had the right to train their students as manual craftsmen, who then worked as dental therapists after an examination.

Apart from the facts that Fr. J. RINGELMANN (1776–1854) was the first lecturer of odontology in Würzburg, and that he had never stood out as a research scientist, he became the first teacher of odontology in a historical dimension in Germany. In those days, all of the dentists in Germany and Austria came from Vienna. In May 1884, the Royal Ministry of Saxony commissioned HESSE to work out a status and a budget for the foundation of an odontological institute at Leipzig University. On October 16th, 1884, the same HESSE was appointed extraordinary professor and lecturer of odontology. He became, at the same time, the director of the institute that had been founded in Goethestraße 5 in Leipzig by special permission of the Saxon Ministry of Culture. Although odontology presented itself in most European countries with a gradually clearly defined field of work at the turn of this century, forensic medicine, up to that time and even later, was fighting for a place in medicine.

Although independent odontological treatises on forensic topics are scattered in the special literature, a turning point in the systematic collection of forensic odontology literature was only reached in the year 1862, when PFEFFERMANN published a short survey on forensic odontology in his book, *Easy Description of the Complete Odontology*.

1.6 Survey of Forensic Medicine

Ambroise Paré (1517–1590) can be regarded as the first medico-legal officer of a modern mold. A second great name in French forensic medicine is Antoine Louis (1723–1791). A royal decree of King Henry IV of France, of 1603, commissioned his personal physician to appoint two medico-legal officers in each town with a permanent jurisdiction. Another decree of 1692 transfers this right of appointment onto the municipalities. In Heidelberg, Germany, medico-legal reports were given by the medical faculty since 1651. As was mostly the case in other fields, forensic pharmacology was, at the beginning, taught as a secondary occupation by representatives of other subjects. The name forensic medicine was used for the first time around 1700.

In 1740, there were already lectures on forensic medicine at Copenhagen University. During the Great Revolution in France, the first lectures on forensic medicine were given at Dijon Academy. The Prague University, where lectures on forensic medicine had been given since 1785, created a chair in forensic medicine in 1807 that was held by J. BERNT from 1808–1813 (Hajek 1956). Under the influence of Josef BERNT and Peter FRANK, the conception of forensic medicine as a subject was changed, and it led to the foundation of a lectureship in 1804 and subsequently, in 1818, to the foundation of an Institute for Forensic Medicine in Vienna (Haberda 1911). The first professor of forensic medicine in Vienna (Reuter 1954) was VIETZ (1805–1813) (Breitenecker 1965). The first chair of forensic medicine was held by A. SCHAUENSTEIN in Graz, Austria, in 1861. Since 1819, forensic medicine has been part of the medical examination in Denmark (Gormsen 1956). In 1910, forensic medicine first had its own rooms; in 1921, the first institute was built.

In 1832, Rio de Janeiro, the then capital city of Brazil, had the first chair of forensic medicine, which was followed by another one in Bahia (Ribeiro 1933). In 1844, the first lectureship for forensic medicine was assigned in Peru (Avendano de Lima 1960). Until today, there has not been a medico-legal institute there. In 1839, the University of Glasgow, Scotland, established a chair in forensic medicine (Glaister 1928). At the end of the nineteenth century, forensic medicine as an academic subject had a paltry existence in Germany (Rötzscher 1991/3, 1992/3). The statistics of 1889 show that there was not a single chair in forensic medicine in the whole of Germany. When Richard KOCKEL (1865–1934) was appointed extraordinary professor of forensic medicine in Leipzig, Saxony, it marked the beginning of forensic medicine in Leipzig. On May 5, 1900, forensic medicine became an independent institute by appointment of the Royal Saxon Ministry of Culture, and KOCKEL became its first director. He is responsible for the fact that forensic medicine, which had been mandatory since 1901, became part of the medical examination (Holzhausen 1965).

After inquiries at all of the German universities, in Kockel (1928), published the following statistics for forensic medicine: 13 universities had a full-time professor of forensic medicine, 2 universities had a full-time associate professor, 3 universities had a court doctor who did the teaching as a secondary occupation, 1 university had a medical officer, and 5 universities had a pathoanatomist. Out of 24 universities, only 14 had their own forensic institutes. Unlike general medicine, forensic medicine had its roots in its home country, because the jurisdiction differed in every country. In 1955, the first textbook of forensic medicine appeared in Finnish.

Forensic medicine, as we see it, has not been fully developed in the USA. Without doubt, this is because of the coroner system. The field of activity of forensic medicine varies in all 50 states. Recently there have been efforts to introduce the subject of forensic medicine according to the European model. One success so far has been the founding of the American Academy of Forensic Sciences in 1948 (Im Obersteg 1949).

The varying development of medicine, dentistry, forensic medicine, and jurisprudence is the direct result of the economic and, at the same time, political development in Europe. In the feudal states of the Holy Roman Empire, the development of capitalism was made particularly difficult because Germany was divided into 300 sovereign and more than 1,000 more or less sovereign states. In this empire, Austria and Prussia ruled side by side in forensic stomatology from 1862 (Carl 1941).

Approximately at the same time, when forensic medicine endeavored to get its place in general medicine, forensic stomatology broke away from dentistry. In 1862, a short chapter on forensic stomatology appeared in *Fassliche Darstellung der gesamten Zahnheilkunde* by Paul PFEFFERMANN (1862), who signed as a doctor of medicine and surgery, M. Sc. in ophthalmology and stomatology, member of the Viennese Medical Faculty and several learned societies and practicing dentist in Vienna. This chapter consists of 12 pages and is divided into:

- Usefulness of a special forensic stomatology
- Objects of stomatological examinations
- Complications of injuries of teeth
- Survey of injuries
- Criteria of abnormities in injuries
- About the writing of forensic stomatological reports
- Complaints about possible complaints about the dentists themselves
- Set phrases for reports

The four cited forensic stomatological reports deal with a syphilitic infection; an injury of teeth from an affray; together with heavy facial injuries; and stroke with a piece of firewood, and finally with a report on the significance and the curability of bad breath.

1.7 History of Forensic Odontostomatology

Oscar AMOEDO (1863–1945), professor of the *École Odontotechnique* in Paris, was the first to sift through the considerable amount of individual treatments and to publish them in a systematic edition (Amoëdo 1897). He is the founder of forensic stomatology (Amoëdo 1990). In 1921, Marhold publishers in Halle/Saale published the *Handbook of Forensic Odontology with Special Consideration of Dental and Social Techniques* by L. MEIER (1921). In a special part of the journal, *Progress in Dentology*, L. MISCH (1925-1933) published regular articles on forensic odontology, ranging from civil law in dentistry to public legal issues and forensic odontology. A. PALTAUF (1927) wrote, in *Scheffs Handbook of Odontology*, about the tooth from the forensic point of view. He recommends dealing with these questions in the following chapters:

- Injuries of teeth
- Injuries by teeth
- The tooth as part of the individual
- The tooth after death

The Handbook of Forensic Medicine and Scientific Criminology by von Neureiter et al. (1940), being the first in this special field, divides forensic odontology into two groups:

I. Correlation between teeth and diseases resulting from treatment of teeth and those resulting from injuries.

II. Criminological importance of teeth and dentures in wounds caused by impressions and bites of the determination of age and identity in living and dead persons with the help of accurate investigation of the dental status. In 1956, Bohne et al. (1956) published their book: "Forensische Zahnheilkunde".

In 1944, D. Schranz, professor of odontology at Pécs University, Hungary, published *Törvényszéki Stomatologia*, a book on forensic stomatology in Hungarian. The eight chapters are: dental law, injuries in criminal law, injuries in civil law, toxicology of forensic odontology, questions of causal connection, the professional error in dentistry, and postmortal changes.

G. Gustafson, Malmö, published, in 1966, the book *Forensic Odontology* with Staples Press London. In 1967, the Japanese Furuhata and Yamamoto (1967) wrote the book *Forensic Odontology* (Yokosuka City, Japan). In 1968, Harsányi and Szuchovsky (1968) published a supplement for handbooks of odontology in Budapest: *Fejezetek az igazsagügyi Fogorvostan köréböl* (*Chapters from Forensic Stomatology*).

At present, there are specialists all over the world who specially devote themselves to forensic odontology in the stomatological institutes and hospitals. In Oslo, forensic odontology has been taught at the university since the turn of the century, and because of this tradition, a special unit has been established and attending lectures has been made mandatory for future dentists (Ström 1953).

At Japanese dental schools, forensic medicine with its dental implications has been mandatory for decades. Brazil and Cuba used to have special chairs for forensic odontology. The American Academy of Oral Pathology established a committee of forensic stomatologists in 1967 to evaluate important issues of forensic stomatology. M. A. Sadre-Ameli gave lectures on forensic stomatology in Teheran, Iran, from 1968. In the same year, a Forensic Dentistry Study Group was established at the Liverpool School of Dental Surgery, with J. Furness as chairman, G. E. Moore as secretary, and Wood and Cockrell as other members. October 1968 saw the fifth course in forensic dentistry at the Pathological Institute of the Armed Forces in Washington, DC, USA. In April 1968, W. Harvey, Glasgow Dental Hospital and School, gave his first lecture on forensic odontology at the Scottish Detective Training Course (Rötzscher 1993/1).

The universities of the former German Democratic Republic also offered courses in forensic medicine for the students of odontology from the ninth semester (5th year of studies). These were not lectures on forensic stomatology, but special lectures on forensic medicine with particular consideration of dental interests. These courses were given by forensic pathologists.

References

Amoëdo O. (1897): Le râle des dentistes dans l´ identification des victims de la catastrophe du Bazar de la Charité, Paris, 04.05.1897. Dtsch. Mschr. Zahnhk, 10, 1897, p. 550–552

Amoëdo O (1900) Die Zahnheilkunde in der gerichtlichen Medizin, aus dem französischen übersetzt von G. Port. Verlag A. Felix, Leipzig

Avendano de Lima J (1960) Pasado y presente de la medicina legal en et Peru. Rev Méd Lege Colombo 15:39–104

Bohne G, Euler H, Venter R (1956) Venter: Forensische Zahnheilkunde. J. A. Barth, München
Breasted JH (1922) The Edwin Smith-Papyrus, an Egyptian Treatise of the Seventeenth century before Christ. N Y Hist Soc Quart Bull VI(1):5–13
Breitenecker L (1965) 160 Jahre Lehrkanzei für gerichtliche Medizin in Wien. Beitr Gerichtl Med 230:12–43
Brittain RP (1966) Origins of legal Medicine: Leges Barborum (Ursprünge der gerichtlichen Medizin: Leges Barborum). Med Leg J, Canb 34:21–23 [ref. In: Dtsch Zschr Gerichtl Med 60, 8? (1967)]
Carl J (1941) Überblick über die Entstehungsgeschichte der Gerichtsmedizin in Deutschland. Med Diss Münster i Westf
Dérobert (1941) Petit historiqué de la médecine légale en France et à Paris. Paris méd II(44/45):I–VIII
Furuhata T, Yamamoto K (1967) Forensic odontology. Yokosuka City
Geist-Jacobi GP (1905) Geschichte der Zahnheilkunde vom Jahre 3700 v. Chr. bis zur Gegenwart. Tübingen 1896. Handbuch der Geschichte der Medizin III. Band, p 355–392
Glaister J (1928) The evolution, development and application of modern medico-legal methods. Glasgow Med J 109:427–437
Gormsen H (1956) Forensic medicine in Denmark. The academical and practical aspects of the subject. A historical review. Acta Med Leg Soc (Liege) 9(Spec No):77–81
Haberda A (1911) Geschichte der Wiener Lehrkanzel für gerichtliche Medizin. Beitr Gerichtl Med I:1–16
Hajek F (1956) Entwicklung der gerichtlichen Medizin an der Karlsuniversität. Soudni lék 3–10
Harsányi L, Szuchovszky G (1968) Fejezetek az igazsagügyi Fogorvostan köréböl (Chapters from Forensic stomatology). Budapest
Holzhausen G (1965) 550 Jahre Medizinische Fakultät. Wiss Zschr Univ Leipzig, Mathemat. Reihe, pp 73–78
Im Obersteg J (1949) Die gerichtliche Medizin in den USA. Beitr Gerichtl Med XVIII:62–68
Jefimow A (1950) Geschichte der Neuzeit (1789 - 1870), 3. Aufl. Volk und Wissen, Berlin/Leipzig, S 12
Keiser-Nielsen S (1968) Scandinavian society of forensic ontology. News Letter 2:6–9
Kockel R (1928) Alte und neue Wege der gerichtlichen Medizin. (Vortrag auf der 16. Tagung der Deutschen Gesellschaft für gerichtl. Medizin in Graz 192?) Dtsch Zschr gerichtl Med 11:1–13
Meier L (1921) Handbuch der Zahnärztlichen Rechtskunde mit Berücksichtigung der gerichtlichen und sozialen Zahntechnik. Marhold-Verlag, Halle/Saale
Mildner AJ (1964) Die forensische Medizin im Alten Testament der Bibel. Dtsch Med J 15:61–63
Mironow J (1961) Forensic medicine in ancient China. Sudebno-med ekspertiza (Moskwa) 4(44–48)
Misch J (1925–1933) Forensische Zahnheilkunde. Fortschr Zahnhk. Bd. I–IX
Mishulin W (1948) Geschichte des Altertums. Volk und Wissen-Verlag, Berlin/Leipzig, pp 8–46
Nobel G (1909) Zur Geschichte der Zahnteilkunde im Talmud. Med Diss, Leipzig
Paltauf A (1927) Der Zahn in forensischer Beziehung. In: Scheff Handbuch der Zahnheilkunde, III. Bd., 4. Aufl. Urban und Schwarzenberg, Berlin-Wien, S 592
Pfeffermann P (1862) Fassliche Darstellung der gesamten Zahnheilkunde. F. Enke Verlag, Erlangen
Renan E (1864) Mission de Phénícіe. Imprimerie impériale, Paris, p 472–473
Reuter F (1954) Geschichte der Wiener Lehrkanzel für gerichtliche Medizin von 1804–1954. F. Deuticke Verlag, Wien
Ribeiro L (1933) Ein Jahrhundert des Unterrichts in der gerichtlichen Medizin in Brasilien. Arg Med Leg 3:63–81
Rötzscher K (1991/1) History. 1.1 Introduction. Newl IOFOS, Year 13, No.1, p 4
Rötzscher K (1991/2) History. 1.2 Early history, part 1, Newl IOFOS, Year 13, No. 2, p 10
Rötzscher K (1991/3) History. 1.2.1 Early history, part 2. Newl IOFOS, Year 13, No. 3, p 5
Rötzscher K (1991/4) History. 1.3. Middle age. Newl IOFOS, Year 13, No. 4, p 4
Rötzscher K (1992/1) History. 1.4 Renaissance. Newl IOFOS, Year 14, No. 1, p 9
Rötzscher K (1992/2) History. 1.5 New history. Newl IOFOS, Year 14, No. 2, p 7
Rötzscher K (1992/3) History. 1.6 Survey of forensic medicine. Newl IOFOS, Year 14, No. 3, pp 3/4
Rötzscher K (1993/1) 1.7 History of forensic odontostomatology. Newl IOFOS, Year 15, No. 1, p 5
Schmidt O (1953) Gerichtliche Medizin in den ersten geschriebenen Rechten germanischer Stämme. Dtsch Zschr Gerichtl Med 42:121–132
Ström F (1953) Retsodontologi. In: Brinch O (ed) Nordisk Medicinsk-odonto-logisk Haandbog. Kopenhagen
von Neureiter F, Pietrusky F, Schütt E (1940) Handwörterbuch der gerichtlichen Medizin und naturwissenschaftlichen Kriminalistik. J. Springer, Berlin

History of Legal Odontology in Argentina

2

Oscar Heit

2.1 Argentinean Society of Legal Odontology and Forensic Odontologist Association of South America

The legal odontology field in Argentina needs further refinement and research progress. To date, the Argentine judicial system, divided into provinces, has no formal incorporation of expert dentists in medico-legal institutes or medical legal departments.

Associations such as the Argentinean Society of Legal Odontology contribute to training odontolegal experts, standardizing knowledge, and developing best-practices manuals.

The dental specialty recognized by resolution No. 956/2010 of the Argentine Ministry of Health is legal odontology, in the same way that the specialty for medical sciences is legal medicine.

The curriculum of traditional education in dentistry in Argentina does not provide the experience, preparation, and training required to work in this field. Thus, the universities and dental faculties in the country offer postgraduate degrees in the field, awarding the title of Legal Odontology Specialist. It is expected that, in the near future, medico-legal institutes will have legal odontology specialists in their teams.

The legal odontology history in Argentina dates back to the 1930s. In 1920, Prof. Juan Ubaldo Carrea, who was the creator of an identification system to determine the medium size human, published *Odontometrics Test*. He also created his own Rugoscopy System in 1937, extending the work of Prof. López de Leon in Guatemala. The first Professor of Legal Odontology at the Buenos Aires University, in 1920, was Dr. Joaquin Gnecco, who published the book *Legal Odontology* on a collection of classes. In 1932, Prof. Beltran published *Legal Medicine Teaching for Legal and Social Odontology*. He defined legal odontology as the application of dental knowledge in the service of justice and the development of laws correlating to their specialty. Another prominent professor was Dr. Bertini, who published his thesis on *Legal Odontology, Identity and Identification* in 1945. In 1953, Prof. Bloise published his work on *Human Identification by Maxillo-mandibulo-dental System.* Dra. Elida Briñon has been an expert in the courts of Buenos Aires for many years. She has published two books, the first, in 1983, entitled *Legal Odontology and Forensic Practice* and the second, in 2006, *Injuries and Iatrogenic Injuries in Legal Odontology*.

2.2 DVI in Argentina

Argentina is a large country; each province has its own court. Currently, stable teams for disaster victim identification (DVI) have not been established.

O. Heit, Prof. Dr.
Faculty of Science and Technology,
University Autonomous of Entre Ríos,
Entre Ríos, Argentina
e-mail: odheitoscar@hotmail.com

K. Rötzscher (ed.), *Forensic and Legal Dentistry*,
DOI 10.1007/978-3-319-01330-5_2, © Springer International Publishing Switzerland 2014

The Argentinean Society of Legal Dentistry works by forming DVI teams with odontolegal experts in each province. INTERPOL forms are used for mass disasters. Moreover, the Dental Forensic Association of South America works to update manuals of good and best practices for DVI cases in the region. In my province, I have had the opportunity to participate in the identification of two plane crashes and many automobile accidents. In these cases, the number of victims was two to five people. The bodies were mostly carbonized. Identification problems sometimes arise in the absence of antemortem dental records. In cases lacking antemortem data, it has been very useful to use digital photographs of people while they were alive. Comparing photographs of smiling is commonly used for odontolegal identification. However, it is still necessary to use X-rays and written records for more efficient work. To compare dental characteristics antemortem and postmortem, we used the Keiser–Nielsen System, based on valuation of the coincidences, discrepancies, and exclusions.

Since 1995, three dental faculties have postgraduate programs in legal odontology and there is a continuous effort to increase the number of universities able to train additional specialists.

History of Forensic Odontology and DVI in Australia

3

Jane Taylor, Russell Lain, and William O'Reilly

3.1 Introduction

Forensic odontology played a vital and historical role in an Australian homicide in 1934. Known as the *Albury Pyjama Girl Case*, it attracted worldwide interest for many years and illustrated the potential and the importance of dental evidence in the identification process. On the 1st of September of that year, the partly burned and battered body of a young woman clad in pajamas was found in a roadside culvert near Albury, NSW. This discovery led to one of the longest investigations in the history of Australian crime. Two simple errors by a local dentist with no previous experience in forensic odontology, who was called in by the police to examine the teeth of the victim, resulted in a delay in identification for 10 years. When identification by dental comparison was finally achieved in 1944, the crime was quickly solved and the woman's husband was brought to trial for murder. The application of dental science for identification in those days was on an ad hoc basis, and individual dentists, usually with no experience or training in forensic matters, were expected to assist as needed. The Pyjama Girl Case vividly demonstrated the serious consequences of this practice (Brown 1984).

3.2 The Australian Scene

Its directions role has been significantly influenced by the continent's geography, with vast areas of *outback* country ranging from arid deserts to dense rain forests and alpine regions and harsh extremes of climate. Australia has a relatively small but expanding multiracial scattered population, unevenly distributed between isolated groups of nomadic aborigines and large densely populated cosmopolitan cities.

The remoteness of the outback provides opportunity for the commission of serious crimes such as homicide with a relatively low risk of detection, and victims may not be found for a long period of time. The potential for death by misadventure in a wide variety of forms is always present. In any of these situations, isolation, climate, and traumatic mutilation of victims may compound the problem of identification, and scientific methods to achieve it are frequently necessary (Brown 1984).

3.3 The Coronial System

Politically, Australia consists of six sovereign states and one territory, with a national Federal Parliament. The coronial system operates under

J. Taylor, Ass. Prof. (✉) • W. O'Reilly, Ass. Prof.
Department of Oral Health, School of Health Sciences, University of Newcastle, Ourimbah, NSW 2258, Australia
e-mail: jane.taylor@newcastle.edu.au; ohreally1@bigpond.com

R. Lain, Dr.
Department of Oral Surgery and Diagnostic Imaging, Sydney Dental Hospital, 2 Chalmers Street, Surry Hills, NSW 2010, Australia
e-mail: russell.lain@sydney.edu.au

K. Rötzscher (ed.), *Forensic and Legal Dentistry*,
DOI 10.1007/978-3-319-01330-5_3, © Springer International Publishing Switzerland 2014

state law in all of the Australian states. Each state is divided into coronial districts under the jurisdiction of local coroners.

The function of the coroner is to inquire into all deaths and fires as he may deem fit. He is the officer responsible to establish the identity of the deceased and also the cause of death. After satisfying himself on these matters, the coroner may then issue a burial or cremation order and authorize the registration of the death, a certificate of which may then be issued.

He initiates police investigation when evidence suggests that a death may have been associated with the commission of crime. The powers of the coroner are considerable, and in South Australia and Victoria, for example, a state coroner has jurisdiction over the whole state and may overrule a local coroner; these powers extend to committal for trial in the Supreme Court (Brown 1984).

3.4 Services in Forensic Odontology

The agencies in Australia that utilize forensic odontology are the Australian Federal Police, the state police forces, the coroner's offices, the state services in forensic medicine and forensic pathology, and the Department of Transport. The Federal Police may also act as the Australian agency for Interpol.

3.4.1 Investigation of all civilian aircraft accidents

While this department operates closely with local coroners in the investigation of aircraft accident deaths, full autopsies are required to be carried out by consultant pathologists appointed by the department. To assist the pathologists in person identification of deceased victims, consultant odontologists have also been appointed in the following states: Queensland, Victoria, Western Australia, and Tasmania, New South Wales, South Australia, and Northern Territory.

Services in forensic odontology are provided at the state level, each state independently employing expertise according to its requirements.

In Queensland, the service is provided by a specialist on the staff of the University of Queensland Dental School. In Victoria and Western Australia, private dental practitioners are employed on a consultancy basis. In New South Wales, forensic odontological services are provided by regional dentists employed by the State Health Commission. The Northern Territory Police utilize the services of a government dental officer. He is experienced in forensic dentistry. In South Australia, the service is provided by the Forensic Odontology Unit in the University of Adelaide.

In cases of deaths from aircraft accidents, the Federal Department of Aviation (Bureau of Air Safety Investigation) controls civil aviation and is responsible for air safety standards and the enforcement of them. The authority for the responsibility for identification of victims of military aircraft accidents in Australia falls within the province of local state coroners (Brown 1984).

Pounder and Harding (1984) have reported that the first autopsies were conducted in Australia in 1790, one on a victim of inanition (starvation) and the other on the Governor's gamekeeper who was allegedly murdered by Aborigines.

Pounder (1984) reporting on death investigations in the early years (1839–1840) of South Australia indicated that both the coroner and jurors were required to view the body of the victim as part of the inquest procedures. This parallels the system derived from the historical British practice of super visum corporis (*after viewing the body*). Although the stated purpose was for the examination of marks of violence, it is reasonable to surmise that it was also for the formal identification of the victim. This practice remained until 1907. Cordner et al. (1992) have indicated that the first lectures on forensic medicine were held in Melbourne in 1866.

It is not known with certainty when forensic odontology was first used in Australia. A report in the New South Wales Police News in 1943 reported the identification in Melbourne, Victoria, of a murder victim, Bertha Coughlin, in 1923, and of Norman List in 1924, using dental evidence (Anonymous 1943).

This article also mentioned that the identity of three victims of a plane crash in the Dandenong Ranges in 1938 *could only be established by means of the teeth.* Cleland (1944) mentioned the identification of a New Zealand citizen in Western Australia in 1930, although this identification appeared to rely more on circumstantial dental evidence than to be a true dental identification.

From around the early 1960s there was spasmodic but increasing use of dentists to assist police in identification procedures. This was generally an informal arrangement with little or no remuneration, which meant that the dentists providing the services frequently had to complete examinations and prepare reports after hours and at weekends. In the vast majority of cases a single practitioner provided the entire service. Limited training in forensic odontology was available to these dental practitioners, and it is a credit to their dedication and professionalism that the discipline has developed to the high standard and international reputation it enjoys today.

The first regularly cited use of Disaster Victim Identification (DVI) practices in Australia was in response to the crash of a Vickers Viscount aircraft into Botany Bay, adjacent to Sydney Airport, on 30 November 1961, resulting in the death of 15 people. The chief investigating officer, Detective Sergeant WB Ross, realized the challenge that would be faced in identifying the victims and indicated in his final report that he had researched extensively prior to planning recovery and identification procedures.

Ninety-four body parts were recovered over 12 days. All identifications were confirmed by visual recognition by family and friends. Several references to the use of teeth and dentistry are made in the case file. Several of the identification summaries of the victims made reference to *favourable comparison of dental charts.* There is no explanation as to why this comparison was favorable, except in one instance where reference is made that ". [a] *dentist identified the teeth mentioned in the morgue book as that of the deceased.*" There is no indication of what the entries in the morgue book contained or who made them. It would also seem that the dentist making this comparison was the dentist of the victim and not an experienced forensic odontologist (NSW Police Case File).

An outcome from this investigation was the development of a Disaster Victim Identification Form for use by the NSW Police. Detective Sergeant Ross indicated that he modelled these forms on information published by a French police officer in a 1952 edition of the International Criminal Police Review, presumably Pedoussant (1952). Both these forms bear a striking resemblance to the current Interpol DVI forms, and it is reasonable to surmise that they provided the template from which the Interpol forms evolved as both French and Australian police officers attended early Interpol standing committee meetings (Edwards MR, 2007, Commander forensic services, NSW Police (Retired), personal communication).

3.5 Australian Society for Forensic Dentistry

Dentists with a special interest in forensic odontology formed The Australian Society of Forensic Dentistry, now known as the Australian Society of Forensic Odontology (AuSFO) in 1982. In recent years the society has aimed to provide leadership in various aspects of forensic odontology, as demonstrated by the development of the Disaster Victim Identification Practice Guide mentioned above. The group also acts as a forum for meetings, supports research, and coordinates regional training and is the representative body for forensic odontology in Australia.

AuSFO is also the contact point for all national and international requests for provision of forensic odontologists to assist in DVI incidents. The Australian Society of Forensic Dentistry became an incorporated body under Federal Law in 1983. Its constitution provides for affiliation with the Australian Dental Association and the International Organisation for Forensic Odonto-Stomatology (IOFOS).

References

Anonymous (1943) Identification by teeth. New South Wales Police News, 1 Mar, pp. 10–12

Brown KA (1984) Australia. In: Hill IR (ed) Forensic odontology. Its scope and history. Marshgibbon, Bicester, pp. 103–110

Cordner SM, Ranson DL, Singh B (1992) The practice of forensic medicine in Australasia: a review. Aust N Z J Med 22:477–486

Pedoussaut A (1952) Identification in air accidents. Int Crim Police Rev 7(54):3–9

Pounder DJ (1984) Death investigation in early colonial South Australia, 1839–40. Med Sci Law 24(4):273–282

Pounder DJ, Harding HWJ (1984) Forensic services in Australia. Am J Forensic Med Pathol 5(3): 269–278

The Role of Dentists in Indonesian Disaster Victim Identification Operations

4

Peter Sahelangi

4.1 Introduction

Indonesia is the largest archipelago in the world, consisting of five main islands, 17,508 smaller islands, spread across three seismic belts that run throughout this country. The islands of Indonesia are a result of the collision of three major plates in which the Australian-Indian plate in the South, the Eurasia plate in the Northwest, and the Pacific plate in the Northeast are all converging in the region of Southeast Asia (Fig. 4.1).

With a total population of 245,613,043 (July 2010), Indonesia's Muslim community exceeds 182,570,000 – the largest Muslim population in the world. Indonesia is extremely prone to disasters, both natural (e.g., earthquakes, volcanic eruptions, tsunamis, typhoon, high tides, landslides triggered by monsoon rains, hot mud eruptions, rainy season's floods, and dry season's drought) and man-made, and has experienced unique obstacles during national Disaster Victim Identification (DVI) operations at mass casualty sites:

4.2 Religious and Cultural Aspects

Aceh is a special territory (Daerah Istimewa) of Indonesia, located on the northern tip of the island of Sumatra. Its full name is Daerah Istimewa Aceh (1959–2001), Nanggroë Aceh Darussalam (2001–2009), and Aceh (2009–Present). The Aceh province has the highest proportion of Muslims in the country with regional levels of Sharia law. 98 % of the 4,486,570 population was identified as Muslims.

Most of the victims in the Aceh tsunami disaster of December 26, 2004, were Muslim. Their families wished to bury their relatives quickly – within a maximum of 24 h (before the next prayer time). Therefore, there was a great struggle to collect antemortem data, attempting the identification and reconciliation within 24 h.

Most Indonesian people have the culture of religious acceptance (entrusting God's will), as long as religious leaders sanction their action according to Muslim teachings. The shortage of forensic pathologists, forensic odontologists, forensic field facilities, communication, and transportation in DVI operations demands a greater amount of time to conduct the appropriate procedures.

Proposed DVI management recommendations:

- In earliest stages of DVI operations religious leaders should be involved.
- Take profile and dental photos of all victims with simple digital cameras.
- Use field-grade handheld X-ray devices to take radiographs of every victim.

P. Sahelangi, Dr. DFM
Department of Forensic and Medico-Legal
Faculty of Medicine, Hasanuddin University,
Makassar, Indonesia
e-mail: petersahelangi@yahoo.com

K. Rötzscher (ed.), *Forensic and Legal Dentistry*,
DOI 10.1007/978-3-319-01330-5_4, © Springer International Publishing Switzerland 2014

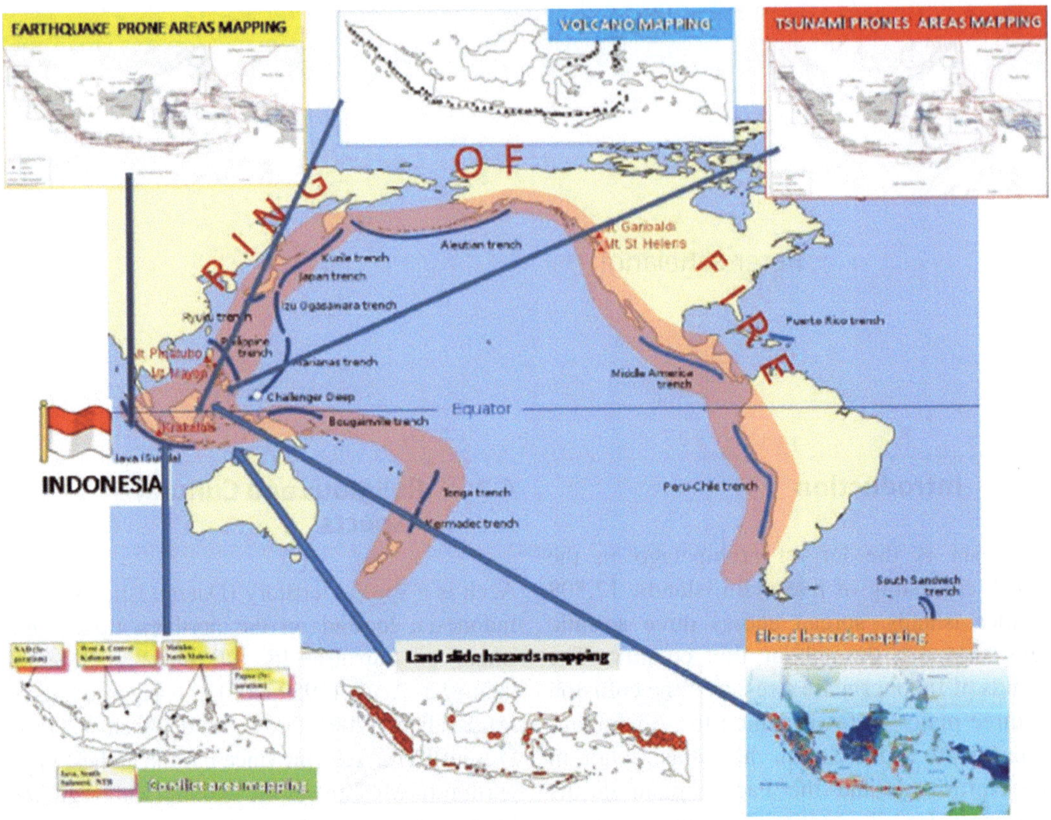

Fig. 4.1 Earthquakes, volcanic eruptions, tsunamis, typhoon, high tides, landslides triggered by monsoon rains, hot mud eruptions, rainy season's floods, and dry season's drought

By adopting such procedures, it is hoped that the identification process can be quicker and more efficient.

How well prepared are we to deal with the worst-case scenarios of this nature? The government and all involved organizations have participated in a discussion to answer this question and, as a result, established a National Standard of Operating Procedure to regulate who will take the responsibility with minimal bureaucracy in the eventuality of a disaster happening in their area.

Dental antemortem data are rare since most Indonesian do not make a regular dentist visit (only a small portion of the population do). No dental chart was available for positive identification of most of the Tsunami victims. Indonesian dentists to this day do not yet use a standardized dental chart (e.g., the dental classification and the symbols used for a correct registration of the various dental treatments) that is useful for the positive identification of disaster victims.

Because Muslims make up the overwhelming majority of Aceh's population, the DVI team was confronted with a problem dealing with the customary religious burial law. The families wished to bury the body of the victims as soon as possible, but the process of identification needed some extra time especially because of the fast-deteriorated body's condition in tropical heat. Since Islamic religious law requires that the burial must take place no later than 24 h after the time of death, the DVI team faced an unrealistic time constraint to properly identify a large number of bodies.

4.3 Recommendations

In future disasters, Religious leader (ustadz, ulama) should get involved at the earliest stage of DVI operations because most Indonesians believe they are obeying God's will according to

Muslim teaching so long as their action is in line with the ustadz's sanction.

- All responder teams are suggested to carry their own digital camera, video camera, and laptop.
- Dentists should bring handheld X-ray apparatus if possible to take onsite dental X-ray of each victim and to record the number on the body tag/label.
- All Indonesian dentist should keep a comprehensive dental record of all their patients following the National Standard of dental record (FDI system) released by the Ministry of Health of Indonesia. All dentists should also familiarize with the contents of *Technical Guidelines for Health Crisis Responses on Disaster* book.
- The Indonesian Dental Association should stress the importance of antemortem dental record and promote the use of it to all dentists in Indonesia, to all 26 University Dentistry Faculties, to all dentistry students, and to the general public at large as well.

4.4 Aceh Tsunami

On Sunday December 26, 2004, at 07.50 AM a big earthquake of 8.9 on the Richter scale occurred off the coast of Indonesia's Aceh province. It was followed 30 min later by a tsunami that razed the entire cities in Aceh west coast to the ground. Within a few minutes all economic and government activities in Aceh province totally ceased. The Indonesian Disaster Victim Identification consisting of 33 police doctors and dentists were dispatched to Aceh utilizing the Chief of Indonesia National Police special airplane. They arrived at the disaster area 24 h later, and shortly after they started organizing their tasks into action.

Indonesia already has guidelines for the management of large number of victims; however, it has come out of the experience gained from transport accidents and from terrorist incidents, and these guidelines are not directly relevant, for example, most natural disaster like tsunami often causes many more deaths than transport accidents or terrorist attacks. It is important for survivors that the bodies of the dead are handled with respect and that the dead are identified so that survivors know what has happened to missing relatives. However, at the same time many people are afraid of what the effect of many dead bodies might be on the living; one belief is that dead bodies are a source of disease. Such a belief can lead to the hasty burial of bodies even before identification has been done. All of the 33 Indonesian Police DVI team tried to do their best to identify the victims, but they often faced difficulties when families of the victims insisted to bury the bodies of their relatives as soon as possible for religious reason within a maximum of 24 h (before the next prayer time). But the situation and condition at the field were not conducive for rapid identification process. The Police DVI team ended up assisting people in the evacuation process. There were a lot obstacles during DVI operation in Aceh such as limitation of transportations, most of the cars were totally destroyed, no gasoline available at all, limitation of field forensic equipments such as refrigeration for preserving human remains, body protection cloths, gloves, boots, non existence body bags (all victims were wrapped in their own *sarong,* a traditional Muslim cloth), no clean water, and no food (response team eat instant noodle every day).

During this difficult identification process, the Indonesian Council of Muslim Leaders (Majelis Ulama Indonesia) issued a decree concerning Aceh Tsunami burial rites:

- The dead are to be simply buried in mass graves, fearing a health risk to the volunteers in the recovery response due to the hot and humid conditions in Aceh that cause rapid decomposition of the bodies.
- The bodies do not need to be cleansed, just placed in body bags in their own clothing.
- No need to separate male and female victims.
- The faces of the victims will be oriented towards Ka'bah Mecca in the West.
- Islamic burial rites (shalat jenazah) should be done after burial.
- All of the victims are declared Syahid Aqirat Death (death caused by disaster).

4.5 Field Management of the DVI Team in Aceh

Every responder's team worked hard immediately after the tsunami hit and tried their best to save the victims. Immediately after deployment the DVI team organized to initiate body's identification tasks in spite of the damaged local conditions and badly destroyed facilities. But due to the shortage of medical personnel, during the first few days, the tasks of the DVI team were often diverted to treating the injured survivors, and at times their manpower was needed to help assist people in the evacuation process. The arrival of huge number of international responders helped speed up rescue and relief missions. The multinational help force and humanitarian aids from abroad along with their sophisticated medical equipments and experienced personnel were able to provide proper medical treatment to the large number of injured survivors that eventually saved their lives.

The responsible institution in charge was not clearly assigned or well organized at that time especially when dealing with such a huge number of dead bodies and injured victims. The situation was in total chaos, while the number of victims increased by the minutes. The chaotic situation was compounded with the destruction of all local hospital facilities and the disappearance of many medical personnel, experts, and nurses who might have lost their lives swept by the tidal waves.

Obtaining antemortem data was impossible since all patients' records were destroyed in the flood.

Because Muslims make up the overwhelming majority of Aceh's population, the DVI team was confronted with a problem dealing with the customary religious burial law. The families wished to bury the body of the victims as soon as possible, but the process of identification needed some extra time especially because of the fast-deteriorated body's condition in tropical heat. Since Islamic religious law requires that the burial must take place no later than 24 h after the time of death, the DVI team faced an unrealistic time constraint to properly identify a large number of bodies.

Reference

Sahelangi P, Novita M (2012) Role of dentists in Indonesian disaster victim identification operations: religious and cultural aspects. J Forensic Odontostomatol 30(Suppl 1): 60–71

Part II

Legal Dentistry

5 Liability in Dentistry: Belgium

Yvo Vermylen

5.1 The Dentist-Patient Relationship

1. The dental contract is a usually unwritten agreement between a dentist and a patient, with on the one hand the dentist's commitment to advice and/or treat the patient and on the other hand the patient's obligation to pay the dental fee.
2. The dental contract is a consensual, reciprocal agreement which must be carried out personally, and it is often characterized by a certain duration.
3. A contract is void if error, deception, or coercion is present: in that case, the contract is not automatically void, but will provide a basis for a claim for annulment. The consent must be given by the contractor.

Incompetent minors, insane persons, and all those who are prohibited to conclude contracts by law cannot enter into contracts. This means that the consent is required from the parent or guardian. Certain minors, intellectually and physically mature, can take decisions in relation with their health, especially if there are no major risks involved, which is almost always the case in the dentistry. This means that for young people under the age of 15 the consent of the parents or guardian must be obtained. Young people often come to the dentist alone with a dental problem. The dentist should in that case contact the parents in order to obtain consent, unless the children have a written consent of the parents. That is a very unreasonable and impractical situation, which in practice is difficult to apply. A young person who is in pain has a right to treatment, and the dentist who should not treat it would be guilty of failure to treat a person in distress. For this reason, it seems logical that in such a case, the treatment should be limited to the problem for which the child consults the dentist and further treatments will be postponed until a consent from the parents is obtained.

Sometimes necessary interventions cannot be performed if the parents do not consent to the treatment. That would be the case with orthodontic treatments. If the orthodontic treatment can be postponed to the moment that the child can give a valid consent (18 years in Belgium), there is not a big problem. If such a treatment will not be possible anymore or with a less favorable outcome, it is in principle possible that a child seeks the assistance of the Public Prosecutor who can send the case to the juvenile court in order to get a court decision. That is very exceptional but not impossible.

Another problem that arises with children is that consent, in case of divorce of the parents, shall be obtained from the parent who has the right of custody, except in emergency situations.

The subject of the contract is the commitment to give, to do or not to do something. Only things that are on the market can be the subject of agreements.

Y. Vermylen, Master of Law
Department of Dentistry, Katholicke Uhiversity
Leuven, Capucijnenvoer 7, 3000, Leuven, Belgium
e-mail: yvovermylen@skynet.be

K. Rötzscher (ed.), *Forensic and Legal Dentistry*,
DOI 10.1007/978-3-319-01330-5_5, © Springer International Publishing Switzerland 2014

A cause is not valid if it is prohibited by law or contrary to public order or public morals. Dental surgery is allowed if it is necessary and therapeutic. What about pure cosmetic or esthetic treatments? Do they have a therapeutic value? Do we have to take only in consideration the physical or functional values? This can be disputed. A human being is concerned not only about physical but also about psychological well-being.

The problem of a patient suffering from an inferiority complex because of strong discolored teeth as a result of tetracyclines or due to heavily filled teeth can only be resolved with porcelain or acrylic veneers.

We can imagine that an intervention is unlawful if the risks of surgery are not in proportion with the therapeutic effects.

A patient has the right to interrupt a treatment unilaterally at any time. This may seem a contradiction at first sight, but it is not because agreements which cover the physical integrity are always revocable.

The revoking of the consent is therefore not a contractual error and does not give rise to damages.

A dentist can also step out of a treatment contract on condition that the health of the patient is not at risk and that he shall ensure that the continuity of the treatment will be guaranteed.

The dental contract is an agreement intuïtu personae, which means that a dentist should carry out the agreed treatment himself and not delegate the treatment without the consent of the patient.

The agreement is automatically terminated by the death of the dentist.

5.2 Obligation of Result or Obligation of Effort

Medicine and dentistry are dominated by an obligation of effort or means: a dentist will use all available means to achieve the best possible outcome, without it being mandatory to achieve a specific result. This is the general rule.

The legal difference between the two is situated in the burden of proof: In an obligation of result the patient only has to prove that the proposed result is not achieved, while with an obligation of effort the creditor must prove that the dentist has not acted as a competent, prudent, and diligent dentist (placed in the same circumstances).

That proof is much more difficult for the patient. He must prove that the dentist acted in a negligent, unscientific way.

In order to know whether or not we have to deal with an obligation of result:

- An obligation of result can be derived from a breach of a statutory requirement or prohibition.
- One can also look at the clauses of the contract or to what is agreed between the contracting parties.
- An obligation of result can be derived from the non-aleatory nature of the treatment. If there are no unforeseen factors to influence the treatment or affect the end result and when we may assume that we almost always get a positive result if we treat the patient lege artis, we may have of an obligation of result.

5.3 Fault

When something goes wrong during treatment and causes damage and if there is a causal relation between the fault and the damage, liability is possible.

The patient has the burden of proof and that is not always easy. He often does not even know that an error was made, and sometimes the damage appears many years after the treatment.

Each patient may expect that his/her dentist is competent, skilled, and experienced in the field of dentistry. This distinguishes him/her from the *ordinary* man who does not have these skills. He should not be world champion or the best specialist in that field of dentistry, but someone who meets the *normal standards of good practice.*

The standard of care is measured through objective, external, and impersonal criteria and compared with the behavior of a *standard dentist* with the same qualifications under the same circumstances.[1] It does not take into account subjective data such as age, sex, intelligence, and character. A dentist must be aware of his/her limits, and if he has no sufficient basic knowledge to perform a certain treatment, it is appropriate to refer the patient to a specialist or another colleague or to first acquire the specific technique. A dentist who performs a surgery which belongs to a recognized specialization in dentistry will be assessed according to the standard of care of that specialty. In Belgium there are two dental specialties recognized: orthodontics and periodontology. Since a general dentist received during his/her training the basic knowledge of orthodontics and periodontology, he may also exercise these subareas of dentistry on the condition that he meets the standards of care that are required for these specialties. A general dentist who performs endodontic or prosthetic treatments will not be compared with the dentists who followed additional training in this area of dentistry at the universities (which are not (yet) been officially recognized as a specialty) but with the *standard general dentist.* A lack of experience cannot be relied upon as a defense if something goes wrong. That means that a newly graduated dental professional or just starting up specialist must fulfill the same standards as his/her colleagues nor can an older dentist rely on the fact that he did not kept up with new treatment techniques.

That standard of care is not determined by the dental profession. It will be the privilege of the judge to decide what a dentist *ought to do.*

A dentist, who has to appear before court in a case where an endodontic file was swallowed, cannot argue that a rubber dam is not widely used in the region (country) where he practices.

The judge will take into account certain circumstances of time and place. That can be when a dentist performs an extraction on a bedridden patient without the necessary infrastructure (difficult circumstances, no accurate lightning) or when the treatment is urgent and life threatening.

The court will take into account the acquirements of science at the time of the surgery. The court will never rely on new scientific insights that were published after the disputed intervention.

5.4 Fault or Complication

The problem with dental and medical treatments is to determine if we are dealing with a fault or a complication and that is not always obvious.

Complications can be linked to the patient, the treatment, or the practitioner.

A patient can be allergic for some products (chrome-cobalt or adrenaline).

There are always risks that are inherent to the treatment. If adrenaline enters a blood vessel during injection of the local anesthetic, he may get tachycardia or syncope. This has no serious consequences for a healthy patient, but might have damaging consequences for a patient with a hidden or existing heart disease.

Practitioner-related complications are mostly the consequence of a lack of experience or incompetence, and in these cases we have to think more in terms of fault.

A judge will decide a case based on the provided evidence if a fault has been made.

In some cases, the burden of proof will be facilitated if the judge has a strong suspicion, deduced from known facts, that a fault has been committed. In that case, the burden of proof will shift to the practitioner.

A dead certainty is not necessary in civil cases, and a judicial certainty is enough (that means that there is such a strong degree of certainty that the judge does not have to consider the opposite anymore, even if it is still theoretical possible).

5.5 Admitting a Fault: Possible?

A dentist who recognizes that he committed a fault during treatment does not recognize liability. A dentist must deal honestly with his/her

[1] In Bolam versus Friern Hospital Management Committee (UK) the judge said it like this: "where you get a situation which involves the use of some special skill or competence, then the test as to whether there has been negligence or not is not the test of the man on the Clapham omnibus because he has not got that special skill. The test is the standard of the ordinary skilled man exercising and professing to have that special skill".

patient and inform him/her when something went wrong during treatment.

Recognizing liability by the practitioner should be avoided, even if that recognition does not bind the insurer. The patient has still the burden of proof, and he will only get compensation for damages from the insurer when he succeeds.

5.6 Installing a Legal Action

The prescription period of a medical error has a double limitation period: the legal action expires at 5 years. It starts to run from the day following the date on which the injured party discovers that something went wrong. No claim for damages can be installed 20 years after the date of the committed error.

5.7 What Can Go Wrong in Dentistry?

A typical treatment can be divided into several phases: the diagnosis and the medical history, the consent of the patient, the treatment itself, and the aftercare.

5.7.1 Diagnosis and Medical History

Before a dentist starts a treatment, he shall obtain a medical and dental anamnesis about the general health of the patient. That can be done with a standard form given to the patient who will answer all the questions. After completion the form is discussed with the patient to make sure that all questions are answered and understood.

This form must be at all times up-to-date and is an entire part of the dental dossier.

If not, the dentist can be held liable for all the damage that may occur.

The dentist shall use all necessary means to arrive at a correct diagnosis.

The use of diagnostic means should be in accordance with the level of difficulty.

Overdiagnosing could also be an error and lead to adverse effects for a patient (such as excessive exposure to X-ray radiation), but if necessary, the patient must be referred to a specialist for additional investigations (cone-beam CT). That means that all relevant clinical, diagnostic, and anamnestic information, related to the dental problem, must be included.

5.7.2 The Informed Consent

Each patient has a right to self-determination and the right to physical integrity. Without consent, a dentist commits battery and can be held liable for practicing illegal dentistry.

Medical and dental treatments are carried out by a person who has the legal authority to do so and require the consent of the patient.

In the United States, this problem of consent for treatment was for the first time raised by judge Cardozo in 1914 stating that: "Every human being of adult years and sound mind has the right to determine what shall be done with his/her own body, and a surgeon who performs an operation without his/her patient's consent commits an assault, for which he is liable in damages".[2]

In principle consent must be given for each treatment. In simple, low-risk diagnostic or therapeutic treatments, consent is assumed.

The consent shall be given by the patient himself. For children or people suffering from mental illness, the permission is given by the parent(s) or guardian.

The consent may be given in different ways: implicitly or explicitly.

For complex treatments a written consent form might be desirable, but it must be made in such a way that it is specifically made for the patient and takes into account all possible relevant problems (at least in Belgium).

[2] Schloendorff v Society of New York Hospital, 105 NE 92, 93, 1914.

Consent, however, is not enough. It must be an *informed* consent.

The information is given by the dentist in, for the patient, understandable terms.

The information must be given timely and to a conscious patient.[3]

A dentist shall not start with a complex treatment immediately if there is no urgent reason to do so. He shall give the patient the time to reflect on it and possibly to go for a second opinion.

Questions of the patient must be answered in good faith, and a well-informed patient will be better focused and cooperative during treatment.

- Information must be supplied on the various aspects of the intervention, on diagnostics, the nature and scope of the treatment, the risks of the treatment, and the consequences of non-treatment. The obligation is not limited to the preoperative phase, but should also be insured for the postoperative phase.
- The usefulness of a treatment should be indicated.
- The possible adverse effects and the risks of an operation must also be included.
- *How much information should we give about risks? All risks or only the relevant risks?*
- There are four different theories, which can be divided into two groups: the dentist and the patient-bound theory.
- Within the dentist-bound theory, we make a distinction between the individual dentist and the standard dentist criterion.

In the *individual dentist criterion,* every dentist decides how much information he will give to his/her patient, but this criterion will not work and will never be accepted in a Court of Law.

The *standard dentist criterion* or *professional standard theory* means that a dentist will give that specific information that every qualified and careful dentist in the same circumstances of time and place would provide to the patient. This is the rule in most Anglo-Saxon countries.[4]

The *standard or reasonable patient theory means that the dentist has to give all information that a normal, careful, and intelligent patient would like to know.*

An American judge expressed this as follows: ... a risk is material when a reasonable person, in what the physician knows or should know to be the patient's position, would be likely to attach significance to the risk or cluster, or risks in determining whether or not to forego the proposed therapy. This is a step further, taking into account all the data that are important for the individual person.

The *individual patient theory*

A Canadian judge said: *without being questioned disclose to the patient the nature of the proposed operation, its gravity, any material risks and any special or unusual risks attendant upon the performance of the operation.*

In a German case a dentist was convicted by the Oberlandesgericht in Koblenz when a block anesthesia resulted in permanent damage to the inferior alveolar nerve. This is a very seldom risk (1 in 26,722). The Court accepted that very seldom temporary risks must not be told, unless they may have a serious impact on the quality of life. In this case, a singing teacher could no longer perform his/her job in the same way as before.[5]

In Belgium we use the *relevant risk theory.*

A relevant risk can be described as a risk that everyone wants to know.

[3]Ferguson vs Hamilton Civic Hosp. "It is inappropriate for a doctor to explain a procedure and its risks to the patient outside the operation room just before it is to be performed and just after the patient has been given Valium to allay his or her anxiety".

[4]"The duty of the physician to disclose, however, is limited to those disclosures which a reasonable medical practitioner would make under the same or similar circumstances" USA, K[3]ansas. "The test of liability in respect of a doctor's duty to warn his patient of risks inherent in treatment recommended by him was the same as the test applicable to diagnosis and treatmen[4]t, namely that the doctor was required to act in accordance with a practice accepted at the time as proper by a responsible body of medical opinion" UK.

[5]Figgener L (2006) Aktuelle Rechtsprechung zum Zahnärztlichen Haftpflichtrecht, ZNN 5:5–10.

Light to relatively heavy risks which occur very seldom (less than 1 %) are only provided if they are life threatening or have a serious impact on the quality of life.

Life-threatening risks must always be indicated.

The possibility of temporary damage to the lingual and lower alveolar nerve when an embedded wisdom tooth must be extracted should be told.

The permanent damage occurs only in 0.36–0.6 % of the cases and must not be told to the patient.

The burden of proof that enough information is given differs from country to country.

France and Italy shift the burden of proof to the dentist.

In Belgium it is the patient who has the burden of proof, and even if the patients can prove the lack of information, he still must prove that he would not have given his/her consent to the treatment if he should have known it in time.

5.7.3 Therapeutic Exception and the Right *Not to Know*

These are two exceptions of the obligation to get an informed consent.

A therapeutic exception means that a medical practitioner has the possibility to withhold certain information (risks involved with an operation) if he is afraid that a patient will refuse to undergo a vital intervention. In that case the burden of proof rests on the surgeon, who must prove that he consulted at least one other colleague about this decision/situation prior to the surgery.

A patient can ask the surgeon/dentist not to be informed about possible risks. But the surgeon has a duty to warn the patient if these risks are life threatening or may have a serious impact on the quality of life.

5.7.4 Treatment

During a treatment, a lot of things can go wrong. In many cases, the damage is recoverable, and sometimes it is irreparable.

5.7.5 Follow-Up or Aftercare

Aftercare is an integral part of the treatment.

It is the duty of the practitioner to give all necessary instructions in terms of medication, possible postoperative complications, and the need for regular recalls.

5.8 The Causal Connection Between Damage and Fault and the Remoteness of Damage

A causal connection exists when it can be proved that, in the absence of the error, the damage would not have occurred.

It is sufficient that there is a necessary relationship between the error and the injury.

The burden of proof of the existence of a causal link is on the patient.

That burden can be relieved and based on common knowledge. If an endodontic file is detected in the lungs of a patient, the judge may assume that something went wrong during the endodontic treatment. In that case, the burden of proof shifts to the practitioner. It is a little bit the same as the *res ipsa loquitur* (the case speaks for itself) rule in Common Law jurisdictions.

A preexisting condition may lead to the conclusion that the sustained damages would have happened anyway also without the error. That is the case when the patient is suffering from an evolutionary process that cannot be stopped (e.g., a terminal cancer or terminal periodontitis). If the health condition is not terminal but in evolution, there will be a moment that the evolutionary process will catch up with the damage. From that moment the duty to compensate for the damage comes to an end. They are called overtaking causes in the legal literature.

The fault of a third party or from the patient himself can lead to a split liability, because there is a combination of errors.

Damage in malpractice cases must be *foreseeable* and that is agreed upon in all jurisdictions to decide that liability is at stake. That is the key question in deciding liability.

The equivalence theory: Belgium and France. This theory argues that each conduct, which is a condition for the occurrence of the concrete reprehensible event, is considered a cause. If that cause is ignored, then the accident would not have occurred in the same way. The cause must be the *conditio sine qua non.* There is no distinction made between the different causes, and each cause is equivalent, how tiny that cause may be (culpa levis).

Too remote, adequate, and proximate are terms used to see that justice is done in a malpractice case. The calculation of the compensation for damage must be legally accurate and should not contain items that are not related to the malpractice. Only *proximate, adequate, direct,* and not too remote causes will be considered so that socially undesirable consequences are avoided. This is the standard procedure in Common Law.

5.9 Dental Damage

Without damage there will be no liability, while it is possible that there is liability without fault (no-fault liability). The Civil Code (Articles 1382–1386 of the Civil Code) gives no definition of what damage really is.

Damage is a static concept, while compensation is a dynamic concept.

The most classical legal definition of damage is the negative outcome of a comparison between two conditions: the current status of the victim after the tort and the hypothetical situation in which he would have stayed if the unlawful act or omission did not exist. Damage is, in fact, the disadvantage or loss that is suffered by the victim of an unlawful act.

The compensation for damages is a dynamic concept, namely, the restoration of the victim in the situation in which he would have stayed if the tort was not committed. That can be done by medical/dental treatments or by pecuniary compensation. Restoration of the damage has a priority to pecuniary compensation.

Damage must be certain, personal, and legal. The burden of proof is on the patient.

To correctly evaluate the dental damage, the patient must necessarily find the assistance of a dentist.

Both parties in a dispute must contribute to the proof. The burden of proof should be distributed on the basis of good faith in carrying out agreements. A dentist, who is the defendant in a procedure against him, can easier provide the exact data of a case than his/her patient.

The role of the judge consists of a neutrality: He must adhere to the facts submitted by the parties, and he must ascertain equality of the parties in court. The judge can request that certain supporting documents be submitted; even if these documents are in the possession of a third party. The evidence of the damage can be delivered with all means of law.

If the existence of the damage is established, the judge must budget it. Only the existence must be sure, not its size. If the extent of the damage cannot be budgeted correctly, the judge will do it ex aequo et bono.

Hypothetical damage may not be reimbursed. The liable will only have to pay damages if it is certain that the assets or the moral condition of the victim is affected. It must not be an absolute certainty, and a legal or moral certainty is sufficient. Damage can also occur at a later time. That is often the case with medical malpractice.

5.9.1 Integral Compensation for Damages

Besides the damage for the degradation of the physical integrity, there is also moral and esthetical damage, travel costs, temporary and permanent impairment (invalidity), and temporary or permanent incapacity to work.

5.9.2 Loss of a Chance

The damage must be compensated, provided that the opportunity is real and that the loss of the chance is established. The compensation should be in proportion to the degree of probability.

In some recent judgments of the Court of Cassation, the application of the loss of a chance is apparently undermined. It must be certain that the loss of a chance (and the injury suffered as a result of that) is due to a mistake and a causal connection between the fault and the damage must be demonstrated. If the injury is not related to the error or would have happened anyway, even in the absence of the error, there is no reason for compensation of damages.

5.9.3 Reservation for the Future

It is often impossible to predict the future evolution of an injury. The condition can sometimes seem consolidated, but experience has shown that in some cases an aggravation can occur after a lapse of time (even years). This could be the case with a possible root resorption or obliteration after luxation. It is then of the utmost importance that a reservation is made for the future evolution. Only in this way can we be certain that the possibility to assess the aggravation later if it effectively occurs is safeguarded.

Insurers are opposed to such a reservation because they cannot file the dossier and they have problems to evaluate which reserves to foresee for the future. If a victim cannot get a reservation for future damages, he will never get a complete and integral compensation and that is exactly what the law requires.

In some cases an insurer may try to circumvent this by taking into account the reservations and by increasing the compensation for damages.

5.9.4 Budgeting the Damage

The judge will budget the damage at the actual price at the time of his/her decision. It must be an integral compensation for damages. The damage must be calculated in *concreto*. It has to be the exact price paid for the treatment and not an average price suggested by the dental expert.

He will take into account increases in the price of the treatments, with monetary inflation and with an increased life expectancy and all the circumstances specific to the person of the victim.

The courts do not take into account facts happening after the unlawful act or omission, which have led to an increase of the damage, if there is no causal relationship with the tort.

The compensation is integral, correct and objective, all the damage, not more, but also not less. Only the error of the victim may reduce the amount of the compensation.

5.9.5 Compensation or Reparation

Reparation is the first choice the Court of Cassation ruled that the injured party is entitled to seek recovery if it is possible or requested by the injured and/or offered by the liable party.

In many cases, however, reparation does not cover all the damage. The placement of a crown or implant will never be as good as a natural tooth. The victim is doomed to live with an ersatz. Additional damages on top of the reparation are sometimes awarded to the victim.

5.9.6 The Duty to Limit the Sustained Damage

The insured person must take all reasonable steps to reduce the damage. There is not a general obligation to do so, but he shall take all reasonable and necessary measures to avoid that the damage will grow. The Court of Cassation says in the following way: "Whereas the injured person is in principle entitled to full compensation for his/her injury, he is not required to limit the damage as much as possible, but he only has to take reasonable measures to limit the damage, and he is only required to do so if that is consistent with the attitude of a reasonable and prudent person." If he does not do so, he will not receive full compensation.

On the other end, a victim taking measures that are excessive, extravagant, and overshooting the target will also not get full compensation. He will only receive a compensation which corresponds to the full compensation applicable to his/her damage.

5.9.7 Preexisting Condition

The preexisting condition is a concept that in fact can be divided into three assumptions: the predisposition to injury, the aggravation of the preexisting condition, and the advancing of the injury.

Predestination to injury. There is the existence of negative characteristics with a potential to cause greater damage than one would expect in a normal person: classical examples of this are the man with the egg skull or the patient with hemophilia.

In that case, the preexisting condition is not taken into account and all damage incurred must be integrally reimbursed. Cassation argues that the fact that a pathological predisposition of a person has contributed to the injury does not relieve the obligation of the contributor to reimburse the full damage, except when it comes to effects that, even without the tort, would have occurred. *The tortfeasor must take the victim as he find him/her.*

The second assumption is about the *advancing of the injury.* Acceleration of the injury is a dynamic process. An existing eye disease will in case of an accident lead to quicker blindness, or a dormant cancer may result in earlier death of the victim than normal. In these cases, there is no obligation to provide full compensation for the injury because the damage would have occurred even without error of the contributor. The only thing that must be determined is the exact moment when the injury from the accident would be overtaken by the evolving situation. From that moment on all compensation for damages comes to an end.

Aggravation of preexisting condition. We have a health condition, which is not perfect, but the condition is static and not evolving. The earlier damage is stopped by a treatment. In dentistry, this might be a tooth which has already been filled.

The Court of Cassation stated that: *In case of an injury caused by a wrongful act or omission, all effects contributing to the damage will be taken into account including those related to the already existing weaknesses.*

5.10 Procedures to Get Compensation

5.10.1 Registration of the Dental Damage

The law foresees that the patient - victim has the burden of proof of his/her damage. Since he is a layman when it comes to describe the exact dental damage he must turn to his dentist for a damage report.

5.10.2 Report of the Treating Dentist

The patient's dentist has the duty to ascertain that all damages are recorded.

He will make a report and take radiographs and photographs.

The report should contain the following:

Identity of the dentist.

Identity of the patient.

A thorough medical and dental anamnesis.

The exact date of the accident (date and time).

Exact moment of the dental investigation. This is important for the prognosis of injuries (time elapsed between accident and treatment).

Exact place of the accident and a description of what happened (the nature of the accident can tell us what kind of traumata we may expect).

5.10.3 Clinical Investigation

Extraoral examination

Intraoral examination

Fractures of the jaws and the alveolar bone

Damage of the parodontium – soft tissues – lips and gingiva

Damage of the temporomandibular joints

Damage to the teeth – cracks, pulp exposure, and crown or root fracture

Tests of vitality, percussion, and mobility

5.10.4 Radiology

Not only panoramic but also apical X-rays. Details are important and X-rays from different angles give better results.

5.10.5 Photographs

One photograph can tell us more than a thousand words. Photographs are very important for the exact registration of the dental damage.

5.10.6 Treatment Plan

First aid: emergency treatment often in a hospital and specific dental treatments at the dental clinic of the treating dentist.

Treatments performed

5.10.7 Costs

A dentist shall take only temporary measures in such a way that the esthetics and the functionality of the patient are restored. In the event of an accident it is not always clear who will be held liable. The definite treatments (crowns, bridges) can be postponed till the moment that liability is established, unless the patient insist to have a definitive solution as soon as possible and will take the risk that he will not be compensated for his/her damage by a third party.

In the event of battery, where the offender could not be identified, the victim has a problem.

A judicial inquiry must identify the offender.

If there is no liability of a third party, the patient can probably find another way to compensate for the damages: a personal insurance, an accident at work, the insurance of a school or sport club, and a travel insurance.

5.10.8 Prognosis to the Future

The dentist proposes a treatment plan for the future, including the costs and the life expectancy of these restorations. There is an agreement that crowns and bridges have life expectancy of 15 years, fillings 5 years, frame prosthesis 12 years, etc.

5.11 Investigation by the Dental Advisor of the Insurance Company

If the third part has an insurance, the victim will be asked to undergo a dental examination by the dental advisor of the insurance company.

He defends in an objective way the interests of the insurance company: Is the report of the treating dentist correct, is there a causal connection between the accident and the claimed damage, and how can this be done in the most fair, accurate, and appropriate way.

There is no contradiction between an objective advice and defending the interests of the insurer. It is not in the interest of the insurer if the dental advisor should minimize the budgeting of the sustained damage. When he does so and when the insurer refuses to settle the case based on the report of his/her dental advisor, the victim may start a judicial procedure. If it then becomes clear that minimizing the damage was not correct, the judicial procedure could have been avoided. The insurer will have a lot of extra costs such as the costs of the expert witness, his/her own lawyer, and the lawyer of the victim, the costs of his/her dental advisor, and the costs of the procedure.

5.12 Out of Court Settlements

5.12.1 Settlement Between Parties

Many cases will be solved out of court by a settlement between the parties. That does not mean that mutual concessions must be done about the extent of the damage. That would not be fair. It excludes the costs of a judicial procedure and it is much faster.

5.12.2 Medical Amicably Expertise (MAE)

If the two parties cannot reach an agreement, a medical amicably expertise can be organized. It is a contractual investigation but it has the same value as a judicial expertise. It is less formal than a judicial expertise and it is in general faster.

This form of settlement of disputes can be very interesting on condition that both parties agree on the nomination of a third, jointly chosen expert. If they do not agree about the third expert, then the third expert will be nominated by the courts. It is the task of this third expert to decide all points of disagreement and to make a final report.

5.12.3 Judicial Procedure

The judge can appoint an expert witness, but before doing so he must be sure that such an investigation is necessary and opportune and cannot be solved with other less expensive means.

The judge can appoint any expert with the necessary qualifications to fulfill the mission. There is no official list of experts, although officious lists exist.

Dental experts investigate the available evidence and give a technical advice based on their findings. The judge decides the value of the evidence, but he has to recognize the strength of the evidence. This means that parts of the report may not be used out of the context of the report nor can he add anything to the report that is not mentioned or dispute the existence of the facts of the case. The advice is not binding, so the judge can decide to follow or not the report of the expert.

Dental experts can be challenged if they have too close relations with one of the parties. An expert who has any knowledge of a possible challenge will warn the parties or refuse his/her mission. In that case another expert will be assigned.

The judge describes the exact mission of the expert, the name and address of the expert, and the monetary provision of the expert. The judge will be kept informed at regular times about the evolution of the proceedings of the expertise.

The expert will convoke all parties to be present at the first meeting. Each party has to present at that meeting all pieces of evidence. All parties have the duty to cooperate with the expert.

The expert will discuss the clauses of his/her mission with the parties. If both parties agree some extra investigations can be added to the mission. He will hear and question the parties. If some specific further investigations are necessary, he will supervise these investigations and make sure that all parties can be present at these investigations, unless they agree that these investigations can be carried out without their assistance. He will decide iff further meetings are necessary. He will also give an estimation of the cost of the proceedings.

The expert has to finish his/her investigation in a reasonable period, and he shall only give his/her permission to a prolongation if it is absolutely necessary and if all parties agree.

When the dossier is complete he will write a provisional report (which contains already an advice) and send it to all parties, who have the possibility to make their remarks within a certain time. The expert must answer these remarks in a motivated way and if necessary change his/her conclusions.

He will then make a final report with his/her conclusions. He will send the report to the judge with all pieces of evidence and at the same time a copy of the final report to the parties.

5.13 Compensation for Iatrogenic Damage in Belgium

- The fund of medical accidents and its procedure[6]

5.13.1 Benefits for All Parties: Victim, Practitioner, and Insurance Company

The burden of proof is difficult for the patient. He sometimes does not know who to hold liable for the damages if it was a multidisciplinary treatment. Was it a complication or a fault? Is there a causal connection? Was the information sufficient to consent?

The practitioner is confronted today with more claim-minded patients. A claim leads to negative publicity and a damaged reputation and may result in defensive medicine (refusal of treatments and overdiagnosis)

Insurance companies will raise the premiums of the liability insurances or limit the coverage of the insurance.

It may also lead to statistical studies and preventive measures.

[6] The Law of 31 march 2010 on Compensation for accidents during medical treatment.

5.13.2 Principles

It is a two-way system: the patient has the choice between a court procedure or a procedure according to this law. He can change from one system to another at any time but not anymore after the proclamation of a final verdict by the Fund or a Court of Law.

The initiative to investigate the case comes from the FUND of Medical Accidents (FMA).

The procedure is in theory free for the patient and the practitioner and fast. The aim is that the procedure should be concluded within 6 months.

5.13.3 Fault Insurance and *No-Fault* Insurance

The FMA investigates the case and establishes liability or not and will provide compensation for damages in some cases without any fault, but only under some very specific conditions: it has to be abnormal, unforeseeable damage, taking into account the actual position of science, the actual condition of the patient, and the objective predictable evolution of his/her condition.

A therapeutic failure or wrong diagnosis is no medical accidents. The practitioner has no obligation of result, and if no fault is found, the practitioner goes free (necrosis of a tooth, fracture of an endodontic file, nervous problems after a block anesthesia). A wrong diagnosis will not lead to liability if he has used all possible diagnostic means.

5.13.4 Exclusions

This law goes not over medical experiments, pure esthetic treatments, or damage already paid for in one way or another.

5.13.5 Procedure

The patient has to request an investigation by the FMA by sending a registered letter, describing what happened, the name of the practitioner, and a description of the damage. The FMA will investigate the case if receivable and give an advice within 6 months. If the claim is not receivable, the patient can bring his/her case to a Court of Law.

5.13.6 Investigation by the FMA

The FMA collects all the information from all parties and shall if necessary (complicated case) organize an expertise before an impartial dental expert. Parties can be assisted by lawyers and dental advisors, and the cost of investigation is advanced by the FMA.

The advice of the FMA is not binding, but it can be used later in a Court of Law.

The costs for the assistance in the procedure (lawyers, medical/dental advisors) are not yet regulated by the law.

5.13.7 Advice of the FMA

That advice should be given within 6 months. It is sent to all parties.

If no liability is withhold, the patient can bring the case to court.

If liability is withhold, the FMA will ask the insurer to do a proposal.

The compensation for damages is complete and integral, including also moral, esthetic damage and incapacitation, and also the loss of a chance on a better outcome is covered.

5.13.8 Case When FMA Pays the Patient from the Fund

(a) A medical accident with no liability but under certain conditions, which are 25 % invalidity, 6 months unable to work, great loss of quality of life, and when the patient dies.

5.13.9 Further Conditions

The accident is not a normal evolution of the existing condition of the patient, that it is abnormal, not foreseeable or not predictable or if the damage could have been avoided taking into account the highest level of actual science and if it was not an accident caused by a defective product.

(b) A medical accident with liability and no or insufficient insurance:

It starts a claim against the practitioner.

(c) If insurer makes a proposal that is obviously insufficient:

It starts a claim against the insurer and/or practitioner.

(d) If liability and the specific conditions for no liability are met:

It starts a claim against the practitioner and/or the insurer.

5.13.10 After the Advice of the FMA

The advice is sent to all parties and the insurer is asked to do a proposal if the FMA withholds liability.

- The insurer can immediately dispute the liability of the practitioner.
- If the insurer does not react within 90 days, he will receive a registered letter from the FMA. If there is no reaction within a month, it is accepted that the insurer does not accept the liability advice of the FMA.
- In both instances, the patient can bring the case before the Court of Law.

The insurer sends a proposal to the patient (also to all other parties).

The patient has 90 days to accept that proposal.

If no reaction, the patient receives a registered letter from the FMA, and if there is still no reaction, the case is closed.

He can ask the FMA if the compensation is sufficient. If not, the FMA will pay the compensation to the patient and start a procedure against the insurer in a Court of Law.

The patient accepts the proposal: he will be paid within a month.

6 Aspects of Swiss Dental Law

Bernhard Knell

The Constitution of the Swiss Confederation distinguishes in the 3rd Title, 2nd Chapter, 10th Section between Civil Law (Art. 1221), Criminal Law (Art. 1231), and Metrology (Art. 125).

Legislation in the field of civil law and civil procedural law is a federal matter. This also applies to criminal law and criminal procedural law. For the organization and the jurisdiction of the courts in civil cases, the cantons are responsible, unless the law indicates otherwise. In criminal law, the cantons also have jurisdiction for the organization and jurisdiction of the courts; in addition, it is responsible for the criminal and law enforcement measures, unless the law indicates otherwise.

On September 1, 2007, the new Federal Law on Medical Profession (MedBG) and on July 1, 2008 the new cantonal Health Act of the Canton of Zurich (GesG) including the new medical regulations (MedBV) came into effect replacing the existing ones.

The following list of topics is based largely on the Health Act (GesG) of the Canton of Zurich, fact sheets of the Association of Cantonal Dentists of Switzerland (VKZS), and the Vademecum "independent professional practice as a dentist/doctor in the Canton of Zurich" of the Health Department of the Canton of Zurich.

6.1 The Independent Dentist

The Swiss dentist is allowed to practice he/her profession based on a federal certificate of proficiency and a cantonal permit to practice. He/her is either in a self-employed freelancer position or works as an assistant to a professional dentist (mostly for postgraduate education or training), in a legal entity or private practice, for example, a dental center. For the unaffiliated practice, a license from the Cantonal Health Department is required. The cantonal permit is granted when the following conditions are met:

(a) A Swiss federal or Swiss federally recognized foreign diploma
(b) Trustworthiness
(c) The physical and mental condition for the flawless fulfillment of the services offered

Permits for professional practice are granted for the period of 10 years. For professionals older than 70 years of age, the permits are limited to a maximum of 3 years.

6.2 Professional Obligations of Unaffiliated Dentists

The professional duties of a dentist are outlined in Article 40 MedBG. Since Article 40 MedBG includes general clauses requiring interpretation,

B. Knell, Dr. med. dent.
Forensic Odontostomatology, Institute of Forensic Medicine, University of Zurich, Zurich, Switzerland

Forensic Dentistry, Center for Dental Medicine, University of Zurich, Zurich, Switzerland
e-mail: bknell@swissonline.ch

K. Rötzscher (ed.), *Forensic and Legal Dentistry*,
DOI 10.1007/978-3-319-01330-5_6, © Springer International Publishing Switzerland 2014

the cantons remain relatively free within the framework set by the Federal Law to specify the following duties.

6.3 Duty of Care

The dentist is liable for any breach of due diligence on work performed. The dentist is generally per se not liable for the dangers and risks of his medical action or resulting ailments. His profession can entail risks for his patients, and for these cases, the Legal Liability Bill (BGE 120 lb 413 et seq.) can be implemented. Generally, the burden of proof for any liability rests with the patient.

The relationship between dentist and patient is of a private nature, and in Switzerland, it is part of the provisions of the Code of Obligations (Art. 394, et seq. (OR)). It therefore follows that the dentist is liable vis-à-vis the patient for diligent workmanship during the ordinary limited period of 10 years after completion of treatment.

Positively formulated: If the dentist performs his work carefully and according to Swiss standards, then there is no liability in case of failure of treatment.

For damage caused to the patient through improper dental treatment, the dentist is obligated to pay compensation. Therefore, the patient has to prove the breach of duty of care by the dentist and the causal connection between the infringement and the damage. On the other hand, the responsibility of the dentist is to provide possible exculpatory evidence to prove that he/her is not at fault (Raschein 1991).

To date, the Federal Court had not had to comment on the requirements concerning the duty of care in his professional practice, because in the few cases assessed there was no obvious violation of fundamental duties of care. The Federal Court has repeatedly expressed the importance of performing diligent services.

The principles developed for medical treatment apply mutatis mutandis to the dental treatment.

In a recent ruling (BGE 133 III 229, February 2007), the Federal Court extensively addressed the topic of the physician's liability and the legal qualification of the doctor's order: According to Article 398 para. 2 CO, the contractor (physician) is obligated to perform a careful and diligent service. It is the peculiarity of this profession that the doctor is obligated to work towards his goal in the best interest of his patient, which however does not mean that this set goal can be fulfilled or even guaranteed, as success as such is not the component of the doctor's duty.

The scope of the medical duty of care depends on objective criteria. Each case must be taken on its own merits which include the type of intervention or treatment, the risks involved, the measure of discretion for possible treatment, the means and time that the physician has at his disposal, as well as his training and performance. The breach of duty, possibly a "malpractice," legally means a nonperformance or poor performance of the contract. Should a patient suffer an injury and by fault of the doctor, then the patient is entitled to compensation. The burden of proof for any proceedings against the dentist lies with the injured party.

The importance of thorough and conscientious treatment is vital to avoid any possible malpractice suits. This includes practice infrastructure which allows the dentist to treat his patients with up-to-date standard in science and technology (§ 14 GesG). The infrastructure must be maintained and the processes of practice so designed that employees work under proper hygienic conditions (source: Vademecum Department of Health Canton of Zurich (GDZH)).

Duty of care also includes the knowledge of one's own limits and capabilities. It also only allows one to carry out medical tasks for which one is trained. Further, the duties shall be confined to the dental field. According to the definition of § 20 MedBV, this includes all treatment of the masticatory system, taking into account the relationship to general diseases and health of the whole organism. Thus, should one have the appropriate skills, it is permitted to interact with acupuncture on body parts outside of the mouth and jaw area, provided this ultimately aids in the treatment of diseases of the masticatory system.

By contrast, for example, the injection of Botox or liposuction is prohibited. Also, the dispensing/prescribing of drugs must be limited to the standard in dentistry.

The issuing of prescriptions for other drugs (such as Dormicum) is prohibited, also for his own use (GDZH).

In the event of failure, the following procedure by the arbitral panels of Zurich has proven effective: Should a filling or crown fall out during the first 3 years after completion of treatment and one suspects this to have happened due to poor workmanship, then the work must be improved free of charge, redone, or the complete amount paid refunded.

After more than 3 years, the fault of the manufacturer is often no longer definable. The arbitration will usually decide on a pro rata refund of 10 % per year after completion of treatment (i.e., in the fourth year 60 % of the fee and in the ninth year 10 % of the fee) (Vademecum GDZH).

6.4 Further Education

Article 40 lit. b MedBG obligates dentists to a lifelong training. Article 41 MedBG delegates the monitoring of the compliance to the professional obligations to the cantons. Until specifications come from the Federal Council, it is understood that the interpretation of the training guidelines is defined by the professional association. The contract between the professional association of dentists in Switzerland SSO and the insurance providers requires the training of 80 h per year to be completed. This includes 30 h of self-study not requiring proof and 50 h in the form of scientific and/or practice-relevant conferences, courses, lectures, seminars, etc. which have to be completed and documented.

6.5 Medical Confidentiality

6.5.1 Terminology

Medical confidentiality and professional secrecy mean the same thing, namely, that they are interchangeable (Martin and Guillod 2000).

6.5.2 Principle

The patient, i.e., a particular person in a medical or dental practice is the beneficiary of the doctor-patient confidentiality clause – the doctor is the guardian. The patient's existing files on diagnoses, treatment, billing, etc. are protected and can be allocated to that person.

According to the Zurich Health Law § 15 para. 2 GesG, data can be transferred within the collective practice. A transfer is only prohibited if the patient explicitly opposes.

6.5.3 Legal Basis

The doctor-patient confidentiality clause has been regulated in Article 321 of the Criminal Code (StGB) and in the Canton of Zurich in § 15 GesG since 2007:

- Those bound to the confidentiality clause are exclusively the practice owner and his assistants.
- A release of medical confidentiality is only possible either by the patient himself/herself or by a supervisory authority (Health Department).
- In case of a breach of patient confidentiality, fines of up to some CHF 10,000 or imprisonment between 3 days and 3 years is possible. Normally, the courts have interpreted the protection of patient confidentiality with tight guidelines. The patient confidentiality in Switzerland is in contrast to France not of the absolute character, as already indicated in the section principle. Depending on the situation, it may be in the interest of other persons or the general public to forward information which is otherwise protected under the confidentiality clause (Martin and Guillod 2000).

The following recommendations, which also concern patient privacy, were published in a pamphlet by the Health Department of the Canton of Zurich and are based on comments from experts and the few existing court decisions.

Dental support assistants are persons who help the dental practitioner in his profession. These are assistant dentists, dental hygienists, dental assistants, secretaries, and internal dental technicians and internal accountants. For the so-called third-party representatives (such as external dental technicians, external accountants, trustees, debt collection agencies, computer providers), the law is also controversial, and there are no precedent decisions, which either include or exclude this group of people from the medical confidentiality clause. As a precaution, it can be assumed that a representative party is not automatically included in the confidentiality clause. Not included in the confidentiality clause are all persons outside of this narrow circle, for example, practice successor, collection agencies, banks, lenders, and tax authorities. The responsible practice owner and his assistants are prohibited to give any insight into any patient's data, except when a particular patient allows for a particular third party, a limited or full insight of his data, or if the Health Department has released the practice owner and his assistants from the professional confidentiality. Data protection is regulated by the Federal Law on Privacy (DSG). The requirements of DSG apply to doctors and dentists and are only subsidiary of the Criminal Code (StGB). If in doubt, the more stringent regulations under the Criminal Code apply instead of the DSG. The DSG, however, has jurisdiction in full for dental prosthetics and dental hygiene practices, which are not under the Criminal Code.

6.6 Measures

6.6.1 Obtaining the Exemption from the Confidentiality

Normally, the dentist is released from the doctor-patient confidentiality clause by the patient himself/herself. This can be verbally (*I agree with the transfer*) or in writing (*I agree with external debt collection in XYZ*). A request for termination of the confidentiality clause (e.g., in the dispute or collection case) must be made in Zurich by the Health Department. Depending on the canton, different procedures are implemented. This could be the Chief Medical officer, the Director of the Health Department or a Health Council (Martin and Guillod 2000).

6.6.2 Dissemination of Information to Third Parties on a "Need-to-Know" Basis

The patient data to be transferred should quantitatively be limited to the essentials. The dental technician can make a crown on the basis of initials or the name (Mrs. H. Smith) and does not need the complete address or date of birth. For referral of a wisdom tooth extraction, the whole medical history is not needed. The successor (doctor) has to make a new medical history, risk analysis, and patient information in each case.

The trustee may conduct sales statistics, turnover-based payments, or value-added tax invoices on the basis of patient numbers, and the tax office is satisfied with initials.

6.6.3 Contractual Arrangements with "Third Parties"

Authorized third parties (dental technicians, IT support) must be personally briefed on the confidentiality clause, if they happen to see confidential data. The number of contact partners must be kept as small as possible. (This has to be handled with special caution when commissioning large laboratories or in combination with dental insurance agencies or IT support.)

6.7 List of Problems

Change of Employees
: Interns and employees on a trial basis have to be instructed as well.

Practice Exchange, Second Opinion
: The transfer of medical data and X-ray images is normally given directly to the patient and not transferred from practice to practice. A corresponding entry must be made in the medical record.

Successor
: Each patient must agree that the medical records be transferred to the successor. Otherwise, the obligation to keep the records for 10 years remains with the former owner.

Disposal of Data

Controlled destruction of documents after 10-year storage period; controlled destruction of hard disks in computer hardware changes

IT

Paperless practices and digital medical records are also problematic. This is because practice partner, business partner, and clinic manager have access to protected data; whole files are transferred via the Internet without anonymity to third parties; and databases cannot be completely erased in any circumstances. When building a database, the concept of how to keep the issue of patient confidentiality must be kept in mind, for example, databases must be strictly separated by practice owners. Exceptions to the confidentiality clause are mentioned in §15 para. 3 GesG:

Persons working in the public health sector are not bound to the confidentiality clause if the report:

(a) Unusual deaths, such as accident, crime, or malpractice, including its long-term effects and suicide
(b) Perceptions that indicate the intentional spread of dangerous communicable diseases in humans and animals

They are authorized to act without explicit permission:

(a) In reporting to the competent authorities, any perceptions relating to a crime or offence against life and limb, public health, or sexual integrity
(b) To help the investigating authorities in the identification of bodies (Knell and Bussmann 1999)

6.8 Duty of Disclosure

6.8.1 Legal Framework

Dental briefing is basic and indispensable in presenting the proposal of the medical/dental treatment to the patient (Wiegand, Manual, p. 119). In addition to the traditional responsibility of the dentist in cases of malpractice, the cases of insufficient medical briefing are increasing.

It is my experience as a longtime expert on legal protection insurances that there is a notable increase of legal cases in Switzerland due to insufficient medical briefing. The Federal Court has compensation claims in which no treatment error was detected (Wiegand, education p.150). This ruling was heavily criticized, but the Federal Supreme Court has upheld it since 1979, and it has been fortified in the more recent decisions for the following reason: Medical interventions are to be judged as unlawful if not based on a medical reason. The preliminary consent of the patient is considered a justification. This is however true if the patient has been adequately informed of the intended intervention. However, the information should be communicated in such a way as not to cause health anxiety for the patient. In this respect, the jurisdiction of the Swiss Federal Court is less strict than that of the German Federal Supreme Court, which does not permit any exceptions from the obligation to inform the patient (Raschein 1991).

The doctor has to prove that he/her has adequately informed the patient and that the patient has consented to the proposed treatment. In some cases, it can be assumed that the patient would have hypothetically consented, if he/her had been informed in the proper manner (source: SSO Internum 1/2008, p.14).

6.8.2 Briefing of the Patient

Dentists have to inform their patient on their own accord in an enlightening and comprehensive manner regarding:

(a) The examinations and the diagnoses
(b) The proposed and other possible treatments
(c) The risks and side effects
(d) The expected development of the medical/dental situation with or without the proposed treatment
(e) The costs

In the medical record, there has to be a note concerning the content and date of the medical briefing.

This briefing can in certain cases be invoiced in reference to the listed prices in 4011. If the patient has accepted this charge, it can also be used as evidence that the briefing has taken place (source: SSO Internum 4/2000).

6.8.3 Implementation of the Briefing

In the following discussion, Dürr Brunner and Haffter are repeatedly quoted regarding medical confidentiality in a brochure of the Winterthur Versicherungen (1996):

- The dentist shall personally perform the medical briefing. This is because only the dentist can usually guarantee a comprehensible briefing for the patient and, thus, protect himself/herself against subsequent law suits. According to Swiss jurisprudence, it is in principle permissible for a doctor to delegate the patient briefing to another doctor. If a patient's treatment however is performed by different specialists, each of them has to meet the briefing requirements for his part of the treatment (Wiegand/Abegglen, education p. 190).
- The patient is the sole recipient of the medical briefing. This principle is fully applicable also to minors or incapacitated patients, as long as they are of sound mind; otherwise, a legal custodian is required (BGE 114 Ia 350 et seq.).
- In contrast to German law, the Swiss courts have never had to deal with the factor of correct timing of a briefing. Although a correct timing of the briefing is also not possible according to German law, the factors for determining the correct briefing time depend on the case in question, the urgency of the procedure, and the size of the anticipated risks.

The more urgent the treatment, the more justifiable the delay of explanation, the greater the risk, the sooner the patient has to be informed (Eisner, explanations, p. 68).

In 2003 the Federal Court decided – except for emergencies – that for normal risk operations, the patient has to have given his consent at least 1 day prior to surgery and for serious operations at least 3 days prior to surgery. This is to give the patient sufficient time to make his decisions in terms of informed consent or to revoke the decision after careful consideration (BGE 4P.265/2002).

- Basically, the medical briefing can be given orally or/and in written form, as in Swiss contractual law the freedom of form prevails. De facto, this principle is, however, limited by the fact that only a written explanation using a formula established by the doctrine and jurisprudence of substantive requirements is not sufficient. This, therefore, requires that the briefing always be done verbally as well.
- Although the informed consent discussion is the best method of clarification, the therapist could have a problem bringing evidence in a court of law. Thus, the question arises as to the appropriate form of evidence. It may be assumed that a sufficiently well-documented medical history will be recognized by the courts as suitable evidence. Otherwise, the dentist has no fair chance to prove the taking place of and content of a medical briefing conversation. Simply, the general statement in the medical record, "the patient had been informed of the planned therapy and its complications," is not enough!
- The patient can refuse the whole or parts of the briefing. This is affirmed by both the Swiss Federal Court (BGE 105 II 288) and the German Federal Supreme Court. There has to be an explicit statement made to that effect or a behavior indicating a refusal by the patient (Raschein 1991).

6.9 Documentation Requirements

6.9.1 Principles and Guidelines for Keeping a Medical History

The legal basis for keeping a medical history derives from the civil law (Code of Obligations, OR). It can be deduced from Article 400 that the dentist has to be able to account for his actions on request at all times (Sigrist et al. 2010). The keeping of a medical history by the dentist is a professional duty (§ 13 para. 1 GesG).

The medical history has to contain all essential information of the diagnosis and treatment.

Important in the history are the records pertaining to the clinical and technical studies, the treatment briefing, the actual treatment (i.e., surgery, medication) and follow-up, treatment completion, billing, and possibly all required correspondence (e.g., insurance, certificates).

There are no binding rules on the scope and content of a medical history. The records have to be complete and true and may not be subsequently altered. Such manipulations are seen as a form of forgery. The patient record may be kept in written or electronic form. If an electronic record form is chosen, the entries in the patient record have to be dated, unchangeable, and available at all times (§ 13 para. 2 GesG).

6.9.2 Publication of the Clinical History and Radiographs

Patients are entitled to a copy of the medical history and any related documents including the original X-ray images (Vademecum Health GDZH). The original of the medical history should not be handed out. Patients are entitled to a copy of the patient record, which may need to be further commented on. The handing over of the patient record can be restricted with regard to the legitimate interests of third parties (§ 13 para. 4 GesG).

If the dentist hands out the original of the medical history, then the patient has to free the dentist from any obligation of storing it. The forwarding of X-rays to a successor doctor for the continuing treatment is not automatic due to the data protection laws. Either there is a written authorization from the patient that the forwarding is permitted or the X-ray documents are sent with an accompanying letter (indicating the sent documents) directly to the patient. It is then the patient's responsibility to send the documents on to the next dentist (Dr. iur. A. Weber, SSO, personal communication, 2003).

6.9.3 Practice Transfer

In a practice, the doctor-patient confidentiality remains in effect between predecessor and new dentist, this being the reason why patient documentation cannot be passed on automatically.

The patient is best informed jointly by the predecessor and successor in either a letter or flyer concerning the imminent change of owners and the planned transfer of the documents. The patient then has a period of 1–2-month time to consent to the transfer of his medical history to the successor. The letter also states that no response assumes agreement to the transfer of records (source: SSO Internum 2/2009, p.66).

6.9.4 Obligation to Store Records

The patient records have to be kept for 10 years after the last treatment (§ 13 para 3 GesG).

The storage requirement applies to the dentist and his successor, if the dentist dies prematurely.

6.10 FOCH

The FOCH (Forensic Odontologist Switzerland) was founded in November 1997. The primary goal was to have enough qualified dentists in situations of natural catastrophes and disasters to identify victims. The dentists working at legal and medical institutes, but primarily dentists in private practices, meet twice a year in Zurich for training and experience. Most members are consultants at legal institutes, and their deputies come from all parts of Switzerland.

The FOCH is a member of the Medical Section of the Swiss Society of Legal Medicine (SGRM) and the International Organisation for Forensic Odonto-Stomatology (IOFOS) since 2004.

References

Dürr Brunner C, Haffter S (1996) Arzthaftung – insbesondere bei Verletzung der Aufklärungspflicht. Versicherung, Winterthur

Knell B, Bussmann D (1999) Zahnärztliche Identifizierung – Schweigepflicht im Rahmen der Identifizierung von unbekannten Toten. Schweiz Monatsschr Zahnmed 109:1279–1286

Martin J, Guillod O (2000) Arztgeheimnis. Schweiz Monatsschr Zahnmed 110:1197–1202

Raschein R (1991) Die rechtliche Stellung des Zahnarztes. Schweiz Monatsschr Zahnmed 101:1033–1036

Sigrist et al. (2010) Lecture Notes doctor-patient-law. Homepage of the IRM (Institute of Legal Medicine); St. Gallen, Switzerland

Dental Law in France

7

Charles Georget

7.1 The Relation Between Dentist and Patient

7.1.1 Introduction

The relation between the dental surgeon and the patient changes as science becomes more and more efficient and as the medical technology sharpens. The Medias often make announcement effects. The medical act is therefore magnified and successful, but the complications and even the failures are eluded. The medical risk is not accepted as it used to be. The *sacred* link that used to exist between the patient and his practitioner has weakened facing the medical consumerism that tends to set in.

For a few years, the responsibility of the practitioner has been getting inexorably heavier and heavier.

7.1.2 History

When France institutes the Napoleonic Civil Code in 1804, *the physician, in the practice of his profession, is not subjected to any responsibility concerning prescriptions and the performance of his art.* Therefore, there is no responsibility until the judgment delivered on the 18 June 1835, which creates the medical responsibility. As a result, this responsibility becomes punishable or almost punishable according to the Articles 1382 and 1383 of the French Civil Code for "… *any fault from the person who, regardless of his situation or profession, causes harm to another, and there is no exception made for the physician.*" If this medical malpractice is at first applied as a general legal liability, it then becomes only applied for the most serious faults.

The Mercier judgment of 20 May 1936 acknowledges the existence of a real agreement between the practitioner and his patient:

"*A real agreement is created between the physician and his patient which includes, for the practitioner, the obvious commitment to cure the patient, that is to say to provide him not only any care support, but conscientious and careful one, and subjected to exceptional circumstances, in compliance with established science. The violation, even involuntary, of this contractual obligation is punished by the same nature of responsibility, also contractual.*" (Cass. Civ., May 20, 1936: D. 1936)

From that day on, the medical responsibility based on the Article 1147 of the French Civil Code becomes a contract.

The physician provides care to a patient that accepts it. It constitutes an agreement.

The punishable medical responsibility has therefore become contractual. This does not mean that the responsibility has diminished. The nonperformance of contractual obligations is reprehensible if it causes harm to the patient.

C. Georget, DDS, PhD
University of Nancy, Nancy, France
e-mail: georget.charles@wanadoo.fr

K. Rötzscher (ed.), *Forensic and Legal Dentistry*,
DOI 10.1007/978-3-319-01330-5_7, © Springer International Publishing Switzerland 2014

Art. 1147 (French Civil Code)

A debtor shall be ordered to pay damages, if there is occasion, either by reason of the nonperformance of the obligation or by reason of delay in performing, whenever he does not prove that the nonperformance comes from an external cause which may not be ascribed to him, although there is no bad faith on his part.

Art. 1382 (French Civil Code)

Any act whatever of man, which causes damage to another, obliges the one by whose fault it occurred, to compensate it.

Art. 1383 (French Civil Code)

Everyone is liable for the damage he causes not only by his intentional act but also by his negligent conduct or by his imprudence.

The law of the 4th of March 2002 relating to the patient's rights states unequivocal articles, and among them is the *Article L. 1110-5, first paragraph, of the French Public Health Code* which enacts that: "Any person, given her health and the emergency response that it requires, must receive the most appropriate care and the most efficient therapies that guarantee the best health security in terms of proven medical knowledge. Acts of prevention, investigation or treatment should not, in the state of medical knowledge, make her take disproportionate risks compare to benefits."

Reading this new article of the French Public Health Code, conscientious and careful care, in compliance with established science of the 1936 judgment, are stated with even more strength with terms qualifying *appropriate* care, requiring *assuring the best security regarding the known medical knowledge* and again, *not put at risk in a disproportionate way compared to the expected benefit.* The formulation is more suitable for the modern needs of science and medical practice, but it can be added to the 1936 judgment.

A real agreement between the practitioner and his patient still exists.

Art. 1147 (French Civil Code)

A debtor shall be ordered to pay damages, if there is occasion, either by reason of the nonperformance of the obligation or by reason of delay in performing, whenever he does not prove that the nonperformance comes from an external cause which may not be ascribed to him, although there is no bad faith on his part.

Art. 1382 (French Civil Code)

Any act whatever of man, which causes damage to another, obliges the one by whose fault it occurred, to compensate it.

Art. 1383 (French Civil Code)

Everyone is liable for the damage he causes not only by his intentional act but also by his negligent conduct or by his imprudence.

7.1.3 Formation of the Medical Agreement

The medical act is based on an agreement. The physician provides care to a patient that accepts it. It constitutes a will contract.

7.1.3.1 Nature of the Agreement

This bilateral agreement is established between the contracting parties binding themselves mutually towards each other (Article 1102 of the French Civil Code) in return for payment either by a direct payment of the deeds by the patient or by a third-party payer (Article 1106 of the French Civil Code).

This agreement is concluded on an intuit personae basis, which emphasizes the patient's liberty of choice who chooses the practitioner for who he is. This choice is made based on the practitioner himself. This choice gives the practitioner the obligation to provide himself care to the patient, except in cases provided by law.

There does not need to be a fault for the patient to be able to withdraw from the agreement binding him to the practitioner.

The practitioner can withdraw from the agreement without having to justify himself. However, the latter must make sure this does not cause any harm to the patient and must ensure the continuity of the care already given by another practitioner.

Art. 1102 (French Civil Code)

A contract is synallagmatic or bilateral where the contracting parties bind themselves mutually towards each other.

Art. 1105 (French Civil Code)

A contract of benevolence is one by which one of the parties procures a purely gratuitous advantage to the other.

Art. 1106 (French Civil Code)

A contract for value is one which obliges each party to transfer or do something.

7.1.4 Care Agreement

Only by existing, the agreement is a source of obligations for the practitioner. The practitioner does not commit himself to cure the patient but at least to provide conscientious, careful care in compliance with established science.

These obligations of means, caution, and diligence must be respected, or they will be punished by a responsibility also contractual. These exist in addition to the requirement of obtaining the consent of the patient before undertaking a treatment.

In France, medical agreement and medical responsibility are intimately related.

In 1967, the Supreme Court of Appeal enacts a judgment specifically regarding the dental practice. *The agreement between the dental surgeon and his patient leads the former to the obligation of providing care to the latter in compliance with the dental practice rules and established science.* There is care agreement, a term that Bery thinks is only meant for conventions aimed at proper therapeutic acts.

7.1.4.1 Validity of the Agreement

Several requisites are essential for the validity of an agreement: the consent of the party who binds himself, the absence of defect of consent, the capacity to contract the existence of a definite object, and a lawful cause.

- The patient's consent is needed in every case. This legal obligation is also an obligation of the dental surgeons' Code of Conduct (Article R 4127–236).
- It has to be a free and informed consent.
- The consent cannot contain any defects. The patient cannot be misled or abused to be persuaded to sign the agreement (Article 1109 of the French Civil Code).
- The civil capacity is required in the medical agreement. Any person may enter into a contract, unless he/she has been declared incapable by law. Non-emancipated minors, adults protected by law for mental reasons, cannot enter into the contract alone.
- The object must be certain. In dental surgery, the object is represented by the care considered.
- The cause must be lawful. It must not be against good character and public order (Article 1108 of the French Civil Code).

An obligation is therefore required: before entering into the contract, the patient must know the content of the agreement. To this end, he shall have received prior information.

Art. 1108 (French Civil Code)

Four requisites are essential for the validity of an agreement:

The consent of the party who binds himself

His capacity to contract

A definite object which forms the subject matter of the undertaking

A lawful cause in the obligation

Art. 1109 (French Civil Code)

There is no valid consent, where the consent was given only by error or where it was extorted by duress or abused by deception.

7.1.4.2 Patient Information

The practitioner must receive the free and informed consent of his patient before undertaking a treatment.

In order to decide freely, the patient must be acquainted. The practitioner therefore has the duty to give reliable information (Article R 4127–236 of the dental surgeons' Code of Conduct).

The law of the 4th of March 2002, the Kouchner law, applies this right for information of the patient. *Everyone is entitled to be informed about his/her state of health...* (Article 1111–2, French Public Health Code).

Right for Informed Consent

Everyone who can contract can consent. It is the adult patient able to express his will, the parents of the minor patient, or the person having the parental authority or the guardian of the orphan. In case of difficulty, the guardian body or the guardianship judge has to consent.

7.1.4.3 Information Issuance

It is issued during an interview. It can be either written or oral.

7.1.4.4 Information Content

The information must be simple, clear, loyal, appropriate, and complete in order to be understood by the patient.

Article R 4127-236 of the Code of Conduct of the dental surgeons:

The consent of the person under examination or cared for is sought in every case, according to the conditions defined in the Article L 1111-2 and followings.

When the patient, able to express his will, refuses investigations or the suggested treatment, the dental surgeon must respect this refusal after having informed him of the consequences.

When it is impossible to receive in due time the consent of the legal guardian of a minor or of a lawfully protected adult, the dental surgeon must nevertheless, in case of emergency, provide the care he considers as necessary.

The information is about the diagnosis, the therapeutic, the surgical techniques, the medical supervision, and the prognosis.

The information explains the goal of the treatment and its particularities, sets out the possibilities of alternative treatments, and warns about the limited future of some treatments. The patient must be informed of the possible consequences of the interventions. The law of the 4th of March 2002 (Article 1111-2 of the French Public Health Code) specifies that *the information must also be about the usual or serious predictable risks.* This does not question the information upon exceptional risks.

He is also informed of the predictable consequences in case of refusal. The patient is therefore able to decide freely.

Participation of the Patient in the Selection of Therapeutic Act

Before starting any treatment, the dental surgeon must offer every therapeutic solution possible adapted to each case. For each therapeutic, the chances of success and risks of failure must be explained.

7.1.4.5 Information Deficiency

Deficient information causes a lack of informed consent which may later be responsible for a loss of opportunity.

7.1.4.6 Non-issuance of Information

The non-issuance of information is punishable under the Article 1147 of the French Civil Code.

7.1.4.7 Exception to the Duty to Inform

The two exceptions preventing the information concern the emergency response and the patient who does not want to know the diagnosis or prognosis. The law therefore recognizes the right not to know, contrary to the right for information.

7.1.4.8 Evidence of Information

In the event of a dispute, the practitioner must provide the evidence that the information has indeed been issued to the patient. This evidence is provided by any written or oral means.

7.1.4.9 Economic Information: The Estimate

The estimate gives technical and financial information.

Every patient must be informed of the fees of the acts he has to pay partially or completely. He must be informed of the conditions of the healthcare coverage by the health insurance funds.

In France, the estimate is an ordinal obligation (Article R 4127-240 of the Code of Conduct of dental surgeons). *When the dental surgeon is led to offer an expensive treatment, he first draws up a written estimate that he gives to his patient.*

It is also a conventional obligation between the dental surgeons and the health insurance funds (order of the 14th of June 2006 and amendment #2 of the 16th of April 2012).

The dental surgeon must give to the insured party a written descriptive estimate. It notably entails:

- The precise and detailed description of the considered treatment and/or the equipment used
- The total of the fees corresponding to the treatment given
- The total of the basis of reimbursement

The estimate drawn up in duplicate must be signed and dated by the practitioner and the insured party or his guardian. This estimate is the property of the insured party who can dispose of it.

When prosthetic works have to be made, a period of 8–15 days must elapse to allow time for reflection to the patient.

As far as aesthetic medicine is concerned, a period of 15 days must elapse between the issuance of the detailed estimate and the intervention.

The conservation of a copy of the estimate signed by the patient constitutes an evidence of the consent about the financial clauses of the contract. The estimate gives evidence of the agreement about the treatment.

In France, disputes often arise when paying the fees of prosthesis not fully reimbursed by the health insurance funds and additional healthcare cover. The patients do not hesitate to look for a flaw in order to be exempted from paying partially or completely the fees. The signed estimate is often the only written proof usable to resolve the litigation during an ordinal conciliation or a legal action.

7.1.4.10 Economic Information: Costs

The practitioner must inform the patient, the consumer of care, of the prices charged. The Article 1111-3 of the French Public Health Code states that *the healthcare professional must also display in a visible and legible way in his waiting room or his office the information relating to his fees, including the extra fees he may charge.*

7.1.4.11 Information Regarding the Aesthetic Acts

The information is written, complete, and exhaustive. It is about every serious risk related to the act and every consequence possible.

7.1.4.12 Acquisition of the Consent

The consent must be acquired to confirm the contract. It can either be oral or written.

Once confirmed, the consent is not a blank document. It is not acquired once and for all. It must be renewed tacitly or explicitly in case of long-term care or when modifications occur during the treatment, for example.

As far as the prosthesis is concerned, the estimate can be considered as a kind of consent.

7.1.5 Performance of the Contract

Once the consent is acquired, the practitioner commits to apply every useful and appropriate means to cure his patient. He is bound by an obligation of means which is composed of human means (conscience and attention) and scientific means (care in compliance with established science). Some practices such as plastic surgery elude from this obligation of classic means. It is a reinforced obligation of means close to the obligation of result that would then apply.

7.1.6 Obligation of Means

7.1.6.1 Obligations of Means Related to Medical Science and Technique

The dental surgeon who has accepted to provide care to a patient commits to provide him informed care in compliance with established science, either in person or when his conscience asks him to, calling on another dental surgeon or physician (Article R 4127-233 of the Code of Conduct of dental surgeons).

The most precise diagnosis must be established. If he considered it to be necessary, the practitioner may ask a competent third party for help.

The Articles R 4127-232 to R 4127-244 of the Code of Conduct of dental surgeons deal with the duties of the dental surgeons towards the patients.

With regard to the therapeutic indication, the dental surgeon is free to prescribe anything he finds the most appropriate in the present circumstances. He must limit his prescriptions and his actions to what is necessary to the quality and efficiency of the care (Article R 4127-238 of the Code of Conduct of the dental surgeons).

The medical act is performed on the basis of the obligation to ensure informed care and in compliance with the established science. Thus, the patient is not subjected to the care provided by the practitioner but is a real player of his own care, an interlocutor taken into consideration.

The monitoring may be blamed particularly after surgical acts such as tooth extraction or implant placement. The means of this monitoring must be applied to ensure the patient supervision. The attending practitioner is responsible for the monitoring of his patient.

7.1.6.2 Ethical and Moral Obligations

The Code of Conduct endeavors to remind the practitioner of ethical points related to obligations of means and confidentiality.

Professional confidentiality is essential for every dental surgeon, except for legislative exemption. Confidentiality covers everything that became known by the dental surgeon in his professional practice, that is to say not only what he has been told but also what he saw, heard, or understood (Article R 4127-206).

Professional confidentiality ensures to the patient that what he says will not be repeated. The relation between the practitioner and his patient is reinforced under cover of the law.

7.1.6.3 Obligation of Medical Humanism

The dental surgeon must care for every patient with the same conscience, regardless of their origin, customs, family circumstances, affiliation or non-affiliation to a determined ethnic, nation or religion, disability, health status, reputation, or the feelings he may experience for them (Article R 4127-211). This humanist obligation concerns the means that must be applied to ensure with the same conscience and the same attention the safeguard of the whole population's health.

7.1.7 Reinforced Obligation of Means

Aesthetic acts are not therapeutic, nor curative, nor urgent, nor compulsory. Their request is often linked to a psychological need. These acts concern tooth whitening, ceramic veneer implant prosthetic, orthodontic, and implanting treatments. This is why the dental surgeons are empowered to perform hyaluronic acid injections for cosmetic purposes on the lips, cheeks, and chin. In this regard, the patient is not a sick person, and the practitioner is subjected to a reinforced obligation of means close to the obligation of result.

It is essential not to aggravate the initial clinical situation. Concerning the plastic surgery, the uncertainty of the results must lead the surgeon to recommend against doing the surgery.

An obligation of non-aggravation exists, knowing that the consequences of the surgery must not exceed the initial disgrace.

7.1.7.1 Obligation of Result

The obligation of result concerning the conception and the supplying of prosthesis is necessary for the dental surgeon. There is failure to comply with this obligation when the dental appliances given do not provide the service that the patient may legitimately expect from them (Cass. Civ., 23rd of November 2004, 03-12.146, Dalloz 2005, IR, p17, note). It is not about prosthetic indication, prosthetic placement, or adaptation which is about the obligation of means, just like any other medical act.

The obligation of result also applies to acts of radiology for which ones the quality (incidence, contrast, clarity, artifacts, etc.) makes the X-ray unreadable or impossible to interpret. However, the diagnosis provided from a good quality X-ray is subjected to an obligation of means.

7.1.7.2 Obligation of Security Result

The dental surgeon must answer to an obligation of security result for every procedure and equipment he uses (sterilization, packaging, etc.), the drugs he prescribes, and the medical measures he places in the mouth (fixed and removable dental prosthesis, implant, etc.) either about the manufacturing technique or about the poor design or about an anomaly of the equipment.

Conclusion

In France, the civil legislation, the Code of Conduct, and the conventions with the health insurance funds supervise the medical contract and the obligations that go along with it. Consequently, the points of references are not always easy to gauge at first sight.

The law is generalist. On the contrary, the jurisprudence that recounts precise points is fragmented. The dental Code of Conduct and the conventions do not really clarify the notion of contracts.

However, the Act of the 4th of March 2002 bears a perceptible improvement. It proclaims with strength and with a formulation more adapted to the current medical practice, the sense of the judgment of the 20th march 1936.

The Act of the 4th of March 2002 also and mainly sanctions the right for information. *Every individual has the right to be informed of his state of health* (Article 1111-2 of the Public Health Code).

Eventually, the evolution of the society shows nowadays that the patient is a consumer of care. The relations established up to this point have changed. It is a reality of society which has become a legal reality. The practitioner must be aware of this.

7.2 The Dental Record

7.2.1 Introduction

A patient record in odontology shows several interesting and even important aspects. It contains every detail about the patient. It also gives information about the patient's history, his state of health and dental status along the years, the care provided, the diagnosis, the prognosis, and the acts of prevention. A patient record guarantees a good knowledge of the patient and minimizes the existing or possible risks.

The texts of the law of the 4th of March 2002 do not contain the words *medical record* but emphasizes on the *information concerning the health*. The healthcare professionals therefore compelled by law and by the code of conduct to constitute a medical record are expected to do so. The healthcare professionals who were not compelled to do so still are not.

The law of the 4th of March 2002 does not create a general obligation.

One must yet understand that the existence of a medical record is a quality and security guarantee of the care (Cardona and Fasquel 2004). It complies with the duty of information. A well-kept record enables to ease disputes and to favor the continuity of the care most of the time.

It also constitutes an element of evidence in the context of a dispute. This may be the object that shows that the practitioner has fulfilled his obligations.

7.2.2 The Dental Surgeon's Obligations

7.2.2.1 Obligations to the Civil Law

In France, the dental surgeon is not subjected to any obligations regarding the keeping of a medical record under the general legislation. If the practitioner wishes to keep such a record for every patient of his, no rule describes the contents of this record.

However, the Article 2262 of the French Civil Code enacts that any action becomes time barred after 30 years. The same applies to the medical responsibility. In the event of a dispute, the dental surgeon who has made a dental record may submit it in court. It is an important element in order to establish the responsibility.

The dental surgeon must therefore keep his adult patient's record for 30 years. As far as a minor patient is concerned, the practitioner must keep the record for 30 years added to the number of years passing between the facts and the patient's majority. In the event of the practitioner's death, the heirs receiving the inheritance have to keep the records during the appropriate period of time. Besides, they must repair the damages caused by the practitioner until they become time barred.

The practitioners must ensure the respect of the records' confidentiality, regardless of their form.

The patients or his assignees have a right of access to the information held in the medical record. The practitioner has the right to communicate to his patient only the information he considers as relevant.

Art. 2262 (French Civil Code)

All claims, in rem as well as in personam, are prescribed by 30 years, without the person who alleges that prescription being obliged to adduce a title or a plea resulting from bad faith being allowed to be set up against him.

7.2.2.2 Moral Obligations

The Code of Conduct of the dental surgeons does not oblige the dental surgeon to keep a medical record.

If the practitioner wants to keep such records, the Code of Conduct states in the Article R 4127-208 that *in order to respect the professional confidentiality, every dental surgeon must ensure the protection against any indiscretion of the clinical records, computer documents, and materials that he may have or use regarding his patients.*

The only real obligation concerns the establishment of the estimate as written in the Article R 4127-240. *When the dental surgeon is led to suggest an expensive treatment, he writes beforehand an estimate which he gives to his patient.*

The last point of the Code of Conduct concerns the case of a patient who expresses his intention to change of practitioner. The Article R 4127-264 enacts that the dental surgeon must give him the necessary information to ensure a good continuity and the quality of the care.

7.2.2.3 Obligations to the Health Insurance Funds

According to the Professional Recommendations and References Department of the ANAES – The Patient Record in Odontology – (2000), the X-rays are an integral part of the record, and they may, for practical reasons, be filed elsewhere. In that case, they must have the same identification number than the patient's record. If the patient has asked for his X-rays, it is recommended either to keep a duplicate of these X-rays or to ask the patient to sign a receipt describing the issued views and the issuing date. The Medical Record in Odontology (2004).

Towards the Social Security, the registered dental surgeons have to date and identify the patients' X-rays. When the practitioner uses a digital radiography system, he must print at least one view corresponding to the invoicing of the radiography cession (nomenclature of professional acts).

7.2.3 The Patient's Record in Odontology

7.2.3.1 Administrative Data

In France, it is only recommended to keep a record for each patient. The constitution of the record enables a rational quality exercise. Its updating offers a good knowledge of the patient. The record must comply with these requests. It must therefore contain a minimum of data.

The medical record should enable to identify the patient without any risk of confusion. Every practitioner has the possibility to fill his record as he wants but the Agency for Accreditation and Evaluation in Health (A.N.A.E.S) recommends taking as an example a list defined by the DSIO norm published by the AFNOR.

Consultant's name	Essential
Last name	Essential
First name	Essential
Symbol to signal homonymouses	Preferable
Civil title: Mrs, Miss, Mr	Preferable
Sex	Essential
Date of birth	Essential
Place of birth	Essential
Complete address	Essential
Telephone – home	Essential
Telephone – professional	Preferable
Social Security number	Essential
Head of the household's code	Preferable
Profession	Preferable
Date of the first appointment	Essential
Date of the last appointment	Preferable
Codification of the reimbursement fund	Preferable
Last and first names of the insured party	Preferable
Codification of the additional healthcare cover	Preferable
Guardian, trustee, third-party payer	Essential
Correspondent	Essential

List published by the AFNOR and recommended by the ANAES (2000)

A.N.A.E.S, Agency for Accreditation and Evaluation in Health; **D.S.I.O**, Standard Data for the Ontological Computer Science; **A.F.N.O.R**, French Association for Normalization; **H.A.S**, The missions of the ANAES have been transferred to the HAS, created in 2005.

7.2.3.2 Clinical Data

The patient's record holds information about his state of health and habits. It specifies the state of the orofacial sphere. It contains data about the history of the diagnosis and prevention acts and the care provided.

Reasons for Consultation

The reason for the consultation is written down. It enables to remember the patient's request.

Medical Anamnesis

The medical anamnesis influences the caring for the patient. It is not enough to do it only once and take it for granted after that. As health events may happen, it must be updated regularly. The anamnesis is done either by an interview with notes or by a written questionnaire. If the latter is chosen, it must be completed by an oral interview made by the practitioner. This interview checks the answers given to the questionnaire and specifies the patient's state of health. It determines the medical risks.

Odontological Anamnesis

It draws up the balance sheet of the care provided in other dental offices before the caring by the new practitioner. Every previous oral event is written down, and the potential X-rays and medical reports and any other useful document given by the patient are read and filed.

Clinical Examination

It must be complete and includes an extraoral examination and an intraoral examination. The dental examination often goes along with the carrying out of an oral pattern.

Further Examinations

Examinations useful to the carrying out of the diagnosis and the treatment plan complete the clinical examination. They are the radiographic examinations, possibly the carrying out of dental study model, and if necessary biological analysis. Every other examination considered as essential must be conducted.

Diagnosis

It is recommended to write down in detail the diagnosis in the record.

Exchanges of Views with Other Healthcare Professionals

It is advised to keep every communication related to the patient. Every important oral indication given by another healthcare professional must be duplicated by a written one.

Treatment Plan

The practitioner commits himself into giving informed care in compliance with the established science. It is therefore recommended to write down a treatment plan and to show it to the patient.

The detailed treatment plan is registered in the record. It can be altered, but the modifications as well as the initial plan will be explained to the patient who will then agree or disagree to it. A descriptive estimate based on the treatment plan is written.

Treatments

During the course of the appointments, it is desirable that the practitioner writes down the acts performed and the prescriptions issued. Asking the patient if he has had a reaction to the drugs and materials used during the previous session is an act of prudence. Every reaction shall be written down on the care record.

Therapeutic Follow-Up

The ANAES recommends the implementation of a therapeutic follow-up of which modes must be explained to the patient (follow-up frequency, follow-up examinations).

Prevention

It is recommended to establish for every patient an individualized schedule of the acts of prevention.

Documents to Be Kept in the Record

It is essential to keep the X-rays that could be given to the patient in exchange for a receipt. If a record of agreement to the care has been written, it shall be added to the record. The same applies to the estimates, the prescriptions, and the certificates. As far as security is concerned, every prosthetic continuation sheet and incident report of any kind shall be filed.

7.2.4 Emergency Care

With a patient unknown from the practitioner, precautions must be taken in order to prevent any risk.

Before any act is undertaken, it is necessary to proceed to the complete medical and odontological anamnesis. It is recommended to have the interview written down and to complete it with the patient. The administrative record can be reduced to the minimum.

7.2.5 The Materialization of the Record

No standardization is requested. The recommendations made notably are that the record must be clear, readable, and updated. The record may exist on paper or on computer. The record's presentation must be progressive. Regardless of the chosen material, this care record must be protected to ensure the confidentiality and to respect the professional confidentiality (premises or piece of furniture not accessible to the public and securing of computer data). Every computer file must be declared to the National Commission for Data Protection and Liberties (CNIL) before being used.

Conclusion

Unlike the healthcare facilities, no legal text makes the self-employed dental surgeon settled in the city keep a patient record.

It is certain that dental surgeons keep records. They are more or less elaborated, but they can at least be a use of keeping the invoicing of the acts. They write down at least the patient's contact details.

Good record keeping enables a global caring for the patient and to be reminded of the whole clinical record. It helps to plan the acts, to explain, and to talk about the treatments with the patient. By existing, the records contribute to the administrative management.

At the request of the patient, it makes the communication of information about him easier.

Finally, in case of extreme necessity, this record will allow to collect antemortem data in order to identify the person.

References

ANAES (2000) The patient record in odontology. The Professional Recommendations and References Department

The Medical Record in Odontology (2004) Medical law and identification applied to odontology magazine, September 2004, pp 53–56

Cardona J, Fasquel D (2004) The medical record and social security: medical law and identification applied to odontology magazine, September 2004, pp 43–47

8 Dentist's Responsibility and Jurisprudence in Norway and Other Nordic Countries

Tore Solheim

8.1 Introduction

The dentist's professional responsibility can be divided into that according to either criminal law or civil law (jurisprudence). Criminal responsibility is regulated by laws whereby you risk punishment, either as a fine or by jail sentencing, if you break the law.

Civil responsibility is a responsibility towards other persons, bodies, or organizations. No criminal law is broken, but it may originate as a disagreement between the dentist and other parties, usually the patient, often involving economic aspects. It may also be an accident, and the victim, usually the patient, may demand economic compensation. Other cases may involve a missed diagnosis or a treatment that does not fulfill the patient's wishes. The civil responsibility may also be directed towards the Dental Association where malpractice or ethical conduct may be the issue. Finally, it may be against colleagues or coworkers if disagreement arises.

In other Nordic countries, the dentists' responsibilities are comparable to those in Norway; however, the exact laws and regulations may vary.

T. Solheim, Prof. (em) Dr. odont.
Institute of Oral Biology, Pathology and Forensic Odontology, University Oslo, Oslo, Norway
e-mail: tore.solheim@odont.uio.no

8.2 Criminal Law

Criminal law was intended to be a superheading, now as it is printed it may need a text. I suggest: "A number of laws may be broken whereby the dentist risk punishment. The most important is the Penal Code 2005 and the Health Personnel Law 1999. However, there are also other laws which will not be discussed here. These include laws on criminal proceedings, prescription of medicine, book keeping and taxation, working environment and working time, health and social preparedness in case of war and alternative treament of diseases.

8.3 Penal Code 2005

This law regulates the entire population of the country. Certain paragraphs, however, may be more relevant to dentists. The law states that assault is a criminal offence. If a patient has not consented to treatment, then the dentist is seen to have committed an assault. It is thus important that the patient is informed about treatment to be performed and gives his consent. He should also be given the opportunity to refuse a treatment at any time. This is further explained under special laws.

This law also confers the duty of confidentiality to employers in public services, including dentists. All health personnel, inclusive private practitioners, are governed by the *Health Personnel Law* which also requires the duty of confidentiality.

K. Rötzscher (ed.), *Forensic and Legal Dentistry*,
DOI 10.1007/978-3-319-01330-5_8,

However, the punishment of a breach of the law may for them be more severe according to the Penal Code, 6 months versus 3 months.

According to the Penal Code, misappropriation of funds is a criminal offence, and dentists found to be benefitting from illegal earnings may thus be punished according to the Penal code.

The Penal Code and also the Law on Child Protection state that a health worker is released from the duty of confidentiality in cases of suspected child abuse.

8.4 Health Personnel Law 1999

This law is directed towards all personnel providing health care. It is therefore rather general and not specific for dentists. From 1980 until 1999 there existed a law specific for dentists and physicians. The old law afforded a number of rights to the dentists, and in reality the monopoly held by dentists has disappeared with the new law. The new law only has duties the dentist and other health personnel must follow.

We, as dentists, have an ethical obligation to be responsible. Auxiliary personnel may be used if appropriate to the task in question. It is obligatory to provide emergency treatment. It is obligatory to abstain from alcohol and other narcotics during work. It is also forbidden to accept gifts given during the course of work. Advertisements should be responsible, reasonable, and sober. Attests and declarations should be objective.

When starting to practice it is necessary to file a report with the local community. It is also obligatory to have medical indemnity insurance.

It is a general rule that the personnel must maintain confidentiality regarding treatment and patient information. However, if the patient may give his consent the information may be passed on to others. After the death of the patient information may be given if valid reasons exist. Information may also be given to other healthcare professionals who are treating the patient, unless the patient objects. If an examination is performed in the capacity as an expert in a court, then it is acceptable to provide the court with information as long as the patient has been informed of the role of the dentist and the reason for the examination.

According to this law a record must be kept for each patient. The content of the record is subject to regulation (Regulation of Record Keeping 2000). It must be clear who has written the record. The patient may see his record and can ask to have it corrected if it is wrong. If the patient does not object the record may be transferred to another practitioner. Electronic records may be used, and the health authorities may have access to the records in case of dispute concerning authorization.

Authorization may be given not only to dentists but also to dental hygienists, dental health secretaries, and dental technicians. Authorization is normally lost when the dentist is 75 years of age. It may be temporarily or permanently lost if the dentist has a serious mental disease and physical disability, uses alcohol or narcotics, has been out of practice over a long period, or be guilty of malpractice or misconduct. The dentist may be given a warning. In case of violation of the law, the sentence may be a fine or up to 3 months prison sentence. A Committee for Health Personnel may examine the case if the dentist does not agree with the reaction from the health authorities.

In Sweden a patient security law affords specific rights to the authorized personnel. It is not specific to dentists; however, it is stated that following injection of local anesthesia, only authorized personnel may examine or give treatment to the patient.

In Iceland there is a special but relatively short law for dentists.

8.5 Regulation of Record Keeping 2000

This regulation is given according to the Health Personnel Law. It should in detail describe what a record should contain. However, it is only given in general terms for all health personnel, and again it is rather unspecific for dentists. Many of the paragraphs are only relevant for hospitals.

It is stated that the record should be written only in Norwegian, Swedish, or Danish. English is not acceptable in the record. The record should be written up immediately following treatment completion. It should be dated and signed so that there is accountability.

The record should contain information so that the patient can be identified. Also, if the patient does not have the competency to agree to a treatment it should be recorded who has this right on behalf of the patient. In addition to consultation and treatments, instruction and advices should be recorded.

8.6 Insurance

According to the Health Personnel Law, the dentist must have insurance. This was previously covered by private insurance companies. Now the state insurance company "Norsk Pasientskadeerstatning," Norwegian state patient injury compensation, is responsible for the insurance in all medical treatments. The dentist must renew this insurance each year, and the insurance premium is according to type of treatment and hours spent in practice. This insurance pays for any injuries, no matter if the dentist may be reproached or not.

8.7 Patient's Rights Law 1999

According to this law, the patient has the right to necessary – and emergency – help. He has also the right to an evaluation of his condition and to freely choose the hospital as well as the dentist. Necessary information allowing the patient to understand his situation must be given. If he does not want this information, he has the right to refuse.

The patient has the right to accept help with his health. He may also withdraw his consent at any time. The consent may be silent by the fact that the patient sits in the chair. However, he must constantly be oriented about what is going to be done and given the possibility to refuse. In the case of incompetent patients, his will should never the less be respected as far as possible. It is a strong restriction to cases where a patient must be treated against his will. The patient can gain access to his own record and can ask for correction or deletion. Complaints about rights not obtained can be sent to the county physician, and a patient's ombudsman may help the patient to obtain his rights.

8.8 Dental Jurisprudence: Civil Law

No laws are broken, but there is a disagreement between the dentist and another party, most often the patient, but it may also be other colleagues or the Dental Association. Few laws regulate this. However, as there often arises a question of economic compensation, a law exists (2001) concerning compensation for patient's injuries. It was validated for public health services in 2003 and for private health service in 2009. This law gives *objective* responsibilities for damages during medical (inclusive dental) treatment. Similar laws have been in use in Sweden and Finland a greater number of years. In Denmark or Iceland still *culpa or negligent responsibility is applied.* When damage occurs in the practice under *objective liability,* the dentist is responsible in all cases even if he cannot be accused of having been negligent. Of course he must have insurance that covers this eventuality. Previously Norwegian dentists were insured by private companies. Currently a state-run company, "Norsk pasientskade erstatning," has assumed all medical insurance responsibility. The cost of the insurance has accordingly increased two- to five-fold. As patients become more acquainted with their rights, the cost will probably rise even more.

8.9 Law on Compensation for Patient Damages (2001)

This law covers damages due to failure in rendering health aid even where blame does not fall on the dentist. This is called objective responsibility. In addition it covers technical equipment failure and infections. Vaccination and responsibilities according to general rules of compensation are also included. These may be according to subjective or culpa responsibilities.

The insurance does not cover responsibilities below 5,000 Norwegian kroner (about Euro 670). If the damage was inflicted knowingly, the insurance can claim legal remedy from the dentist. All health providers must notify "Norsk pasientskadeforsikring" each year and pay the fee according to the type of aid and amount of hours worked.

Any claim must be submitted in writing, and if this is delivered to the dentist he must immediately send it to the insurance company. The company decides whether and how much compensation is to be paid. Both dentist and patient must be notified of the result. Complaints about the result may be sent to the Patient Damage Committee who has the power to change the decision.

8.10 Complaints About Dental Treatment

If a patient is dissatisfied with the dental treatment given, he may file a complaint to the Complaint Committee within the Norwegian Dental Association. It must be in writing, and the committee will examine the case and suggest a solution. This solution is limited to either a full refund or, if possible, a free renewal of the work carried out.

A more official route for a complaint is to the county physician. He will decide the action to be taken. If the problem is serious or difficult it may be forwarded to the Directorate of Health. If the dentist is found to be negligent he may be given a warning or a temporary or permanent withdrawal of the license to prescribe medicine or to practice.

If the patient demands compensation for damage or suffering, he must send the complaint to *Norsk pasientskadeerstatning*. The complaint will then be dealt with according to the practice described above. It is also possible to file a complaint against a dentist to the Consumers' Association or to the Competition Authority of the State if the question concerns the competition or price.

8.11 Ethical Rules of the Norwegian Dental Association

The Dental Association makes efforts to improve the ethics of their members and have set up a number of ethical rules or guidelines for dentists. They have also an Ethical Committee to be consulted when ethical problems arise.

It is stated that the considerations regarding the patient's health must be superior to all other considerations. It is necessary that the dentist practice in accordance with science and experience. He must update his knowledge and be familiar with laws and regulations for his practice.

The dentist must keep records according to laws and regulations and must maintain professional confidentiality. He has a duty to inform his patients about fees according to laws and regulations.

A patient must be free to choose a dentist, but a dentist may also refuse to treat a patient if valid reasons exist. A dentist must give emergency help to patients in need and must in addition to treatment also provide advice and instruction. Unnecessary and unreasonably expensive treatment must not be given. The treatment must be based on informed consent.

All treatment must be completed unless interrupted by the patient. Patients should be referred to other dentists with more suitable competence if necessary. If the dentist finds changes to the general health of the patients, the patient's permanent physician should be informed.

The dentist must help the patient to obtain their rights according to the law, but must not help the patient to obtain undue advantages, economic or otherwise.

In relation to colleagues, a dentist should give support and help. He should not unduly criticize the work of his colleagues. However, the patient's health must supersede this. Disagreement must be kept on a professional level and not be publicized in such a way as to damage a colleague's reputation.

If professional or ethical failure is discovered it should be taken up directly with the colleague in a careful way. It could also be brought before the local dental association or a superior person. When a patient is referred to a specialist, the specialist should, following completion of treatment, provide the referring dentist with an orientation about the diagnosis and treatment. No further treatment should be given. Likewise if emergency treatment is given, the patient's dentist should be given an orientation and no further treatment should be given.

A dentist must practice under his own name and be able to provide evidence that he is member of the Dental Association. Advertisements must not be incorrect or misleading. Patients must not be contacted unless an agreement has been established. Any official publication must have a general form, and he must not make statements that contradict with views held by the Dental Association. If the dentist has a different opinion, it must be made clear that this is his own opinion and not that of the Dental Association.

If a dentist violates the ethical rules the Dental Association may react with a criticism or give a warning. If serious, the dentist may be asked to pay a fine or be excluded from the Dental Association with eventual publication of the case.

8.12 What May the Dentist Be Held Responsible for?

Following an accident it is the dentist according to the law responsible even if it was an accident that could easily happen. Clearly the dentist is held responsible in cases of malpractice. It is, however, more difficult to ascertain with whom the responsibility rests when regular treatment does not lead to the expected result. The insurance will not pay in all such cases.

It may often be the situation that no formal ethical rules are broken. The dentist and the patient may disagree about what is ethical or not. In these cases it may also be very difficult to decide what is right or wrong.

The dentist will always be responsible for injuries due to accidents. If these occur after gross negligence or on purpose, the insurance company may take regress from the dentist. Examples of injuries that may occur are foreign objects in the trachea or esophagus and severing the lingual artery, both of which may be life threatening. Accidental jaw fractures, or severed lingual nerve or mandibular nerve occurring in the course an operation, are also severe injuries. Less severe damages are artificial perforation of the pulp during tooth preparation or instrument fracture in the root canal during root canal treatment. In addition, fillings or crowns may be loosened during preparation or extractions.

The opinion of what really constitutes malpractice may be very subjective. It is reasonable to say that small deviation from normal is natural. It is impossible for a dentist to give optimal treatment 100 % of the time. One case may also be more difficult than another. A specialist should also be able to provide a more ideal treatment than a general practitioner. Therefore, the patient may sometimes have to accept a treatment which is suboptimal.

One reason for the result to be suboptimal may be that the dentist has chosen a treatment according to sound professional assessment, which later did not give the expected result. In these cases the dentist cannot be responsible. However, if the treatment was chosen based on lack of knowledge or poor clinical judgment, the dentist will be responsible.

It may also be bad if a diagnosis has not been made or a necessary treatment is not given. Failure of making a diagnosis which should result in treatment is serious. If this did not lead to consequences for the patient, then the dentist will not be held accountable. If, however, this leads to negative consequences, for example, undiagnosed caries which later resulted in pulp involvement requiring root canal treatment, then the dentist will be held responsible.

8.13 Concluding Remarks

The dentist's responsibility may be about the same in all countries. The laws may vary somewhat in the different Nordic countries, but may vary more between other countries. Also the way it is handled by lawyers and insurance companies may vary. The main difference may be in that in most countries only culpa responsibility applies. The patient must be able to prove that the dentist has been negligent in some way before he can get any economic compensation. In three of the Nordic countries objective liability or no fault liability is the rule according to the law.

The discussion may be who is most close to carry the burden of an accident? It may for the patient have unbearable consequences both in suffering and economics. The dentist may have insurance for this so it is easier for him to carry the consequences. He is also the one who has contributed to the accident and may have been more or less negligent.

For the dentist, it may be an advantage that he does need to be engaged in a nerve-wrecking process of proving or disproving his negligence. An accident has happened, and it may only be fair that the patient has the right of economic compensation regardless of the dentist being negligent or not. The issue of negligence need not be explored or discussed at all. The only disadvantage is that the insurance fee increases considerably. For the dentist it may not mean so much as he may increase his fees to cover this. Maybe in the future, other countries also will adopt this practice.

References

Ethical rules of the Norwegian Dental Association. http://www.tannlegeforeningen.no/storypg.aspx?id=676&MenuNode=634257788832825451&zone=70

Health personnel law (1999). http://www.lovdata.no/cgi-wift/wiftldles?doc=/app/gratis/www/docroot/all/tl-19990702-064-0.html&emne=helsepersonell*&&

Insurance/Patient injury compensation (2001). http://www.lovdata.no/cgi-wift/wiftldles?doc=/app/gratis/www/docroot/all/nl-20010615-053.html&emne=pasientskade*%20%2b%20erstatning*&&

Law on Compensation for Patient Damages (2001): http://www.lovdata.no/cgi-wift/wiftldles?doc=/app/gratis/www/docroot/all/nl-20010615-053.html&emne=pasientskade*%20%2b%20erstatning*&&

Patient's Rights Law (1999). http://www.lovdata.no/cgi-wift/wiftloksok?base=QNL&sys=1&felt=emne&emne=Lov+om+pasientrettigheter&button=S%F8k&PROS=02

Penal code (2005). http://www.lovdata.no/cgi-wift/wiftldles?doc=/app/gratis/www/docroot/all/nl-20050520-028.html&emne=STRAFFELOV*&&

Regulation of Record Keeping (2000). http://www.lovdata.no/cgi-wift/wiftldles?doc=/app/gratis/www/docroot/for/sf/ho/ho-20001221-1385.html&emne=pasientjournal*&&

Dental Law in Finland

9

Hannu Mäkelä

9.1 Public Dental Care

According to the law of social affairs and health, public dental care provides compulsory dental treatment for the population up to the age of 18 years without payment. The dental care of the population older than the age of 18 years varies, depending on the capacity of the home municipality, such that small communities often are able to better provide for their citizens, even up to 100 % of dental care, than larger communities. However, waiting lines are not avoidable. There is legislation to guarantee that waiting times are kept within acceptable limits. Any dental treatment must begin within 3 months after a dental check-up. Another delay of 3 months is allowed if the dental condition of a patient would not adversely affect the patient's health.

9.2 Private Dental Care

The cap between the request for and the offer of dental treatment is bridged by cooperation with the private sector. Municipalities have made agreements with private dentists so that those patients will have their dental treatment subvented. Many patients prefer direct consultation with private practitioners. The costs of private dental treatments are paid by the national illness insurance in preset conditions. Private dentists mainly practice in cities.

9.3 Free Choice of Practitioners

A patient has a right to freely choose their practitioner; in the future, even throughout Europe. At the moment, a patient can freely choose a dental practitioner in a public dental care center. Later, patients can freely choose the entire dental care center in a community or in the entire country. Because of the role of the European Union (EU), a patient will have compensated dental care in the EU with the same conditions as those in Finland. However, costs will be compensated according the regulations in Finland.

A "ping-pong effect" caused by the continuation of dental treatment is not desirable, therefore, a patient should stay in a chosen dental office at least a year, for example.

9.4 Documentation

The documentation of dental care is regulated by the Ministry of Social Affairs and Health. Thorough documentation is also an elementary step in dental care. A treatment without documentation actually is not processed.

Nowadays the documentation is mainly computer based. This is a helpful way to obtain a complete documentation in a clearly readable

H. Mäkelä, DDS, PhD
LtCol res Finnish Air Force MC, Havutie 12,
FIN-40950 Muurame, Finnland
e-mail: hannu.makela@pp5.net.fi

K. Rötzscher (ed.), *Forensic and Legal Dentistry*,
DOI 10.1007/978-3-319-01330-5_9, © Springer International Publishing Switzerland 2014

and universally understandable form for forensic purposes. These days, X-rays are also mostly in digital form as well, so they can be quickly sent to investigating authorities around the world.

The Ministry of Social Affairs and Health coordinates the national dental care. A statistical evaluation of dental care results for administrative procedures, quality control, and scientific, especially epidemiological, research of dentistry requires computerization.

The future plan is for the entire health care system in Finland to be placed in a national central database. There is an essential problem of how all of the computer programs will communicate with each other. There are many different computer programs for dental care on the market, and the wound point is the common contact point.

For forensic purposes, it is essential that computer programs include a feature to gather information for the identification according to findings, not personalities. If a program would be able to list patients in a dental office, e.g., those with implants, or with some type of prosthetic work, the identification procedure would be more effective.

9.5 Privacy

Privacy in dental care is nowadays a serious matter. In Finland, there is special legislation for data protection. Private life is protected by the constitution and should be inviolable. Because of the law for data protection, patients are allowed to control the use of their personal data. They decide who is allowed to see and work with their records. A dental staff is obliged to inform patients about the patients' rights. Patients are authorized to regularly obtain information regarding who is involved with their personal data. The dental staff is only authorized to handle the dental data of a patient as a member participating in dental care.

9.6 Health Care Insurance

All Finnish citizens and people living permanently in Finland are insured by the national illness insurance. A patient can obtain dental treatment in the public dental care sector or in a private sector. Payments in the public dental care sector are limited by a legal act and the rest of the cost is carried by the community. In the private sector, a patient obtains a partial refund of costs from the national illness insurance.

9.7 Malpractice, Evaluation of Dental Damage

If a patient is not satisfied with their dental care, the patient first contacts their practitioner and informs the practitioner about the problems around or unsatisfying results of the dental care. If possible, the problem will resolved at this level. The problem is frequently a lack of information. In the public sector, the superior of the dental clinic and the patient ombudsman will also be notified.

In Finland, every dental practitioner must have liability insurance for malpractice and complications in dental care. In the public sector, the organization handles the insurance and a private practitioner will have a personal agreement with an insurance company. In accusations of malpractice or evaluation of dental damage, all documents, x-rays, casts, etc. are collected from the practitioner or clinic. An experienced dentist will be ordered, as an expert, to reexamine the whole chain of dental treatment, beginning from the first dental check-up, over the subsequent dental treatment, to the end result. The experienced dentist will give their opinion if the case is a complication arising from the risk of dental therapy or malpractice. This opinion can be the basis for an insurance payment.

The National Supervisory Authority for Welfare and Health is an authority that supervises all medical professions. After earning a dental degree from a university, an authorization is granted to practice as a dentist. This authority also supervises dental care in Finland, ensuring that the dentists are qualified and that dental care is available to everybody who needs it. The capability of dental professionals must be on a qualified level, if there is a remarkable disability in professional skills, the authorization can be restricted or even cancelled.

Patients who are not satisfied with the dental treatment they have received may possibly revise their dental care. If a patient cannot reach a solution with their dental practitioner regarding a dental matter with complication, they contact the Finnish Patient Insurance Center. This center, set up by the insurance companies, is charged with the practical handling of cases with complications or malpractice. After getting a report from a patient, this center requests a statement.

Forensic Odontology in the United Kingdom

10

Ian R. Hill and James Hardy

10.1 Introduction

Despite the historical record, the United Kingdom, like other countries, was slow to recognize the value of forensic odontology as an adjunct to legal proceedings. Increased recognition of the benefits bestowed by the subject largely results from the efforts of Scandinavian workers and the Federation Dentaire International (FDI). By promoting forensic odontology in the academic environment, the FDI and its contributors did much to underscore its claims to academic respectability. This has led to its acceptance in assisting the legal process in many countries, although it remains a minority speciality. Like other jurisdictions, British courts have recognized that dental expertise can be useful in resolving legal questions. However, it has to be accepted that it is an adjunct to these proceedings, and not a prime mover. Trial by experts is not liked by the courts; they prefer a system in which all of the evidence placed before them is considered in context, and not in isolation. Only in that way can a true determination of the issues be made. It is this dislike, or perhaps concern that experts could usurp the role of the court, that has been an impediment to the acceptance of the expert in trials. However, despite these misgivings, forensic odontology is widely accepted by all of the UK courts. Increasing sophistication in the methodologies available means that the value placed on the subject has increased. The courts have recognized this and are much more demanding of those who would claim that they are experts. This is quite different from some aspects of an editorial in *The Lancet* for 15 December 1951, which reported that "teeth have often played a distinctive part in reconstructing crime" (Anon 1951).

The writer's enthusiasm hid the fact that at that time there were few practitioners, they worked in isolation, and there was no recognized training.

Obviously, there is a need for those professing special knowledge to prove that they are thus qualified, and this means that those aspiring to be forensic odontologists have to acquire the requisite knowledge. Those who have been accredited must show evidence of continuing professional development. Much of the impetus for the provision of educational facilities in the United Kingdom has come from the British Association for Forensic Odontology, which was founded in 1982, with the aid of IOFOS, the FDI, and the British Dental Association (Hill et al. 1984).

At the present time (2013), the United Kingdom is in the fortunate position of having sufficient forensic odontologists to meet the

I.R. Hill, OBE, MA, MD, PhD, MRCPath, FFFLM, MRAeS, LDS (✉)
International Organisation for Forensic Odontostomatology – IOFOS, London, UK
e-mail: irhill@mail.com

J. Hardy, OStJ, BDS (Lon), MSc, MGDSRCS (Eng), MGDSRCS (Ed), LDSRCS (Eng), Dip F Od, Dip FHID
Criminolgy Department, Portsmouth University, Portsmouth, UK
e-mail: jojhardy@gmail.com

K. Rötzscher (ed.), *Forensic and Legal Dentistry*,
DOI 10.1007/978-3-319-01330-5_10,

needs of HM coroners, procurators fiscal, the police, UK Disaster Victim Identification Teams (UKDVI), and other disaster management organizations and social services. The United Kingdom at present has a reserve pool of qualified and accredited forensic odontologists resulting from the numbers of dental practitioners attending the Diploma in Forensic Odontology courses, MSc courses in Forensic Odontology, and other related courses in recent years. However, the outlook for the future training of forensic odontologists in the United Kingdom is uncertain due to the recent termination of a number of these recognized courses.

10.2 Dental Law in the United Kingdom

10.2.1 The Legal Basis of Expert Evidence

The conditions governing the provision of expert evidence in UK courts reside in the complex web of laws of evidence. These have a common law ancestry, and this sometimes predisposes them to some criticism. As Keane (1994, pp. 1–3 and 15–18) says, "the modern law of evidence remains essentially a case-law subject, built on common law principles and overlaid with a statutory veneer." Not surprisingly, this leaves the laws open to challenge, especially where admissibility is concerned. The details of these conflicts and the law itself are outwith the scope of this book, suffice it to say that the primary object is to provide a forum wherein a fair assessment of admissible evidence is made. If evidence is to be admitted, it must be relevant, and not excluded by any rule of the law of evidence. A consequence of this is that, no matter how relevant some evidence is, it may be excluded. An out-of-court statement about the case, such as an admission of guilt by a third party, would be excluded under the rule of hearsay. Lay people sometimes find these rules hard to accept, believing that they can be inimical to the search for justice.

Many countries have adopted the English system of justice, which is based on a Common Law approach, and is characterized by an adversarial approach to the judicial process, as opposed to the inquisitorial system used in Roman Law jurisdictions. Variations do exist in the way that the English system operates in different countries, as is seen in the United Kingdom, where England, Wales, and Ireland are essentially the same, but Scottish Law is an amalgam of English Law and Continental Law resulting from its alliances with France. Even where the systems are similar, such as in Ireland, it must be remembered that they are separate systems (Spencer 1990). There is much reciprocity between the English and the Scottish systems, with decisions finding their way into one another's deliberations. Similarly, there is a free flow of experts across the boundary. English and Scottish laws have influenced the legal systems in many countries, especially those in the British Commonwealth and the United States, but they are sovereign states; thus, they are not bound by British decisions and have their own law and procedures. There is also some reciprocity between decisions made in Australia, New Zealand, and Canada and the law in the United Kingdom.

While these differences are important, reflecting cultural and procedural demands, they do not materially affect the way in which forensic odontologists work; Scotland may demand that two odontologists examine the case. In practice, a free flow of experts operates across the border, and there is unanimity in their approach, with common professional development, standards, and methodologies. There are though differences in the court structure, and those working in Scotland are required to add to their statements the words that they testify on soul and conscience. Although the differences are largely procedural and therefore not relevant to the practice of making a forensic examination or the principles underlying the basis of opinion, they are important. There are also differences in procedure in the civil, criminal, coroner, and sheriff's courts, and forensic odontologists should be aware of the differences. A lack of awareness of the matter of the proceedings.

10.3 Training

As a subject and speciality, forensic dentistry in the United Kingdom has always taken a low priority in the undergraduate teaching curriculum in dental schools. Indeed at undergraduate level, teaching tends to be opportunistic, with little formal recognition. Similarly in the past, postgraduate education was sporadic. The first serious attempt to address the problem of this lack of training was the introduction in 1984 of the postgraduate Diploma in Forensic Odontology (Dip F Od) course run at the London Hospital Medical College. This was a day release course that proved to be extremely popular. The course extended over three 10-week terms at the end of which the students sat a written examination, had a viva, and gave a presentation of an original research project conducted by themselves. This was a highly successful course. After 4 years, it closed and, following a few years break, moved to the University of Hertfordshire where it continued to run for a further 4 years.

For several years, an MSc course in forensic odontology was run at the University of Cardiff in Wales under the direction of Professor David Whitaker. Following his retirement, Dr. Cath Adams continued to run the course for several years in Cardiff. More recently, the course has been run at the University of Glamorgan, although now 2013 the last intake of students is undergoing training. There are no plans to enroll more students for future courses at the University of Glamorgan.

The Centre for Forensic and Legal Medicine at the University of Dundee has recently started accepting students for their Master of Forensic Odontology course, a 1-year full-time postgraduate degree course. This is not, however, a route to dental registration nor does it accord the right to practice forensic odontology in the United Kingdom.

While there are a number of other educational institutions in the United Kingdom offering courses in allied forensic disciplines, e.g., the Society Apothecaries, none of which purport to qualify those attending to become forensic odontologists.

The UK armed forces have a tri-service dental branch Navy (Royal Navy, Army, and Royal Air Force), providing a tri-service Dental Identification Team (DIT). In recent years, team members have been very active in assisting with the postmortem identifications of members of UK armed forces killed in Iraq and Afghanistan. Team members have deployed to Iraq as part of a forensic investigation team. A number of team members deployed to Thailand in 2004/2005 to assist with the identification of victims of the Asian Tsunami.

The UK armed forces dental services are subscribers to the NATO STANAG 2464 that is involved with the provision of military dental field identification services. DIT members undergo frequent refresher training in order to keep their skills up-to-date and ready for deployment.

10.4 Accreditation of Forensic Odontologists in the United Kingdom

For many years in the United Kingdom, there was no accreditation process for forensic odontologists. Police, coroners, procurators fiscal, lawyers, or any investigating authority requiring the service of a forensic odontologist for identification or criminal casework would contact a local general dental practitioner or hospital-based specialist and request them to perform the necessary service. In the majority of cases, there was little evidence base for their selection, convenience and locality being the usual criteria.

The British Association for Forensic Odontology (BAFO) was aware of this unsatisfactory arrangement and, in response, drew up a register of forensic odontologists from its members. The register was divided in two: an *A* list gave details of the more experienced members, while a *B* list provided details of less experienced BAFO members but who wished to be considered for work. These lists were circulated to police, coroners, and procurators fiscal and published on the BAFO website.

In 1999, the Council for the Registration of Forensic Practitioners (CRFP) was established in the United Kingdom in response to concerns about miscarriages of justice in which deficient scientific evidence was implicated and to promote public confidence in forensic practice in the United Kingdom. Without a credible professional register, both public confidence and the credibility of evidence given in court could be greatly affected. Forensic odontologists were encouraged to register with the CRFP. BAFO had a very large part to play in drawing up the guidelines for acceptance onto the register, and several BAFO members were co-opted onto the CRFP accreditation board. Unfortunately, on 31 March 2009, the CRFP ceased to exist.

Since this time, BAFO has been working closely with the Forensic Regulator, the National Police Improvement Agency (NPIA), and the Serious Organised Crime Agency (SOCA), UK police, and other agencies to set up a system of accreditation for forensic odontologists in the United Kingdom. While the process for accreditation of UK forensic odontologists is still being developed, it is envisaged that the NPIA and eventually SOCA will hold the details of these accredited forensic odontologists and will advise their use by the various judicial agencies. BAFO will continue to be responsible for the accreditation and reaccreditation process for UK-based forensic odontologists.

In order for a forensic odontologist to be accredited and to practice in the United Kingdom, they must hold a recognized dental qualification and be registered with the General Dental Council.

10.5 Bite Mark Guidelines

BAFO members undertaking bite mark/mark cases adhere closely to the BAFO Bite Mark Guidelines. These guidelines emerged following discussions by the BAFO Committee at its meeting on 1 May 2004. They are based on a draft document prepared by Dr. D R Sheasby and Professor D G MacDonald (Glasgow) and on separate submissions from Dr. G T Craig (Sheffield), Dr. Graham Ritchie (Suffolk), and Professor D K Whittaker (Cardiff).

The guidelines are intended to reflect what the BAFO committee regards as current good practice in the area of bite mark investigation and analysis. While adherence to the guidelines is of course not mandatory, BAFO members engaging in bite marks cases might reasonably expect that their existence will be known to the courts. The adoption of these guidelines by individual BAFO members is voluntary, and BAFO disclaims any liability that may arise in connection with their use.

10.6 UK Disaster Victim Identification (UKDVI) Team

Before 2005, there were no formal arrangements for disaster victim identification in the United Kingdom. Assistance could be provided by the Royal Air Force Department of Aviation Pathology and Forensic Medicine if the legal authorities in charge of the disaster wished. This department was formed in the 1950s in the wake of the Comet accidents and gave assistance to the civil authorities under the auspices of the Aid to the Civil Powers Act. Teams were sent to a range of incidents over the years, and technical advice was given on a number of occasions. The shortcomings of the lack of a national team were discussed after the sinking of the Herald of Free Enterprise at Zeebrugge in 1985, after which meetings were held with officials of the Home Office. The concept of a national team was dismissed because it was felt that the local police authorities were the best people to carry out the task. Further discussions were held after the Marchioness disaster in 1989, but to no avail. Thus, unlike many other countries prior to the tragic events in the Indian Ocean region in December 2004 when the tsunami struck, taking the lives of hundreds of thousands of innocent victims, it is fair to say that the United Kingdom had no truly nationally coordinated response to DVI. There were a number of very committed and experienced individuals but very little appreciation, outside those few, of what the work entailed. Some development had already taken place following the Marchioness disaster in 1989 to establish national standards, but it was not until the spring in 2005 that the Association of Chief Police Officers (ACPO) was commissioned by HM Government to create a UK capability. Much of the credit for establishing and running a tailor-made course for police officers must go to Professor Sue Black, head of the Centre for Anatomy and Human Identification at the College of Life Sciences at Dundee University. Professor Black developed an online course to train 500 police officers over a 2-year period in the procedures they would be expected to perform when called to take part in a mass disaster response. Once the students had satisfactorily completed their online course, they were eligible to attend a 4-day residential course at the University of Dundee. The practical element of the course taught the techniques of strip searching and documenting their findings using cadaver material. In a final exercise, they were required to demonstrate the techniques they had learned and present their findings to an Identification Commission chaired by the procurator fiscal. The importance of this development was emphasized by the events in London in July 2005, which highlighted how vulnerable we all are. There was no shortage of appropriately qualified pathologists and forensic odontologists who could be called upon to assist in the aftermath of a disaster; it was the fact that there was no coordination with the police and other agencies that caused the difficulties. Following the 2005 initiative, an immense amount of work has been undertaken by training teams to work in disaster situations, standardizing the methodologies involved and creating a greater understanding of the problems involved. Perhaps the most important aspect of this work is that it emphasized the fact that identification is a multidisciplinary task, in which all of the available information is used to establish an identity. The UKDVI team is now internationally recognized through INTERPOL as being one of the world's leaders in this field of expertise.

A number of BAFO members have been heavily involved in advising UKDVI on the role and function of the forensic odontologist in the disaster situation and have been responsible for drawing up the best practice guidelines for use by members of the team. Many BAFO forensic odontologists and dental care professionals (DCPs) are members of the UKDVI team and take part in training exercises on a regular basis.

10.7 The Legal Basis of Expert Evidence

The conditions governing the provision of expert evidence in UK courts reside in the complex web of laws of evidence. These have a common law ancestry, and this sometimes predisposes them to some criticism. As Keane (1994, pp. 1–3 and 15–18) says, "the modern law of evidence remains essentially a case-law subject, built on common law principles and overlaid with a statutory veneer." Not surprisingly this leaves the laws open to challenge, especially where admissibility is concerned. The details of these conflicts and the law itself are outwith the scope of this book, suffice it to say that the primary object is to provide a forum wherein a fair assessment of admissible evidence is made. If evidence is to be admitted, it must be relevant, and not excluded by any rule of the law of evidence. A consequence of this is that, no matter how relevant some evidence is, it may be excluded. An out-of-court statement about the case, such as an admission of guilt by a third party, would be excluded under the rule of hearsay. Lay people sometimes find these rules hard to accept, believing that they can be inimical to the search for justice.

Many countries have adopted the English system of justice, which is based on a Common Law approach, and is characterized by an adversarial approach to the judicial process, as opposed to the inquisitorial system used in Roman Law jurisdictions. Variations do exist in the way that the English system operates in different countries, as is seen in the United Kingdom, where England, Wales, and Ireland are essentially the same, but Scottish Law is an amalgam of English Law and Continental Law resulting from its alliances with France. Even where the systems are similar, such as in Ireland, it must be remembered that they are separate systems (Spencer 1990). There is much reciprocity between the English and the Scottish systems, with decisions finding their way into one another's deliberations. Similarly there is a free flow of experts across the boundary. English and Scottish laws have influenced the legal systems in many countries, especially those in the British Commonwealth and the United States, but they are sovereign states, thus they are not bound by British decisions, and have their own law and procedures. There is also some reciprocity between decisions made in Australia, New Zealand, and Canada and the law in the United Kingdom.

While these differences are important, reflecting cultural and procedural demands, they do not materially affect the way in which forensic odontologists work; Scotland may demand that two odontologists examine the case. In practice a free flow of experts operates across the border, and there is unanimity in their approach, with common professional development, standards, and methodologies. There are though differences in the court structure, and those working in Scotland are required to add to their statements the words that they testify on soul and conscience. Although the differences are largely procedural and therefore not relevant to the practice of making a forensic examination or the principles underlying the basis of opinion, they are important. There are also differences in procedure in the civil, criminal, coroners and sheriff's courts, and forensic odontologists should be aware of the differences. A lack of awareness of the nature of the proceedings can detract from an expert's reception and may affect the quality of any evidence given.

Historically, Scottish approaches to forensic medicine were superior to those in England and Wales, as indeed were those in most European countries. It has been said that England and Wales lagged 200 years behind continental Europe. Despite the differences between Britain and the rest of Europe, this did not produce the dissimilar outcomes in criminal trials claimed by some commentators (Clark and Crawford 1994; Crawford 1994). It is though salutary to learn that continental Europe was making progress in forensic medicine in the thirteenth century and that textbooks were being produced long before the United Kingdom put the subject on the curricula of medical schools. Forensic odontology dates back to AD 49, but in the United Kingdom it has had a sporadic life in undergraduate teaching.

The origins of expert and evolution of expert witnesses are closely allied to the development of the jury system, which has been highly influential. Originally, members of the community with knowledge of the details of the offence were called upon to act as jurors, but this became a body of people who lacked such knowledge. Witnesses became more important as purveyors of facts in trials, but that was all that was expected. The juries were there to infer from the evidence presented to the court. Some witnesses were called because they had special knowledge. They were able to help the court by providing information which was beyond the understanding of ordinary people. These experts had derived their specialist knowledge by virtue of their skills and experience, something which was beyond the scope of the general public. One important feature of their acceptability to the courts was that they need not have had direct familiarity with the crime (Eigen 1994). This is a particularly important feature of *t*heir acceptability, one which has a resonance today: they were essentially witnesses for the courts. It has taken many years to achieve today's degree of sophistication, and as the history of forensic odontology shows, recognition has only grudgingly been accorded. What is particularly disappointing is that some authors of textbooks on the expert witness seem to be unaware of the history and role of forensic odontology. Robertson and Vignaux (1995, p. 202) said that forensic scientists generally only use methods that have a tried and tested evidence base that are fully accepted by the relevant field, adding that occasionally odontologists attempt to apply their knowledge to forensic scientific problems. It is disappointing that a text designed to analyze the field of the expert witness and reduce misunderstandings should be so fundamentally flawed. While the case load is smaller than some specialities, forensic odontological evidence is used regularly in many courts worldwide and has been for many years.

From the earliest inception, the expert witness has been differentiated from the witness to fact in that he/she is allowed to express an opinion about the findings, and not just a statement of the events. The expert's task is to explain evidence, so that those who do not have specialist knowledge can understand the information placed before them. Exceptionally other witnesses may be allowed to express an opinion on matters that do not demand specialist knowledge, as a way of conveying those facts that they have personally observed. There are two reasons for this. Firstly, while any fact that a witness can prove is relevant, their opinion is not. Opinions of a non-expert do not have any probative value and are usually sufficiently irrelevant to a subject not calling for such expertise. Secondly, the general rule prevents witnesses from usurping the role of the trial (Keane 1994, p. 398). This has long been an important feature of the administration of justice that the accused should be tried by their peers and not by specialist witnesses.

In recent years, the role of the expert witness has been challenged in a number of jurisdictions, mostly because the quality of the evidence has been found wanting. In the adversarial process, the practice of opposing the word of an expert is an integral part of the trial, and this has proved to be a way of testing the authority of the evidence. Unfortunately, there have been occasions when the bearing of a witness has proved more powerful than the validity of what is being stated. The confident, self-possessed witness may be very convincing, whereas the quiet, rather diffident individual may not be to the detriment of justice. Not surprisingly, the courts, who have a delicate relationship with experts, have raised questions about the probity and relevance of their participation in hearings. Added to this is the profusion of variants on the theme of expertise, with America having large numbers of different groups, all of whom claim the special privilege. Other countries have also seen a proliferation of these groups, and it is sometimes felt that the basic objective of the expert witness is to explain matters which cannot be understood by the ordinary man who has not had appropriate training. It is though, those who have made extravagant claims, which cannot be supported by professional knowledge, who have caused the most damage.

While most of these examples have arisen in different fields than forensic odontology, the effect is to create tensions in respect of the role of the expert, and this has been felt in many countries. Moreover, there have been situations in which forensic odontologists have been found wanting in this respect. Injury causation is not an easy field to study, especially when injury timing is involved. One American practitioner made extravagant claims for photographic technology in wound analysis, leading to errors in court proceedings. There have also been disputes about the validity of bite mark evidence and the matching techniques used.

Questions about the validity of expert evidence are not restricted to what may look like the arcane debates of lawyers; there is a genuine need to ensure that what is being offered conforms to the highest levels of professional probity. Not only that, it has to be of value to the courts in their deliberations. English law has been forged by cases which have defined the process, but inevitably there are anomalies and an opportunity for judge-made interpretation. Situations where new discoveries or areas of knowledge are concerned.

Advances in knowledge can prove that what was believed to be true in the past was wrong, or they can set the court on an uncharted path. Despite lay views to the contrary, science is not static. It is constantly changing in the light of new discoveries, thus creating a degree of uncertainty among forensic odontologists, but despite many improvements in the methods used, it is still not possible on many occasions to give an accurate answer. There has to be some uncertainty, so that all that is possible is a guide, and the accuracy of that varies with age. Clearly, the evidence given in nineteenth-century England was wrong, and while this is obviously an extreme example, it does illustrate the principle behind the dilemma facing the courts.

Novel evidence is obviously taxing, because the courts do not have a yardstick to gauge it by, and this is discomfiting. It must be remembered that the law is a reactive subject, responding to circumstances by using precedent as guidance, but occasionally when there is not one it will have to resort to what is known as a legal fiction. This has nothing to do with detective stories and the like. It is a strategy in which the law uses an existing decision as an example and adopts the principle involved, transferring it to another circumstance. Whether or not the same device can be used to declare new knowledge or techniques acceptable to the courts is not known. What it does though is it illustrates some features of the way that the law tries to approach a problem, using lateral thinking, but that is not really enough. The question posed by advances is, are they acceptable or not? Frequent claims for potential miracle cures appear in the media, such as gene therapy, but these do not always materialize, and a rethink has to take place. Thus, as far as genes are concerned, the emphasis has switched from individual genes to genetic pathways, which is quite different from the published exaggerations. What it does not mean is that the basic idea was wholly wrong; it is just that a different route is needed to achieve the objectives. The difference between this and what has been called junk science is stark. In so far as the latter is concerned, this was widely discussed in America in relation to the Bendectin fetal abnormalities trial. It was defined as a situation in which a witness seeks to present grossly fallacious interpretations of scientific data, which Foster and Huber (1997) say is a legal problem, not a scientific one, that is fostered by the adversarial system. This is not wholly accurate, because the individual witness has to be prepared to accept instructions and to give the evidence. Nevertheless, the idea that there may be someone at large who is willing to state something that is at odds with mainstream ideas and is worth cultivating can be a boon to lawyers faced with otherwise overpowering evidence. Science is a cumulative process, which to a large degree is self-correcting. Not every new idea withstands the test of time, but this is different from bad science, which is grossly flawed, and will not pass peer review. Even so, detecting the flawed and differentiating it from the reasonably stated idea that fails can be difficult, especially when the false doctrine is presented in a plausible way by a confident witness. New discoveries and ideas can tax the courts, especially in those areas where there is a rapid shift of knowledge, raising legitimate challenges to the established order.

Inevitably novel evidence taxes the courts because they cannot be certain about its reliability. Not surprisingly they can be cautious in their approach. Forensic odontology has had to face this hurdle by showing that its methodology and theoretical basis were sound, even so there are those who do not fully accept its capabilities. America adopted the Frye test as a means of resolving the difficulties involved in resolving questions of acceptability. Unfortunately, it was not as effective as had been hoped and was subjected to considerable criticism. What it said was that the opinions expressed must have gained general acceptance in the appropriate field, but how could this be achieved? Moreover, where did a respectable new idea find currency? Daubert is claimed to have superseded Frye following William Daubert et al. from Merrell Dow Pharmaceuticals Inc. Briefly, Daubert judges scientific validity on the following criteria:

1. Can the theory be tested, and has it been tested?
2. Has the theory been published and subjected to peer review?
3. Have actual or potential error rates been considered?
4. Is the technique widely accepted in the relevant scientific community?

English courts have shied away from prescriptive concepts like Frye and Daubert, resisting the imposition of additional requirements (Robertson and Vignaux 1995, pp. 202–210; Foster and Huber 1997). In the event, decisions about acceptability tend to be the domain of the trial judge. Despite this Daubert and Frye do offer some guidance about how new ideas should be perceived and tested. Recently medical and dental publications have questioned the veracity of scientific papers following a number of dubious papers (Anon 2012). Inevitably this raises concerns about the reliability of medical and dental science. The extensive debates which are taking place are outwith the scope of this book, but the potential for them to impinge on the role of the forensic odontologist must be borne in mind.

Developments like this create uncertainty, and while this is not by itself a bad thing in that it stimulates research, it does not accord well with the court's need for answers. Lawyers are looking for finite answers to questions, even when these concern complex matters. They want them presented concisely and precisely answered in language the juror and themselves can understand. In forensic odontology, bite marks have stimulated some controversy. Analyzing them involves matching patterns, something which contains elements of subjectivity, despite the advances in the techniques available. Where there are marked individual characteristics, then the diagnosis may be straight forward, but when this is not the case, the task is much harder, and some assessment of the possibility of error has to be made. Currently there is some movement towards international agreement in this field, reducing its uncertainties (Hill 2000). Expert witnesses must acknowledge the existence of any uncertainty, reinforcing their claim of impartiality as witnesses for the court, irrespective of the side instructing them.

Expert witnesses in the United Kingdom have enjoyed immunity from suit for over 400 years, something that was traditionally based on the public interest, in that they were expected to give truthful and fair evidence, without fear of being sued by the losing party. This immunity was lost in 2011, in the case of Jones v Karney, where the expert in a civil case changed her mind after a meeting with the defense expert. There is no reason why experts should agree, but the science has to be right. In civil cases in the United Kingdom, such as when seeking compensation, it is usual for the experts to meet, and if possible agree, but they may not, in which case they are required to give reasons for any disagreement. This occasionally happens in criminal cases. Failures to give professionally sound evidence will be acted upon appropriately by the courts, who may refer the expert to the appropriate licensing authority; in the case of dentistry, this would be the General Dental Council, which adjudicates on matters involved in fitness to practice panel hearings. There have been a number of instances where this has happened in medicine, but the same rules apply to dentists. In R v Day, a psychiatrist was said to have given inadequate evidence, claiming that the accused had a condition called intermittent explosive disorder. He did not tell the court that this was a controversial diagnosis and that it is not recognized in the International Classification of Diseases. He was struck off the medical register (Dyer 2012).

This case, and others, illustrates the perils in not being truthful. Holding an opinion is one side of the argument. Opinions have to be soundly based and supported by evidence. If there is any impediment to its widespread acceptance, then this must be acknowledged, so that the court can make its own judgment. What this means in practical terms is that there must be full disclosure of all of the evidence and its basis, so that no one can be left in any doubt. In the criminal courts, this usually means that all of the prosecution material will be disclosed to the defense, but the latter may not disclose everything to the prosecution; this is a matter which is criticized but accepted within criminal proceedings.

The loss of witness immunity was viewed with dismay by some observers, but it was overdue in that lawyers had shortly before lost their immunity. It was inevitable; all it took was for a suitable case to precipitate the action. Support for the English court's removal of professional immunity from suit came from the European Court of Human Rights (Tormey 2012). It had been concerned for some time that granting general immunity was contrary to the concept of justice, despite this though, there were some who felt that the move was inherently flawed, in that experts would be deterred from expressing an opinion. This does not appear to have been the case.

Technically experts should not proffer an opinion on the issue that the court is charged with determining. However, it is increasingly common for them to express opinions that have the effect of doing just that, giving the feeling that prohibition may no longer be operative. This does not mean though that experts can express opinions of guilt or innocence. It is important to remember that juries are not bound to accept an expert's opinion, but they should be directed to do so in the absence of circumstances casting doubt upon it.

Forensic odontologists in the United Kingdom have to work in a complex evidential system, which has developed in response to past decisions made during trials in which the judicial process has been faced with new situations. Inevitably, this can create a feeling that the judicial decision made is arbitrary; a judge refused to admit evidence using the Individual Severity Score, an internationally recognized system designed to give an indication of injury severity, because he did not accept it. Not surprisingly, the potential for this to happen increases any feelings of insecurity a witness may have, making it harder to give precise answers to questions. Nevertheless, the assessments of evidence's admissibility are not ad hoc, being founded upon the need to ensure a fair trial. A rigidly enforceable rule would occasionally mean the exclusion of highly relevant evidence and permit the inclusion of that which is prejudicial (Keane 1994, p. 32). There is always the possibility that if a judge's decision seems to be capricious and exclusion or inclusion of evidence is felt to be pivotal, an appeal can be made to the higher court.

Dentistry has its basis in biology, arguably the hardest task master because of its capacity for variation, so individual responses to stimuli may differ widely. Characteristically science is a cumulative process, in which new discoveries challenge the existing, demanding reappraisal of existing intelligence, creating uncertainty. Because precise answers are not always possible, despite the needs of the court, the value placed on dental evidence may diminish, but the discomfort felt by venturing a false claim would be far greater. The imperative is that the forensic odontologist's evidence should be an accurate presentation of the findings and their analysis, consistent with the current state of knowledge. Truth may be a philosophically awkward concept, but undoubtedly the courts will be expecting that its expert witnesses adopt a truthful approach to their evidence, acknowledging where fault lines may lie in an incident case. As with other jurisdictions, forensic odontologists are expected to remain within their core of expertise. Some will accept a wider scope of case load than others. Each of them will have to justify their experiential basis; false claims can lead to discomfiting sanctions. No matter how experienced a forensic odontologist is, nor how powerful the dental evidence may be in a particular case, it is only a part of the whole. It has to be seen as a piece of the picture and not the whole. Even though dentitions are infinitely variable, and capable of providing powerful evidence, there can be no absolute guarantee that there will never be a possibility that two sets of teeth will be incontrovertibly distinguishable in isolation.

References

Anon (1951) Forensic importance of teeth. Lancet 258:1127

Anon (2012) Moral decay at GSK reaps record $3billion fine. Lancet 380:2

Clark M, Crawford C (1994) Introduction. In: Clarke M, Crawford C (eds) Legal medicine in history. Cambridge University Press, Cambridge, pp 9–10

Crawford C (1994) Legalising medicine; early modern legal systems and the growth of medico-legal knowledge. In: Clarke M, Crawford C (eds) Legal medicine in history. Cambridge University Press, Cambridge, pp 89–109

Dyer C (2012) Doctor's failing as an expert witness were dangerous court finds. BMJ 345:6

Eigen JP (1994) 'I answer as a physician.' Opinion as fact in pre-McNaughton insanity trials. In: Clarke M, Crawford C (eds) Legal medicine in history. Cambridge University Press, Cambridge, pp 167–168

Foster KR, Huber PW (1997) Judging science: scientific knowledge and the federal courts. MIT Press, London

Hill IR (2000) Evidential value of bitemarks is forensic odontology. In: Willems G (ed) IOFOS millenium symposium. Leuven University Press, pp 93–98

Hill IR, Holt JK et al. (1984) The United Kingdom. In: Hill IR (ed) Forensic Odontology, its scope and history. IOFOS, Marsh Gibbon, pp 216–217

Keane A (1994) The modern law of evidence, 3rd edn. Butterworths, London

Robertson B, Vignaux GA (1995) Interpreting evidence: evaluating forensic science in the courtroom. Wiley, Chichester

Spencer JR (1990) In: Spencer JR (ed) Jackson's machinery of justice, 8th edn. Cambridge University Press, Cambridge, pp 16–17

Tormey WP (2012) Cannabis misinterpretation and misadventure in a coroner's court. Med Sci Law 52:229–230

11 Legal Aspects Related to Healthcare Insurance, Dental Practitioners, and Forensic Odontologists in South Africa

Herman Bernitz

11.1 Healthcare Insurance

Healthcare insurance providers, dental practitioners, and forensic odontologists are highly regulated in South Africa. Healthcare providers are regulated by the Council for Medical Schemes, CMS (Council for Medical Schemes 2010), while dental practitioners and forensic odontologists are regulated by the Health Professions Council of South Africa (HPCSA) (Health Professions Council of South Africa 2013).

The HPCSA and CMS are statutory bodies appointed by the government and are responsible for all aspects of professional and ethical practice by its members and the protection of the public which they serve. The information in this document has been copied verbatim from the relevant chapters published by the responsible councils.

A minority of South Africans have healthcare insurance, which is expensive and restrictive in relation to treatment protocols. The vast majority use government provided services, which are either free or rendered at a minimal cost to the patient. Practitioners have the choice of charging tariffs above the so-called medical aid rates, but patients are then responsible for the accounts rendered. A new health policy known as the National Health Insurance (NHI) (National Health Insurance 2013) is being formulated, but is as yet not in place. The NHI is a financing system that will make sure that *all* citizens of South Africa (and legal long-term residents) are provided with essential health care, regardless of their employment status and ability to make a direct monetary contribution to the NHI Fund. Health care is regarded as a basic human right – this is a widely accepted international principle. This right should not depend on how rich we are or where we happen to live. The right to obtain health care is written into the South African Constitution (Constitution of the Republic of South Africa no 108 of 1996).

11.2 Liability Insurance

It is a statutory requirement that all dental practitioners have some form of dental liability insurance. Insurance packages, related to the level of risk, are offered by the South African Dental Association (SADA) (South African Dental Association 2013). Practitioners may use private companies if they wish.

11.3 Patient Rights and Ethical Values

The patient's rights and core ethical values and standards required of dental practitioners and forensic odontologists include the following:

Respect for persons: "Healthcare practitioners should respect patients as persons and acknowledge their intrinsic worth, dignity,

H. Bernitz, BChD, MSc, Dip Odont, PhD (Pret)
Department of Oral Pathology and Oral Biology, School of Dentistry, University of Pretoria, Pretoria, South Africa
e-mail: bernitz@iafrica.com

K. Rötzscher (ed.), *Forensic and Legal Dentistry*,
DOI 10.1007/978-3-319-01330-5_11, © Springer International Publishing Switzerland 2014

and sense of value" (Health Professions Council of South Africa 2013).

Best interests or well-being: *Non-maleficence*: "Healthcare practitioners should not harm or act against the best interests of patients, even when the interests of the latter conflict with their own self-interest" (Health Professions Council of South Africa 2013).

Best interest or well-being: *Beneficence*: "Healthcare practitioners should act in the best interests of patients even when the interests of the latter conflict with their own personal self-interest" (Health Professions Council of South Africa 2013).

Human rights: "Healthcare practitioners should recognize the human rights of all individuals" (Health Professions Council of South Africa 2013).

Autonomy: "Healthcare practitioners should honor the right of patients to self-determination or to make their own informed choices and to live their lives by their own beliefs, values, and preferences" (Health Professions Council of South Africa 2013).

Integrity: "Healthcare practitioners should incorporate these core ethical values and standards as the foundation for their character and practice as responsible healthcare professionals" (Health Professions Council of South Africa 2013).

Truthfulness: "Healthcare practitioners should regard the truth and truthfulness as the basis of trust in their professional relationships with patients" (Health Professions Council of South Africa 2013).

Confidentiality: "Healthcare practitioners should treat personal or private information as confidential in professional relationships with patients – unless overriding reasons confer a moral or legal right to disclosure" (Health Professions Council of South Africa 2013).

Compassion: "Healthcare practitioners should be sensitive to, and empathize with, the individual and social needs of their patients and seek to create mechanisms for providing comfort and support where appropriate and possible" (Health Professions Council of South Africa 2013).

Tolerance: "Healthcare practitioners should respect the rights of people to have different ethical beliefs as these may arise from deeply held personal, religious, or cultural convictions" (Health Professions Council of South Africa 2013).

Justice: "Healthcare practitioners should treat all individuals and groups in an impartial, fair, and just manner" (Health Professions Council of South Africa 2013).

Professional competence and self-improvement: "Healthcare practitioners should continually endeavor to attain the highest level of knowledge and skills required within their area of practice" (Health Professions Council of South Africa 2013).

Community: "Healthcare practitioners should strive to contribute to the betterment of society at large" (Health Professions Council of South Africa 2013).

11.4 Informed Consent

Healthcare practitioners should:

"Give their patients the information they ask for or need about their condition, its treatment and prognosis" (Health Professions Council of South Africa 2013).

"Give information to their patients in the way they can best understand it. The information must be given in a language that the patient understands and in a manner that takes into account the patient's level of literacy, understanding, values, and belief systems" (Health Professions Council of South Africa 2013).

"Refrain from withholding from their patients any information, investigation, treatment, or procedure; the healthcare practitioner knows would be in the patient's best interests" (Health Professions Council of South Africa 2013).

"Apply the principle of informed consent as an on-going process" (Health Professions Council of South Africa 2013).

"Allow patients access to their medical records" (Health Professions Council of South Africa 2013).

11.5 Patient Confidentiality

Healthcare practitioners should:

"Recognize the right of patients to expect that healthcare practitioners will not disclose any personal and confidential information they acquire in the course of their professional duties, unless they agree to such disclosure, or unless healthcare practitioners have good and overriding reason for doing so (e.g., if disclosure is not made, there is the likelihood of serious harm to an identifiable third party, or there is a public health emergency or any overriding and ethically justified legal requirement)" (Health Professions Council of South Africa 2013).

"Not breach confidentiality without sound reason and without the knowledge of their patients" (Health Professions Council of South Africa 2013).

"When claiming from medical schemes explain to patients the significance of ICD 10 coding and get the permission of patients to breach confidentiality when making a medical scheme claim" (Health Professions Council of South Africa 2013).

11.6 Duties to the Environment (Conservation of Natural Resources)

"Healthcare practitioners should recognize that they have a responsibility to ensure that in the conduct of their affairs they do not in any way contribute to environmental degradation" (Health Professions Council of South Africa 2013).

"Healthcare practitioners should protect the environment and the public by ensuring that healthcare waste is disposed of legally and in an environmentally friendly manner" (Health Professions Council of South Africa 2013).

11.7 Legal Aspects of Dental Expert Investigation

There are four acts that govern the forensic dental examination of suspects and victims, whether postmortem or antemortem. The following acts apply:

- The Human Tissue Act of South Africa (Act 65 of 1983)
- The Inquest Act of South Africa (Act 58 of 1959)
- Criminal Procedure Act of South Africa (Act 51 of 1977 with Amendment Act 9 of 2012)
- National Health Act of South Africa (Act 61 of 2003)

11.8 Right to Complain

Patients have the right to address any malpractice complaints to the HPCSA. They also have the right to complain about healthcare services that either violate their rights to good health or breach ethical standards to have their complaint investigated and to receive a full response thereafter. The following procedure is followed:

"Within seven (7) days of receiving a complaint, the registrar forwards the complaint to the healthcare professional concerned and requests a written explanation from him/her. (*Note that the healthcare professional may refuse or be advised not to provide an explanation, as an explanation may be used as evidence later.*)" (Health Professions Council of South Africa 2013)

"A letter of complaint together with the healthcare professional's explanation (if submitted) is referred to the Professional Board concerned for consideration" (Health Professions Council of South Africa 2013).

"Should the board decide that there are grounds for complaint, a Professional Conduct Committee will hold a professional conduct enquiry, during which oral evidence is presented, often including independent, expert witnesses. (*Note*: *Professional conduct enquiries are open to the public and the media, unless closed at the discretion of the chairperson.*)" (Health Professions Council of South Africa 2013).

"Should the professional conduct enquiry find the healthcare professional guilty of misconduct, the committee's decision is final, unless either party lodges an appeal" (Health Professions Council of South Africa 2013).

"A healthcare professional found guilty of professional misconduct may be subject to the following penalties:

A caution or a reprimand or both

A fine

Suspension for a specified period from practicing his profession

Removal of his name from the relevant register

A compulsory period of professional service

Payment of the costs of the proceedings" (Health Professions Council of South Africa 2013)

11.9 Disaster Victim Identification

Any dental practitioner or forensic odontologist offering his services to victim identification is subject to the four acts mentioned under point 7.

South Africa has a formal DVI team comprised of police officials under the direct supervision of a senior police official. All medical and dental services are *ad hoc*, and the number of volunteers is determined by the size and nature of the disaster. The volunteers are primarily university staff, but when needed, suitably trained private practitioners are included.

References

Constitution of the Republic of South Africa no 108 of (1996) Available from http://www.info.gov.za/documents/constitution/1996/a108-96. Accessed 18 Feb 2013

Council for Medical Schemes (2010) Available from http://www.medicalschemes.com. Accessed 18 Feb 2013

Health Professions Council of South Africa (2013) Health professions act 56 of 1974. Available from http://www.hpcsa.co.za. Accessed 18 Feb 2013

National Health Insurance (2013) Available from http://www.doh.gov.za. Accessed 18 Feb 2013

South African Dental Association (2013) Available from http://www.sada.co.za. Accessed 18 Feb 2013

12 Argentinean Society of Legal Odontology and Forensic Odontologist Association of South America

Oscar Heit

12.1 Argentinean Society of Legal Odontology and Forensic Odontologist Association of South America

The Argentinian Society of Legal Odontology (SADOL) was founded in 1977 in the city of Rosario, province of Santa Fe, Argentina. Its first president was a physician, Oscar Sanchez, and his secretary was an odontologist, Héctor Ceppi.

Because of the political situation in Argentina at that time, SADOL stopped developing. In 1995, however, the Odontologist School of Tucuman's State University presented the first specialist course approved by The National Commission of the Evaluation and Certification Universities, awarding a Legal Expert Odontologist degree, the first in South America. Rosario's Odontology State University followed. In 2001, the Health State Ministry recognized legal odontology as a specialty and published this in the Official Bulletin of November 2001. Ceppi, therefore, started the legacy and today SADOL is a successful society with members all around Argentina. SADOL has had annual meetings since 2005. The sixth meeting was in Buenos Aires in May 2010, at which time, we also paid tribute to Dr. Elida N. Briñón, a pioneer of legal odontology in Argentina. She has been an expert in the courts of Buenos Aires for many years and has published two books: the first in 1983, entitled *Legal Odontology and Forensic Practice*, and the second in 2006, *Injuries and Iatrogenic Injuries in Legal Odontology*. Argentina, Bolivia, Brazil, Paraguay, Peru, and Uruguay were represented at the Buenos Aires 2010 meeting.

The Managerial Commission of SADOL for 2009–2011 was constituted at the May 2009 meeting. The members are Carlos Marcelo Gonzalez (President), Roberto Rivarola (Vice-President), Judith Prado Pagniez (Secretary), Oscar Heit (Treasurer), and Marcelo Luzi (Minutes Secretary and Interinstitutional Relationships).

The Forensic Odontologists Association of South America (AOFS) was recently created and consists of Carlos Marcelo Gonzalez (Argentina; President), Rosario Rovira Gómez (Bolivia; Secretary), Celia Mármol (Paraguay; Treasurer), Ana María Carlos Erazo (Perú; First Vocal), Rhonan Ferreira da Silva (Brazil; Second Vocal), Alicia Picapedra (Uruguay; First Accounting Manager), and Manuel Maurelia (Chile; Second Accounting Manager). AOFS will have its first meeting during the Eighth International Congress of Odontologists of Paraguay, 9–11 September 2010, in Asuncion, the capital of Paraguay's Republic. The main aim of this meeting will be the creation of a disaster victim identification team for South America.

The legal odontology field in Argentina needs further refinement and research progress. The

O. Heit, Prof. Dr.
Faculty of Science and Technology,
University Autonomous of Entre Ríos,
Entre Ríos, Argentina
e-mail: odheitoscar@hotmail.com

K. Rötzscher (ed.), *Forensic and Legal Dentistry*,
DOI 10.1007/978-3-319-01330-5_12, © Springer International Publishing Switzerland 2014

Argentine judicial system, divided into provinces, has, so far, no formal incorporation of expert dentists in medico-legal institutes or medical legal departments.

Since 1995, three dental faculties have postgraduate programs in legal odontology and there is a continuous effort to increase the number of universities able to train additional specialists. Associations such as the Argentinean Society of Legal Odontology contribute to the training of odontolegal experts, standardization of knowledge, and developing best-practices manuals.

12.2 Patient's Rights in Argentina

In Argentina, the Patient's Rights Law in relation to professional health institutions was approved in 2009. Law No. 26,529 governs the exercise of patient's rights: autonomy, information, and clinical documentation (medical history and informed consent). With regard to the obligation to make medical records available to patients, Law No. 26,529 reads: Article 12. – Definition and scope. For the purposes of this law, the medical history is understood to be the complete chronologic record of actions taken by health professionals and allied personnel pertaining to the patient.

The patient has the rights, according to Law No. 26,529: Art. 2 – Patient Rights. The following rights are essential in the relationship between the patient and health professionals or health insurance agents, and any intermediaries:

(a) Assistance. Patients, including children and adolescents, have the right to be assisted by health professionals without prejudice and discrimination regarding their ideology; religious, political, or socio-economic status; race; sex; sexual orientation; or any other condition. The acting health professional may only discharge the duty of care when the patient's care has been actually transferred to another qualified professional.
(b) Treatment with dignity and respect. The patient has the right to receive decent treatment from the health system agents involved, with respect to personal and moral convictions, particularly related to socio-cultural conditions, gender, modesty, and privacy, whatever the condition; this right is extended to the relatives or companions of the patient.
(c) Intimacy. Any health care activity aimed at obtaining, sorting, using, managing, storing, and transmitting information and clinical documentation regarding a patient should observe strict respect for human dignity and autonomy, and be handled under the shelter of privacy because of the same and because of the confidentiality of sensitive data, without prejudice to the provisions contained in Law No. 25,326.
(d) Confidentiality. The patient has the right to be informed about any person involved in the preparation or handling of clinical documentation, and access to the contents of the same, save due reserve, unless expressly provided to the contrary, issued by competent judicial authority or authorization from the patient.
(e) Autonomy of the Will. The patient has the right to accept or reject certain therapies or medical or biological procedures, with or without cause, as well as to subsequently revoke manifestation of the will. Children and adolescents have the right to intervene in the terms of Law No. 26,061 for the purposes of decision making about therapies or medical procedures involving biological specimens or their life or health.
(f) Health Information. The patient has the right to receive necessary health information linked to their health. The right to health information includes the right not to receive such information.
(g) Medical Interconsultation. The patient is entitled to receive health information in writing and to obtain a second opinion about the diagnosis, prognosis, or treatment related to their health.

It is important to establish the difference in principle between the guardian of and the ownership of the medical history. Law No. 26,529 explains:

Section 14. – Ownership. The patient is the holder of their own clinical history. Upon simple request, the patient must be provided a copy thereof, certified by a competent authority of the Healthcare Institution.

Section 18. – Inviolability. Depositories. The history is inviolable. The public or private health care facilities and health professionals, in their capacity as owners of private clinics, are responsible for their custody, assuming the character of trustees of the former, and must implement the necessary means and resources to prevent access to the information contained therein by unauthorized persons.

According to Law No. 26,529, the mandatory archival time for medical records is at least 10 years, as established in the following Article:

Section 18. – The requirement in the preceding paragraph shall govern for a minimum period of 10-year statute of limitations of contractual liability. This period runs from the last performance recorded in the medical record; the depositary shall have the same mode and manner prescribed by regulation.

Attention to the structure and composition of the dental history model is proposed to replace the clinical record, crediting all requirements (seats) with basic clinical, legal, and methodological tools, both for the protection of the professional and the patient. Regarding this issue, Law No. 26,529 establishes the following data necessary in the medical record:

Section 15. – Seats. Without prejudice to the provisions of the preceding Articles and so provided in the rules, the medical record must establish:

(a) The starting date of its preparation
(b) Details identifying the patient and their family
(c) Details identifying any intervening professional specialty
(d) Clear and accurate records of the acts performed by the professionals and assistants involved
(e) Genetic background, physiological and pathological, if any
(f) All medical procedures undertaken or indicated, whether they be prescription drugs and supplies, treatments performed, practices, and complementary major studies related to the presumptive diagnosis and appropriate certainty, proof of involvement of specialists, diagnostics, prognoses, procedures, and any other activities inherently evolving from these, especially medical admissions and discharges

The seats that correspond to the provisions in paragraphs (d), (e), and (f) of this section shall be made on the basis of classifications and universal models adopted and updated by the World Health Organization; the enforcement authority shall be updated by regulation.

The initial medical record is created by the professional, and begins with personal details of the professional and the patient, followed by the record of the anamnesis (dated, and composed of the chief complaint and medical and dental health questionnaires) and the results of the general extraoral physical examination and the intraoral clinical examination.

Complementary examinations (such as models, radiographs, laboratory examination, and photographs), plan and treatment options, fees and payment methods, indications, prescriptions, certificates, abandonment of treatment, and receipts must be included in the medical record.

A demonstration and discussion of a model of dental history that best meets the ethical and legal requirements of dental practice in general medicine is presented.

Informed Consent Law 26,529 defines an adequate dental history as sufficient declaration of intent made by the patient or their legal representatives, if any, issued upon receipt, by the intervening professional, that is clear, accurate, and appropriate with respect to:

(a) The patient's health
(b) The proposed procedure, specifying the desired objectives
(c) The expected benefits of the procedure
(d) The risks, discomfort, and foreseeable adverse effects
(e) Identification of alternative procedures and their risks, benefits, and damages in connection with the proposed procedure
(f) The foreseeable consequences of the failure to complete the proposed procedure or specified alternative
(g) The right that, should the patient suffer an irreversible or incurable disease or when in terminal stage, or the patient has suffered injuries causing the patient to be in the same situation, they may reject surgical procedures, hydration, food, artificial resuscitation, or life support; such measures that are

extraordinary or disproportionate to the prospects of improvement or produce excessive suffering. The patient also has the right to refuse hydration and nutrition procedures when the sole effect of those procedures is to prolong the time the patient is in the irreversible and incurable terminal stage

(h) The right to comprehensive palliative care in the process of their disease

12.3 Injury in Terms of the Penal Code

Crimes against persons in the *Argentine Criminal Code* are discussed in Articles 89–94; the first three articles define each of the three types of injury (described below) and set the basic sentence and the latter three articles refer, respectively, to injuries caused by negligence, incompetence in an art or profession, or deviations from regulations or duties attached to a particular appointment.

The Criminal Code encodes the *damage to the health of people* on a legal basis with progressive severity criminal scales, as:

- Article 89. – Will be imposed a prison sentence of 1 month to 1 year, one who causes another, in the body or health, damage that is not covered by other provisions of this code. [Commonly called minor injury, although the law does not name it as such];
- Article 90. – Will be imposed confinement or prison sentence of 1–6 years, if the injury causes a permanent debilitation of health, in a sense, of an organ, or limb; causes permanent speech difficulty; or if it has endangered the life of the victim or rendered them useless for any work (read: like all overhead) for longer than a month or has caused permanent deformation of the face. [Commonly called serious injury, although the law does not name it as such.];
- Article 91. – Will be imposed confinement or imprisonment of 3–10 years, if the injury causes a physical or mental illness, certainly or probably incurable; permanent futility for speech; the loss of a sense, an organ, a limb, or the use of an organ or member, or of speech or the ability to beget or conceive. [Commonly referred to very serious injury, although the law does not name it as such].

The word organ is used in criminal law to indicate a part or group of parts that make up a particular function; the word sense is understood on the same basis.

Two standards are used for the assessment of damage:

- Chronological or labor standard: refers to the time of disability with respect to employment, and accounts for the disability going beyond affecting those activities that can earn a living, including habitual activities, such as dressing, grooming, etc.
- Dynamic or functional standard: sets an ascending scale in the injury to health.

The teeth have masticatory, phonetics, and aesthetics function, these are to be valued when it comes to dental injuries. Only the masticatory function requires the integrity of the temporomandibular joints, the jaw muscle and the tongue, and salivary secretion. The fact that the damage is reparable with prostheses is irrelevant to the criminal category of injury.

The possibility that the injured person can replace missing teeth with artificial teeth has no influence on the classification of the offense of injury, because the law dispenses recovery of their conditions through denture resources, as with other types of injuries that can be ameliorated with skillful surgery.

The injured person is not always in the employment stage of life. In the case of a child in preschool or an elderly retiree, the time unavailable for daily employment is not a useful parameter and is replaced by the time unavailable for activities such as their usual games in the case of a child or habitual walks in the case of an elderly person. The assessment of injuries should be considered absolutely independent from the type of damage with respect to the person's sex, age, type of work, or economic and social status.

In criminal cases, the odontolegal expert submits a report to the prosecutor regarding the severity of the injury examined, according to the parameters established by law. Some authors have established severity scales that can help develop better valuation standards in legal odontology.

Dentistry and Forensic Odontology in Australia: A Brief Overview

13

Jane Taylor, Russell Lain, and William O'Reilly

13.1 The Practice of Dentistry in Australia

The legal matrix under which forensic odontologists practice in Australia is governed by the civil and criminal framework that affects all Australian citizens and therefore healthcare providers including dentists.

The Commonwealth of Australia was formed in 1901, after the six British colonies agreed to form a federation. The constitution of this new country recognized the common law system and established a federal system of powers and laws. The primary source of these laws was British law. Some laws are federal laws, such as those relating to trade and commerce, defense, external affairs, and immigration; others are concurrent, with individual states and territories making laws independent of or additional to federal powers. If there are inconsistencies between federal and state or territory laws, then federal law prevails.

With respect to dentistry, the federal Health Practitioner Regulation National Law Act 2009 informs the activities of the Dental Board of Australia and prescribes such things as qualifications necessary for registration, conduct of practice, use of titles, and a complaints management system. All states and territories in Australia have additional regulations, specific to the practice of dentistry, in the geographical area in which they practice.

The Dental Board of Australia is 1 of the 14 National Health Practitioner Boards that function under the umbrella of the Australian Health Practitioner Regulation Authority (AHPRA). The board is responsible for the registration of all dentists and paradental practitioners (dental hygienists, oral health therapists, dental therapists, dental prosthetists) in Australia, as well as assessing the qualifications of overseas trained practitioners who wish to practice in Australia. The board also approves accreditation standards for courses of study leading to registrable qualifications. State and Territory Registration and Notification Committees have delegated powers to make certain decisions in their own jurisdictions.

In addition to its registration function, the Dental Board of Australia also has a protective jurisdiction in that it ensures public safety by handling notifications and complaints from the public relating to unprofessional conduct, professional misconduct, and notifiable conduct.

It is important to understand this is a protective and not a punitive jurisdiction and to that end the Dental Board of Australia conducts, as appropriate, inquiries or hearings when there has been a complaint against a practitioner about treatment

J. Taylor, Ass. Prof. (✉) • W. O'Reilly, Ass. Prof.
Department of Oral Health, School of Health Sciences, University of Newcastle, Ourimbah, NSW 2258, Australia
e-mail: jane.taylor@newcastle.edu.au; ohreally1@bigpond.com

R. Lain, Dr.
Department of Oral Surgery and Diagnostic Imaging, Sydney Dental Hospital, 2 Chalmers Street, Surry Hills, NSW 2010, Australia
e-mail: russell.lain@sydney.edu.au

K. Rötzscher (ed.), *Forensic and Legal Dentistry*,
DOI 10.1007/978-3-319-01330-5_13, © Springer International Publishing Switzerland 2014

provided or that there is concern about the appropriateness or standard of treatment provided.

Complaints against a dentist may also be made through either the civil or criminal courts or to other statutory bodies such as the Health Care Complaints Commission. The types of claims made against dentists and oral health practitioners reflect other Western countries, and examples can be found in the Australian Dento-Legal Review.

Duty of care, informed consent, privacy of personal health records, and care delivered to a standard of the majority of professional colleagues are all principles that apply to dental practice in Australia.

The Dental Board of Australia also issues guidelines, policies, and codes in areas such as record keeping, consent, infection control, tooth whitening and bleaching, and conscious sedation. All dentists are expected to comply with these policies and guidelines. Failure to comply may lead to the dentist having orders or conditions placed on their ability to practice and in serious matters where unsatisfactory professional conduct or professional misconduct are proven, the dentist may either be suspended or deregistered.

There are mandatory reporting requirements where a dentist has reasonable cause to be concerned that a colleague may be suffering an impairment that this is reported to the registering authority. Impairment may include a psychological condition or an addiction to alcohol, prescribed medication, or illicit substances. Mandatory reporting also applies to cases of suspected child abuse.

While Australia has a publically funded universal healthcare system, only limited access to dental services is available through Medicare. The majority (over 90 %) of dental care is provided through the private sector in Australia, and as such the profession is considered to be self-regulated. Fees for dental services are thus not mandated or regulated, and although market pressure impacts, practitioners are able to charge a self-determined amount for all services. Complaints related to the levels of fees occur, as does fraud relating to provision of service and fees and the involvement of third-party health insurers.

13.2 Forensic Odontology in Australia

The federal and state systems of laws mentioned previously also impact on the practices of both forensic odontology and Disaster Victim Identification across Australia. Each state and territory in Australia has its own police jurisdiction, which necessitates differing management of forensic odontology services and Disaster Victim Identification according to the relevant legal structure. In addition there is a federal police force, the Australian Federal Police (AFP), whose traditional jurisdiction is enforcement of Commonwealth laws such as those relating to major fraud, border protection, drug importation and trafficking, people smuggling, electronic crime, child protection, and counterterrorism. Since the Bali bombings of 2002, the Forensic Services branch of the AFP have also been involved in managing Australian responses to international incidents (e.g., the Asian tsunami) and also the identification of Australian citizens killed overseas in disasters.

13.3 The Coronial System, Part 2

As a natural consequence of Australia's history, the source of much of Australian law is British law. This brings two principal differences between Australian and Continental European laws.

Firstly, the nature of Australian civil and criminal court procedure is adversarial rather than inquisitorial. The process is aimed at seeking justice – not at seeking truth. Therefore, each party presents witnesses and evidence to the court both to support their version of events and to challenge or discredit their opponent's version of the facts. This feature, along with the presence of a jury in most cases, is at the heart of civil and criminal court procedure in this country.

Secondly, the role of the coroner introduces a legal framework which is different from European law in style and substance. The coronial system originated in Britain circa 1194 and was directed at bringing to the King revenue from shipwrecks, valuables which were discovered by chance, objects which had caused the death of a person and the property of felons.

This administrative role has transformed over time into six roles for the modern coroner: administrative, investigative, preventive, educational, DVI management, and judicial (Waller 1994; Ranson 1996).

The administrative function relates to the recording and management of the processes associated with deaths, both suspicious and natural, as well as running inquests and fire inquiries. The investigative role is now carried out by police, either uniformed or detectives depending on the nature of the death, acting on behalf of the coroner.

The preventive role is relevant in bringing to the attention of the community and relevant authorities such elements as industrial design of motor vehicles, factory equipment, building design, and work practices to avoid future deaths.

The coroner is thus able to make recommendations in relation to public safety. Public education sits beside this preventive role.

The coroner plays an important role in DVI, particularly in relation to the identification of deceased persons, collection of evidence, recording of significant events during the DVI response, and often dealing with families of victims and the media.

It is the judicial role of the coroner which highlights the difference between criminal and coronial procedure in Australia. The coronial court is not adversarial. Coronial courts are not bound by the mandated Rules of Evidence. Hearsay evidence is allowed, so the process is closer to the European inquisitorial or investigating magistrate model.

Finally, it should be noted that apart from public safety concerns, a primary role of a coroner is to detect hidden homicide.

13.4 Coordination and Cooperation

Practices in forensic odontology and DVI are relatively standardized across Australia. Small variations do exist in response to local conditions, but interstate colleagues are easily able to work alongside each other when required. All states routinely use the Interpol F1 and F2 forms for data recording. The guiding principle is adherence to Interpol protocols, wherever possible. This carries through the use of teams of two, quality assurance, terminology, and consistency in documentation and levels of confidence in the identification.

In a tangible development of understanding, the need for consistency in approach at a national and international level, the Australian Society for Forensic Odontology (AuSFO) has developed the Disaster Victim Identification Practice Guide (Taylor 2009, 2010). This guide has gained national and international acceptance as a gold standard guide for the odontology aspects of a DVI incident.

The use of computerized matching programs to assist dental identifications is one area of noted difference between stats in Australia. The national implementation of PlassData® TMDVI System International by the AFP has not resulted, to date, in universal availability of this program for routine forensic odontology casework. In the instance of a DVI incident, however, this software is used by all jurisdictions to assist in incident management. Prior to the roll out of this software, South Australia was the only state to use a computerized program as part of routine casework. This program, called OdontID, was written by a former staff member of the Forensic Odontology Unit (Taylor 1987). The comparison program D.A.V.ID was created in Victoria (Clement et al. 2006; Al-Amad et al. 2007) but was not used in routine casework. Similarly, the program Identic was written by a postgraduate student in New South Wales (Arneman 1991) but was not used routinely.

13.5 Australasian Disaster Victim Identification Committee (ADVIC)

ADVIC is a committee existing under the umbrella of the Australia New Zealand Policing Advisory Agency (Australasian is a term used to denote Australia and New Zealand). As such this is a police-oriented entity and functions in a way not dissimilar to the Interpol DVI Committee. Membership comprises Australian state and territory, the New Zealand DVI commanders, and representatives from the scientific disciplines: pathology, odontology, biology, and mortuary science.

This committee has overseen the development of the Australasian Disaster Victim Identification Standards Manual, which comprehensively addresses police and scientific activities during the management of a DVI incident (ADVIC 2004).

The committee supports state and territory DVI Committees in their activities including training and acts as the representative group for DVI activities in Australia and New Zealand.

13.6 Training and Specialization

Forensic odontology is recognized as a specialist area of practice by the Dental Board of Australia. A number of odontologists in Australia are thus recognized as dental specialists. More recently, forensic odontology has been introduced as a separate stream within the Faculty of Oral and Maxillofacial Pathology in the Royal College of Pathologists of Australasia. A group of founding fellows in forensic odontology now represents the discipline within the college and constitutes a core knowledge and skill base.

This will now provide structured training opportunities and pathways to specialist recognition for future generations of odontologists in Australia.

13.7 DVI Incidents of Note in Australia

Responses to some DVI incidents in Australia have seen the creation of dedicated DVI squads in various states, for example, following the 1977 Granville train accident where 83 victims were identified visually and by means of jewelry and documents; the formal review of this incident saw the NSW Police form a dedicated DVI squad. The Victorian DVI odontology team was formed in 1981, and over 35 dentists volunteered their assistance (Bastiaan 1984).

Dedicated DVI squads now exist within all police jurisdictions within Australia.

Small DVI incidents occur regularly across the vast expanse of Australia. The majority of police jurisdictions choose to manage these incidents according to DVI principles and protocols, recognizing this both as good practice and as valuable training. Examples of such incidents include the Newcastle earthquake in 1989 (13 deceased), the Thredbo landslide in 1997 (18 deceased), the Glenbrook train accident in 1999 (7 deceased), and the 2003 Waterfall train disaster (7 deceased) in new South Wales; the Kew Cottages Hostel fire in 1996 (9 deceased), the Linton bushfires in 1998 (5 deceased), a light plane crash at Myrrhee in 2002 (6 deceased), the Mt. Hotham plane crash in 2005 (3 deceased), a car accident at Donald in 2006 (8 deceased), the Kerang train crash in 2007 (9 victims), and the crash in the Burnley Tunnel in 2007 (3 deceased) in Victoria; the crash of 2 Blackhawk helicopters near Townsville in June 1996 (15 victims), the Childers Backpackers Hostel fire in June 2000 (15 victims), and the Lockhart River plane crash in May 2005 (15 victims) in Queensland.

Larger incidents have included the Ash Wednesday bushfires of 1983 which claimed 47 lives in Victoria and 28 in South Australia. Fourteen of the 22 (64 %) Victorian victims who could not be visually recognized were identified via forensic odontology (Bastiaan 1984). Eight (29 %) of the South Australian victims were identified by dental comparison (Pounder 1985).

South Australia seems to have developed a national reputation as the locale for bizarre murders with the victims of many of these incidents being formally identified by forensic odontology. In what became known as the Truro murders, seven young women were murdered over a 7-week period commencing just before Christmas in 1976. The final set of remains was not located until 2 years after the last murder. Dental records were used to identify five of the victims, with additional corroborative identification information being provided by craniofacial superimposition. It is believed that this series of murders only ceased when the principal offender was killed in a car accident. The public success of this case was one of the reasons why the Forensic Odontology Unit was established.

The DVI case of note in recent memory for Tasmania is the Port Arthur massacre of 1996, where Martin Bryant shot and killed 35 and wounded 19.

Three of these victims were subsequently burnt beyond recognition in a fire set by the gunman in a nearby guest house where he had held them hostage overnight. The identification of these three victims was assisted by odontology evidence. The fire was so extensive and intense that almost 30 kg of debris was collected during the recovery of the bodies to ensure all possible remains were located. One body was so severely incinerated that only fragments of both jaws and a few teeth were able to be located. Two of the victims wore dentures, one a full upper against some remaining lower natural teeth and the other full upper and lower dentures. One full upper denture survived the conflagration. Dental and medical radiographs of the head area were instrumental in confirming the identification of these victims (Taylor et al. 2002). The identification of the other 32 victims was completed by visual recognition by family and friends by means of engraved jewelry and documents found on the deceased.

The largest loss of life in a single incident in recent Australian history occurred on 7 February 2009 in what has become known as the *Black Saturday* bushfires in regional Victoria. The state response required the assistance of forensic specialists from across Australia to identify the 173 victims.

Significant postmortem destruction and commingling of human and animal remains meant that a significant contribution to identification was provided by odontology (Cordner et al. 2011; Lain et al. 2011; Hill et al. 2011).

13.8 Disaster Victim Identification and the Law

All phases of DVI operate in an environment informed by two legal frameworks: firstly, the policing powers that give police the authority to control entry to disaster scenes and public safety associated with these scenes. This carries through the other phases of DVI, with police responsible for the chain of custody of human remains, property, and antemortem data obtained from relatives of missing persons or their dental practitioner. This applies whether the mass casualty is a natural disaster or criminal act. The body of the victim, however, comes under the responsibility of the coroner.

Secondly, coronial law applies. This persists until the body is identified and released by the coroner. Coronial law is very powerful and generally subsumes other laws. The coroner has jurisdiction over anybody entering the state of Australia (see section on Coronial law).

13.9 Conclusions

Forensic odontology and the law sit comfortably together in Australia, with a clear legal framework, which allows for appropriate input by odontologists into the legal process. Forensic odontology has an established role in all of its elements in the civil, criminal, and coronial systems.

In spite of recent advances in rapidity and ability to detect data from very small traces in the field of molecular biology (DNA techniques), odontology and fingerprint techniques remain primary identifying methods, particularly in DVI incidents. Postmortem changes to human tissue and the specific nature of individual mass casualty incidents mean that in many cases, odontology is still able to provide an essential role in the DVI process and routine casework. The technology is traditional, but by no means obsolete.

With the clear pathway for specialist recognition, the future of forensic odontology in Australia is certain and strong.

References

Australasian Disaster Victim Identification Committee (ADVIC) (2004) Australasian disaster victim identification standards manual. Self published

Al-Amad SH, Clement JG, McCullough MJ, Morales A, Hill AJ (2007) Evaluation of two dental identification

computer systems: DAVID and Win ID3. J Forensic Odontostomatol 25(1):23–29
Arneman KMT (1991) Forensic dental identification: towards a simplified computerised system. Thesis submitted for the Master of Science in Dentistry, University of Sydney
Bastiaan RJ (1984) Dental identification of the Victorian bushfire victims. Aust Dent J 29(2):105–110
Clement JG, Winship V, Ceddia J, Al-Amad S, Morales A, Hill AJ (2006) New software for computer-assisted dental-data matching in disaster victim identification and long-term missing persons investigations: "DAVID Web". Forensic Sci Int 159S:S24–S29
Cordner SM, Woodford N, Bassed R (2011) Forensic aspects of the 2009 Victorian Bushfire Disaster. Forensic Sci Int 205:2–7
Hill AJ, Lain R, Hewson I (2011) The role of the forensic odontologist in disaster victim identification: lessons for management. Forensic Sci Int 205:44–47
Lain R, Taylor J, Croker S, Craig P, Graham J (2011) Comparative dental anatomy in disaster victim identification: lessons from the 2009 Victorian Bushfires. Forensic Sci Int 205:36–39
Pounder DJ (1985) The 1983 South Australian bushfire disaster. Am J Forensic Med Pathol 6(1):77–92
Ranson D (1996) Forensic medicine and the law. Melbourne University Press, Melbourne
Taylor JA (1987) "OdontID" – a computer program for dental identification. Advances in medical research. In: Australian Society for Medical Research conference, Adelaide, 27 Feb 1987
Taylor J (2009) Development of the Australian Society Of Forensic Odontology disaster victim identification forensic odontology guide. J Forensic Odontostomatol 27(2):56–63
Taylor J (2010) Developing protocols for disaster victim identification. Lambert Academic Publishing, Saarbrucken
Taylor PTG, Wilson ME, Lyons TJ (2002) Forensic odontology lessons: multishooting incident at Port Arthur, Tasmania. Forensic Sci Int 130:174–182
Waller K (1994) Coronial law and practice in New South Wales. Butterworths, Sydney

Dental Law in the United States of America

14

Joseph P. Graskemper

14.1 Introduction

Dental records have become more and more important with the introduction of more procedures and techniques available to the dentist and the increase legal scrutiny of alleged dental malpractice cases. Dentists no longer simply fill or extract teeth. Today's dentist, with proper training, is able to provide patients with advanced endodontic, periodontics, restorative, and other general and specialist patient care. As techniques and treatments have expanded, so has the risk involved in providing such advancements. With the increase in risk, the chance of a bad result also increases, such that the patient may become dissatisfied and seek legal recourse. In the early 1970s, it was relatively uncommon that a dentist would be sued. With the increase in legal pursuit to remedy an acceptable or bad result, dental records were found to be lacking of basic information needed to defend the dentist. By the 1980s, there was a large movement within the dental community to improve the records kept by dentists regarding their patient treatment. Hence, greater importance has been placed on the information placed in the dental records as well as proper maintenance of dental patient records.

J.P. Graskemper, DDS, JD, DABMM
Stony Brook School of Dental Medicine,
Stony Brook, NY, USA
e-mail: jpgraskemperdds@optonline.net

14.2 The Legal Dental Record

Dental records are legal records documenting the treatment provided for a patient. Therefore, it is very important that dentists learn what information should be entered and how to enter it into the record to withstand legal scrutiny. There is also the professional responsibility to make the patient's dental record confidential and safe, especially with computer-generated (paperless office) dental records. Confidentiality should remain a constant concern with readily transmitted patient information via the Internet. In the United States, the Health Insurance Portability and Accountability Act (HIPAA) of 1996 was passed to protect patient information and enhance the rights of consumers to access their health information.

First and foremost, the dental record is the factual representation of the patient's dental treatments, diagnostics, correspondence, and consultations. The patient's record should contain information that would allow another dentist or an expert witness, if needed, to understand the need for the treatment provided, the manner in which it was performed, and the patient's response and outcome from the treatment provided. It should also contain any pertinent information relative to the treatment being provided (Sandy Sanbar et al. 2010, p. 2). The records should contain comprehensively pertinent dental, medical, or health information about patients, including diagnosis and treatment of diseases (Sandy Sanbar et al. 2010, p. 2). Dental records

K. Rötzscher (ed.), *Forensic and Legal Dentistry*,
DOI 10.1007/978-3-319-01330-5_14, © Springer International Publishing Switzerland 2014

must be direct, concise, clear, complete, and unambiguous. Forensics often look into dental records for identification of a former patient. Hence, the need to be complete cannot be emphasized enough.

14.3 Purpose for Dental Records

The following is a list that shows the many purposes of good dental records:

1. Recording the health status of the patient at the time of the initial examination
2. Recording the treatment provided to the patient
3. Providing legal documentation on behalf of the patient, the courts, third-party payers, or the patient's heirs
4. Providing legal documentation in the defense of legal claims made against the dentist
5. Fulfilling the laws regulating professional services
6. Advancing medical/dental research
7. Contributing to quality assessment and assurance
8. Providing communication among health practitioners
9. Helping identity victims of a mass disaster [or unidentifiable body] (Loomis et al. 2002)

14.4 Record Protocol

In general, most records contain abbreviations that are commonly used in recording patient care. Any abbreviation used should be commonly known within the profession. The abbreviation should be able to be understood by another dentist, including an expert witness, in understanding the care provided. So, any personally created abbreviations used for your own office would probably not be acceptable in proper record keeping. All entries made in a paper chart should be in ink, preferably black since it copies the best, in case copies are needed for the defense of a malpractice claim. Pencil, highlighter, and sticky notes should not be used. If a sticky note is used as a reminder, be sure to remove it when completed or incorporate the information on the note into the record as soon as possible. However, in reality, sticky notes are used in many offices as reminders. Many advise not to use sticky notes in the chart to avoid confusion and inquiries as to why the information was not part of the permanent chart. Hence, do not use them. Personal subjective opinions/feelings/attitudes towards the patient also have no place in the records. As an expert witness, poorly copied, indecipherable records make the defense of a malpractice claim extremely difficult.

Other entries pertaining to the patient that should be made include those regarding the patient's cooperation or noncooperation in the treatment provided, such as poor oral home hygiene, behavior management problems, not following referrals, refusing recommended treatment, cancelling appointments, not showing for appointments, or coming unreasonably late. Continued noncooperating situations affect treatment outcomes and may raise suspicion of malpractice when the desired results are not obtained. These situations all show the patient's contributory or comparative negligence per your jurisdiction. It cannot be stressed enough the importance of recording any patient's noncooperation.

All entries should be dated and signed or initialed. There should be no lines or pages left blank. If this should occur, place a squiggly line through the empty space so as to prevent any additions to the record that would cause suspicion of an altered record. If a mistake is made upon entry, do not white out, scratch out, or try to transfigure the entry. Simply draw a simple line through the entry and make the correct entry. Upon review of your records at a later date, you may find that there is a need to add to the records concerning treatment previously rendered. Do not back date the entry. Rather, enter the current date, mark it *Late Entry*, and then make your entry correctly.

14.5 Electronic Records

Electronic/computerized paperless offices are no longer a thing of the future. In fact, in some countries, electronic records will be required in the near future. This is a great improvement on having paper records and charts. They facilitate effective quality assurance, analysis of practice patterns, and research activities; speed the retrieval of data and expedite billing; reduce the number of lost records; allow for a complete set of backup records at little or no cost; expedite the transfer of data between facilities, regardless of geographic separation; are a proven long-term cost reducer; and, in most cases, are practice enhancers and a public relations tool (Rule 1001 (3) Federal rules of evidence, Supra Note 10). Electronic records provide at least seven major improvements over paper records:

1. A legible record.
2. Standard of care guidelines automatically triggered by diagnosis forces proper sequencing and needed criteria for proper patient care.
3. Electronic prescription alerts and possibly prevents both provider and pharmacist of potentially harmful drug-drug interactions or incompatibilities with the patient's physical or laboratory findings (Pollack 2011).
4. Electronic medical record systems can track ordered laboratory, diagnostic, or imaging tests, alert the provider of abnormal tests, and even notify the patient of the need, or the lack thereof, of future tests, diagnosis, or treatment (Sandy Sanbar et al. 2010, p. 1).
5. Automatically confirm the date and times of all entries and keep a dated and timed log of all individuals, with password protected access, who have accessed the record [audit trail] (Pollack 2002).
6. Automatically generate patient educational materials tailored to the patient's diagnosis and treatment (Sandy Sanbar et al. 2010, pp. 1–2).
7. A well-documented, complete, and unambiguous medical record allows for a much easier and possibly successful defense of a dental malpractice claim.

There are also some concerns regarding electronic records. Critics cite high initial cost, large training investment, hardware crashes and breakdowns, power failures, software glitches, sabotage of the system by disgruntled employees and hackers, unauthorized access, viruses, Trojan horses, reluctance of physicians to use the tightly controlled format for notes, and a host of other real and imagined problems (Evans et al. 1994). There is also the reliability of an electronic record for admissibility in a courtroom. To be admissible as evidence in a courtroom, the electronic records must be reliable. To be reliable, the electronic records must not be alterable upon entry (read-only format), retrievable when needed (backup system), and kept confidential with only authorized password protected, audit-trail worthy entries. As with paper records, electronic records must also be kept in safe storage, per your jurisdiction's requirements, via a secure off-site backup system (Bruckner 1998). Hence, the maintenance of the integrity of the dental record from its origination to its final resting place in storage is of most importance. Many malpractice decisions have been made based on the authentication, completeness, and integrity of the paper or electronic dental record.

14.6 Information in a Dental Record

The dental record must contain all the information pertaining to the patient. Records should include the following information:

1. Specifics, in detail, of the treatment provided
2. Reactions to treatment, adverse and positive
3. Doctor and patient comments (including complaints, resolutions, and patient noncompliance)
4. Radiographs
5. Prescriptions
6. Laboratory authorizations
7. Correspondence and telephone conversations between the patient and other healthcare providers (including cancelled and missed appointments)
8. Consultations requested and reports
9. Informed consent forms
10. A drug and medication log (including any over-the-counter [OTC] drugs or supplements)
11. Financial information and agreements (separate from the treatment records)
12. Demographic information (including place of employment)

13. Medical and dental history (including periodic updates as needed per the patient's needs)
14. Waivers and authorizations
15. Insurance information and claims submitted
16. Contact person in case of emergencies (including information about the primary physician)
17. Other information unique to the specific patient's needs (Sandy Sanbar et al. 2002).

14.7 Release of Dental Records

As with any healthcare records, dental records are requested for various purposes. From a licensing agency investigation, defense of a malpractice lawsuit, to the transferring to another dentist or other healthcare provider at the patient's or other healthcare provider's office request, dental records will be needed to be released. Whenever there is a request for a patient's dental records from the patient, another dental office, attorney, or licensing agency, a signed written authorization from the patient must be had before the release of the dental records. Upon the receipt of the release, most jurisdictions allow a certain time period in which to release that information, either by review, a summary of the records, and/or copies. You normally can charge a reasonable fee for clerical time and/or cost per copy. However, you must not refuse the request in the case of the patient's inability to pay. Never give original records to the patient or anyone else, including your malpractice attorney, unless under court order. People tend to lose things; and, once lost, records may never be found (Graskemper 2011, p. 64).

To disclose patient information without a patient-signed written authorization would be considered a breach of confidentiality or even a breach of privileged information and a violation of the Health Insurance Portability and Accountability Act (HIPAA) (Graskemper 2011, p. 64). Such a disclosure is normally not covered by malpractice insurance. There is a lot of information within the dental record, all of which is considered confidential, while some may be considered privileged. Confidential is the information routinely obtained during the course of treatment, which includes personal medical information and any other personal information obtained. Privileged is the information that is non-healthcare information that is not allowed to be disclosed in a judicial proceeding without permission of the person who supplied the information requested. Privileged information is normally not communicated within the typical dental setting.

There are three waivers under which the dentist may disclose a patient's confidential information:

1. Express waiver: a patient-signed written authorization as discussed.
2. Implied by law: mandated reporting of child abuse
   - Mandated reporting of communicable diseases to a health agency
3. Implied in law: a patient approved referral to another healthcare provider
   - Patients in a teaching facility
   - Most minor information to the parent or legal guardian (Graskemper 2011, p. 64)

Exceptions in which the dentist may disclose information in the dental record in a dental record without the patient's consent include:

1. Defense of a claim challenging the dentist's professional competence in a peer review process
2. Claim for payment of fees
3. Third-party payer relating to fees or services rendered
4. Court order from a police or federal agency as part of a criminal investigation
5. Identification of a dead body
6. To report a legal violation of another healthcare professional, if the dentist reasonably believes it is necessary to disclose the information to comply with Public Health Code (highly communicable disease) (Weber 2001)
7. Sharing information with other healthcare providers for treatment purposes
8. The transfer of patient records involved in practice transition of sale (American Medical Association)

When requesting a valid general release from the patient, it should contain seven items:

1. Patient's name and identifying information
2. Address of the healthcare professional or institution directed to release the information
3. Description of the information to be released
4. Identity of the party to be furnished the information
5. Language authorizing release of the information
6. Signature of the patient or authorized individual
7. (If necessary) the time period for which the release remains valid (American Medical Association)

Upon the receipt of a properly executed release, most jurisdictions allow a limited time period in which the provider must provide the information requested. Some jurisdictions allow the patient to receive the requested information regardless of ability to pay for copies, written summary, clerical time, or outstanding balance.

14.8 Retention

Due to the many various statute of limitations found in different jurisdictions, it is best to retain records indefinitely. However, due to storage of paper records, it is possibly not practical or reasonable to maintain records forever. Hence, retain patient records as long as possible. Normally, 10-year retention of records fulfills most jurisdictions. Some jurisdictions like Massachusetts and California statutes of limitations run from the time the patient discovers or should have discovered the injury that resulted from the dental malpractice (Graskemper 2011, pp. 65–66). Hence, such statutes of limitations dictate the healthcare provider and maintain patient records indefinitely.

14.9 Ownership

Often when patients request their records, they believe that the actual treatment record is theirs. There is little controversy about who owns the tangible [dental] record, that is, the paper, film, or recording that contains the medical information: the healthcare provider, who is responsible for creating, compiling, and maintaining the [dental] record, owns it (Dewitt et al. 1991). However, in most jurisdictions if not all, the patient has rights to the information contained within the dental record.

14.10 Disposal

As time passes and storage becomes a problem financially and/or needed space, destruction of old records could be destroyed per your jurisdiction. It is normally advised that at least 10 years have passed. For minors it is recommended the 10 years or until the patient reaches the age of majority plus the applicable statute of limitations. When disposing of the records, every effort must be taken to protect the confidentiality of the patient. To properly dispose of patient records, it is highly recommended to use a licensed shredding company, with a written receipt/certification for shredding showing the time period of the records, commonly called a Certificate of Destruction.

Besides patient records, there are many other records required of a business to retain and store for future reference, such as employee records, OSHA reports, tax returns, banking statements, accounts receivable, and accounts payable. Be sure to check with your jurisdiction of which records must be retained and for how long.

14.11 Informed Consent

With information readily available to the patient and the ever-improving patient's level of education, communication is in the forefront of risk management in patient care. Patients want more information regarding their treatment to make their own treatment decisions, thus keeping patient autonomy strong and intact. To fulfill this need for knowledge of the patient to better understand their treatment needs and become more involved in their treatment options, informed consent is most important. One of the utmost functions of informed consent is the protection of the patient's right to self-determination to accept the treatment proposed (Schloendorff v. Society of New York Hospital). What is needed to make a proper informed consent? What makes the consent valid? To what extent does the consent apply? These questions are often asked when legal scrutiny is applied in an alleged malpractice lawsuit.

In the 1914 New York case of Schloendorff v Society of New York Hospital: "*Every human being of adult years and sound mind has a right to determine what shall be done with his own body; and a surgeon who performs an operation without his patient's consent commits an assault for which he is liable in damages*" (Schloendorff v. Society of New York Hospital). The term *informed consent* was first used in 1957 by a California appeals court, which explained: "*A physician violates his duty to his patient and subjects himself to liability if he withholds any facts which are necessary to form the basis of an intelligent consent by the patient to the proposed treatment*" (Salgo v. Leland Stanford, Jr et al. 1957). This was emphasized in the 1972 case of Canterbury v. Spence requiring all material risks to be disclosed to the patient (Spence & 464 F2d 772, 783 (DC Cir 1972)). Risks are deemed material when the reasonable person in the patient's position would likely attach significance to the risks in question when deciding whether to proceed with a proposed therapy (Graskemper 2005). Without a proper informed consent, the dentist may be held liable for malpractice and possibly battery.

14.12 The Standard

The standard to which a dentist will be held to may be found in one of two prevalent standards: the professional community standard and the reasonable person standard. Under the community standard, the dentist must inform the patient of those risks that others in the same community are disclosing to their patients. This standard is slowly being replaced by the reasonable person standard due to the fact that if all the community practitioners practice below the standard of care by not properly informing their patients regarding a certain procedure, pockets of substandard care would exist (Graskemper 2011, p. 51). Patients now have easy access to dental care information via the Internet. With such access, patients expect their dentists to fully inform them about the procedure to be done. What is of most importance is that enough information is given to the patient to allow the patient to make an informed decision. And having such information, would a reasonably prudent person undergo the procedure knowing what the patient knew? (Graskemper 2011, p. 51)

It is not imperative to inform the patient of every risk/benefit nuance of the procedure. Risks that are very rare or are of such general knowledge need not be disclosed. However, informed consent is patient and treatment specific (Graskemper 2011, p. 52). Hence, what is told to the 20-year-old patient with good health regarding an extraction of a root-resorbed deciduous tooth and to the 70-year-old patient with extensive medical history including blood thinners and bisphosphanates, regarding an extraction of a fractured root canalled mandibular second molar, will and should be different. Each has different direct and foreseeable risks attached to the extraction procedure. Every patient is entitled to be informed of all directly related and reasonably foreseeable risks.

There are other times in which the dentist may be forced into a situation where an informed consent may not have been given. In such situations, a red light should flash for the dentist to tread carefully and fully document the situation such that there is no miscommunication regarding the lack of an informed consent. If the risks of a bad outcome or possible claim of malpractice are great, the dentist should refuse treatment.

First, there are the *patient set-ups* by which the patient wishes not to be informed. The *patient set-ups* will usually be something similar to:

> "Whatever you say, you're the doctor."
> "You are such a good dentist, I trust you to do what is right."
> "You don't have to tell me, I've had this done before."
> "Just do the best you can, I trust you." (Graskemper 2011, p. 53)

Secondly, there is the situation where the patient is under any type of sedation and the treatment extends beyond that which was expected at the time of treatment plan discussion and obtaining informed consent prior to sedation. Fully document the reason for the further needed treatment and fully inform the patient upon recovery. This does not allow the dentist to extend treatment far beyond that which was intended or not related to previously agreed to treatment prior to sedation. This has been referred to as the *Extension doctrine* (White et al. 2010).

Thirdly, there is the situation where the patient will become unduly stressed by the information and he or she wishes to waiver the information regarding the risks of the procedure, such as a highly dental phobic patient. However, enough information must be given so the patient understands the general nature of the procedure and then waives his or her right to more risk information. Again, fully document such patient waiver.

Fourthly, many jurisdictions recognize a physician's right to withhold information from a patient if disclosure would be harmful to the patient. Perhaps the best-known statement of this principle, commonly known as *therapeutic privilege*, is in the landmark *Canterbury* case (White et al. 2010, p. 5):

It is recognized that patients occasionally become so ill or emotionally distraught on disclosure as to foreclose a rational decision, or complicate or hinder the treatment, or perhaps even pose psychological damage to the patient (Spence and 464 F2d 789 (DC Cir 1972)).

Since this privilege is usually allowed in life-threatening situations where a patient in poor health must decide on a life-threatening surgery and receiving such information may refuse the needed treatment based on the patient's frailty, instability, or perversity. A paternalistic doctor-patient relationship does not fulfill this exception. Dentists normally would not rely on such privilege to withhold information. If the dentist does rely on this exception, he or she will have a heavy burden of proof showing the need to take such exception.

Fifthly, where there is an emergency, either life threatening or the patient is physically unable to give consent, consent is not needed if the delay in obtaining consent would result in substantial risk of further injury or even loss of life (Graskemper 2011, p. 53). This is commonly held up under the various Good Samaritan laws. Under such a statute, consent is waived and protects the dentist from ordinary negligence. It does not protect the dentist from a gross negligence claim: the wanton disregard of reasonable care for the patient.

14.13 Elements of Informed Consent

Informed consent has two aspects: the informed part and the consent part. Each of these has numerous elements to be fulfilled to have a valid informed consent.

The informed part consists of six parts which the dentist is responsible to provide for the patient to be properly and fully informed:

1. The use of understandable terms when explaining the procedure
2. Give reasons or diagnosis prompting the planned procedure
3. What are the benefits, anticipated outcome, and prognosis of the procedure
4. Any reasonable and foreseeable risks that are attached to the procedure
5. Reasonably feasible alternative treatment including no treatment and the accompanying risks and benefits
6. The associated costs of the planned procedure and alternative

I have added costs due to the fact that it is a determining factor for the reasonable person when deciding whether to consent (or not) to a particular dental treatment or its alternative. If a written document is being used, be aware not to simply make a *laundry list* of possible risks. If such a list is used, the words *but not limited to* should be inserted prior to the list of risks. This alerts the patient that there may be other risks, though remote, may be possible. Also available are informed consent videos that fulfill most of the elements. After which, the patient should sign a form acknowledging they viewed and understood the video.

The consent part consists of eight elements to allow the consent to be valid:

1. The consent must be freely given and voluntary.
2. The patient must be given an opportunity to ask questions and have them answered competently and completely.
3. To be informative and understandable, the information part as well as the consent part must be in a language the patient understands. If necessary, provide an interpreter or have the patient bring an interpreter with him or her to the dental appointment. If an interpreter is being used, record the name and relationship to the patient.
4. The person giving the consent must be authorized to make such decisions.
5. Consent must be obtained by the dentist or trained auxiliary personnel (per your jurisdiction).
6. The dentist must be available to answer any patient questions.
7. Some jurisdictions require the consent to be a signed written document for certain invasive procedures. It is highly advisable to obtain a written signed consent for any endodontic, surgical, or other invasive procedures.
8. Consent must not be rushed or coerced (Graskemper 2011, p. 54).

As with any written consent, the patient and a witness should sign and date the document and it should be noted in the chart. The dental assistant or hygienist may inform the patient; however, it is the dentist's responsibility to confirm with the patient that they understood or have any questions regarding the procedure or informed consent, which the dentist must answer. The document commonly will recite that the patient was given an opportunity to ask questions and to receive answers and explanations from the dentist. Nevertheless, it is not the document that is the informed consent. It only documents or memorializes that a discussion between dentist and patient regarding all the elements of the informed consent has taken place prior to treatment being rendered. It is the actual discussion with the patient that is the informed consent.

14.14 Exceptions

All patients do not have the authority to consent to treatment. Most jurisdictions allow patients 18 years of age and over and of sound mind to consent to treatment regardless of who is financially paying for the treatment. As with any major guideline, there are exceptions. A legal guardian may consent for a patient under age or with an incapacity to consent, such as mental retardation, Alzheimer disease, and senility. Grandparents, older siblings, or relatives do not automatically become the legal guardian solely on the fact that they brought the minor or elder patient to the office and stating it is O.K. and consents to treatment. Without a written medical authorization, they do not have authority to consent. If a minor-aged patient presents for treatment without a prior parental approval, the dentist should make a good-faith effort to contact the parent for consent. Proper documentation of the telephone consent must be recorded in the record. If parental contact is unsuccessful, the dentist should either refrain from treatment or proceed in the patient's best interests, if only to temporize to prevent further harm to the patient. This also keeps the ethical concepts of beneficence and malfeasance intact.

Depending on your jurisdiction, there are basically five exceptions to allow a patient under the age of 18 to give their informed consent:

1. Emancipation
2. Married
3. A parent and for their child
4. In an emergency (life and death) situation
5. Pregnant

Based on good-faith effort to verify the exception, the dentist must use caution and must well document such effort.

14.15 Patient's Capacity to Decide

If the patient presents themselves as being of sound mind but the dentist after discussion of the proposed treatment needs to question the ability of the patient to give an informed consent, the dentist must further evaluate the patient's capacity. The main question is: "Does the patient's perceived incapacity compromise his or her decision making?" (Graskemper 2011, p. 56)

To help make a determination of the patient's ability to grant informed consent, the following questions may lead the dentist to making a good-faith effort determination:

1. Does the patient understand the proposed treatment plan and how it would affect him?
2. Does the patient understand that there are options, their differences, and results of the options including no treatment?
3. Does the patient have the ability to clearly choose an option?
4. Does the patient understand the affect of his or her decision on themselves and on others including the responsibilities that attach to the decision being made? (Ozar and Sokol 2002; Graskemper 2011, p. 56)

If the patient's capacity is still questionable, the dentist should ask the patient if they would like someone, usually a family member, to help in the decision-making process. If such a person is involved, be sure to note who the person is, their relationship with the patient (legal guardian?), and how they were involved in the decision making. Again, a good-faith effort by the dentist is paramount to having an informed consent, ethically uphold the patient's autonomy, and maintaining the ethical concepts of malfeasance and beneficence.

14.16 Types of Consent

There are two types of consent: implied consent and express consent. An express consent may be written or oral. It is when the patient acknowledges their consent either by a signed written consent (preferable) or verbally states their consent, which must be properly documented. An express consent must be understandable, direct, positive, and unequivocal. Merely signing a treatment plan or a financial agreement is not an express consent since it does not contain all the elements needed to properly inform the patient. Any invasive procedure should be accompanied with a signed written express consent.

An implied consent may be *by law* or *by action.* Implied consent by law applies to treatment being rendered at an accident. A reasonable person would consent to treatment to prevent further injury or death. Implied consent by action applies to the patient acknowledging their consent by their actions. The patient, by their action or inaction, such as making an appointment, sitting in the dental chair, opens their mouth, allows for anesthetic, allows the treatment, and makes no objection to the treatment being rendered, has given their implied consent. Hence, the dentist may in good faith assume the patient has consented to treatment.

Neither express, implied by law, nor implied by action, consents do not protect the dentist from negligence or claims of dental malpractice. The dentist is still held to the standard of care a reasonably prudent dentist would have done in the same or similar set of circumstances.

14.17 Refusal of Treatment

When a patient refuses treatment, it is highly advised to have the patient sign a written informed refusal indicating the patient's full understanding of the risks associated with his or her refusal to the recommended treatment. This includes the refusal not to seek specialty care when recommended. This prevents the patient from stating in a future alleged malpractice lawsuit that they were not informed of loss of teeth or even death due to their refusal to treat.

14.18 Ethical Crossover

Informed consent is the legal sister to the ethical concept of patient autonomy. Patient autonomy gives the patient or the patient's guardian the right to self-determination as to the course of treatment the patient wants to allow. A patient cannot exercise that right if they are not given a proper informed consent. Hence, the dentist must properly discuss the treatment involved and allow the patient to decide whether they will or will not consent to the treatment.

References

American Medical Association, Patient Confidentiality. http://ama-assn.org/ama/pub/category/print/4610html. Accessed 19 Oct 2010

Bruckner F (1998) The duty to inform, liability to third parties and the duty to warn. J Med Pract Manage 100

Dewitt T et al. (1991) Patient information and confidentiality: treatise on health care law. Matthew Bender

Evans RS et al. (1994) Preventing adverse drug events in hospitalized patients. Ann Pharmacother 28:523

Graskemper JP (2005) Informed consent: a stepping stone in risk management. Compend Contin Educ Dent 26(4):286

Graskemper J (2011) Professional responsibility in dentistry: a practical guide to Law and ethics. Wiley-Blackwell, Ames/Iowa

Loomis GA et al. (2002) If electronic records are so great, why aren't family physicians using them? J Fam Pract 51(7):636–641

Ozar D, Sokol D (2002) Dental ethics at chairside. Georgetown University Press, Washington, DC, p 117

Pollack B (2002) Law and risk management in dental practice. Quintessence Publishing, Chicago, p 137

Pollack B (2011) Law and risk. In: Graskemper JP (ed) Professional responsibility in dentistry: a practical guide to Law and ethics. Wiley-Blackwell, Ames/Iowa, p 61

Rule 1001 (3) Federal rules of evidence, Supra Note 10

Salgo v. Leland Stanford, Jr., Univ. Bd. of Trustees, 317 P. 2d 170, 181 (Cal. App. Ct. 1957

Sandy Sanbar S et al. (2002) Legalmanagement in dental practice. Quintessence Publishing, Chicago, p 137

Sandy Sanbar S et al. (2010) Medical records: paper and electronic, Module 5, Chapter 13. In: Sandy Sanbar S (ed) Legal medicine and medical ethics, 8th edn. Law of Medicine Publication

Schloendorff v. Society of New York Hosp., 105 N.E. 92, 93 (N.Y. 1914)

Canterbury v Spence, 464 F2d 772,783 (DC Cir 1972)

Canterbury v Spence, 464 F2d 789 (DC Cir 1972)

Weber R (2001) Release of records. J Mich Dent Assoc 83(6)

White C et al. (2010) Informed consent to medical and surgical treatment, Module 5, Chapter 11. In: Legal medicine and medical ethics, 8th edn. Law Medicine Publication

Dental Law in Germany

15

Klaus Rötzscher, Günter Seifert, and Rolf Singer

15.1 Preliminary Comments

Knowledge in the field of civil and criminal relationships between dentist and patient is of increasing importance. Any dentist may be asked to testify as a witness, as at expert witness court (*Fifth Title. General provisions relating to the inquiry* §§ *355ff*; *Seventh Title. Evidence of witnesses* §§ *373ff*; *Eighth Title. Evidence by experts.* §§ *402ff CCP*), (§§ *407ff CCP*). In criminal proceedings, the Criminal Procedure is binding (§§ *48*, *72 ff. CCP*). As a consequence, every dentist should acquire knowledge of civil or criminal law to reduce uncertainties or realistically estimate their own situation and to act as an expert interpreting medical facts for the court.

15.2 General Legal Basis

The Dentistry Act (§ *1 para 1 and 3*, *as amended 31 March 1992 ZHG in its form from 16 April 1987* [*BGBl I, S. 1225 ff*]) requires a medical license for activities of prevention, diagnosis, and treatment of anomalies and diseases of the teeth, mouth, and jaw, including the anomalies of tooth positions and the absence of teeth. Approval (permission and obligation) to participate in contractual dental care is based on the admission regulations for (contract) dentists. Registration in the Dentist's Register and a 2-year preparation period are prerequisites for approval (§ *95 para 2 SGB V*, § *3 para 2,3 ZO-Z*). The possibility of double registration of oral and maxillofacial surgeons as doctors and dentists has been confirmed by the Federal Social Court in 1999 (*BSG Kassel, Judgement of 15th November 1999, Az. B 6 KA 15/99 R*). Foreigners from countries within the European Union (EU) are treated as Germans. Exams completed in the member states are recognized in principle.

The temporary pursuit of dentistry requires a revocable permit (§ *1 para 1*, § *13*, *para 1 to 5 ZHG*). Foreign and German dentists who obtained their Ph.D. at a foreign university need a permit to hold this academic title. This is subject to approval (§ *2 para 1 and 3 of the Act on the use of academic degrees*). The foreign origins of the doctorate must be obvious in the academic title (e.g., MUDr. Univ. Prag or Dr. med. dent. Univ. Zagreb) (*VGH München, BayVBl. 1970.185*).

According to § *1 para 4 ZHG*, dentistry is not a free trade. The partial performances in § *5 and 6* of the Dental Act may be delegated. Liability and responsibility for these services remain the dentist's (Linder 1997). The independent

K. Rötzscher, Dr. med. Dr. med. dent. (✉)
German Academy of Forensic Odontostomatology (AKFOS), Wimphelingstraße 7, 67346 Speyer, Germany
e-mail: roetzscher.klaus.dr@t-online.de

G. Seifert, Dr. med. dent.
Orthodontist, Marktplatz 5, 83471 Berchtesgaden, Germany

R. Singer, Univ.-Prof. (em) Dr. med. Dr. med. dent.
Department of Oral and Craniomandibular Surgery, Clinicum Ludwigshafen/Rhein, Kalkofenweg 1, 67227 Frankenthal, Germany

K. Rötzscher (ed.), *Forensic and Legal Dentistry*,
DOI 10.1007/978-3-319-01330-5_15,

activities of employees as dental assistants/helpers (ZAH) or dental specialist assistants/helpers (ZMF) – in the form of an activity on a freelance basis – are not admitted according to the Dentistry Act.

Physicians and dentists need freedom to make professional decisions, as well as the trust of their patients. The law provides no more than a framework. The dental profession can only be performed, according to the professional code of law, "in diagnostic and therapeutic freedom" (Laufs 1996a).

The standard of tomorrow, based on the scientific work of today, has a price, in which many patients are unfortunately not interested. Current medical law seems to be exhausted between the duties of the physician and the rights of patients (Laufs 1996b). Modern medicine must even take risks to ban health risks and open new territory for the benefit of patients. Modern medicine is confronted with a plethora of different ventures because of the exponential growth of scientific knowledge and technology.

"As Critical Counsiliar Committees, the ethic committees support the medical profession in all medical experiments and clinical studies. The ethics committees are expected to protect both, the patient and the doctor" (Laufs 1996b).

15.3 Contract Law

15.3.1 Relationship Between Dentist and Patient

15.3.2 Treatment Contract

If a patient is receiving dental treatment, a treatment contract is conducted between the patient and the dentist. *BGHE of 18.03.1980, Az. VI ZR 247/78*; *VersR 1980, 558* states that "As well as between dentist and private patient there is also a contractual binding between dentist and public health patient, usually in a work delivery form. Basically, the treatment contract is completed with the conclusion of treatment, in case of prosthetic treatment with the inclusion of the necessary restoration" (Tiemann 1982).

15.3.3 Cancellation of the Contract

A contract can be cancelled either by ordinary notice or without notice (dismissal without notice for cause; § *626 BGB*). A termination of the treatment contract is also given if the patient engages the services of another dentist (Figgener 1998). In contrast, the dentist can only terminate the contract if the patient can be treated elsewhere. The cancellation of the treatment contract is only effective if the dentist was informed about it (Tiemann 1982). In case of a contract termination, a proportional payment is due (compensation for damages for termination without notice) (§ *628 para 1 sentence 1 BGB*).

OLG Hamm, Judgement Az. 3 U 9/97 states that "If a dental treatment is characterized by careless work, this justifies the loss of confidence and thus the cancellation of the contract." This may result in loss of fees and compensation for damages and pain.

For example, if the dentist uses a different alloy from that agreed upon in the contract, a breach of the contract is given and entitles the patient to cancel and refuse the treatment fee (§ *628 para 1 BGB p. 2*). *LG Nurnberg-Furth, Judgement Az. 11 S 867/93* states that "Patient and dentist agreed to use only best gold alloy for bridges, but the dentist used a palladium-based alloy. As a consequence the patient was released from paying the treatments cost."

In another example, a dentist's performance was totally inadequate and unacceptable. Despite several attempts, the damages could not be fixed. All treatments had to be repeated by another dentist. *OLG Dusseldorf, Judgement, Az. 8 U 131/93* states that "The patient must accept the attempt to correct any inaccuracies. The dentist was required to refund the fee and to bear the costs caused by his treatment. Additionally, compensation for pain at the amount of Euro 1.780 was admitted."

Additionally, an unexcused absence at a treatment appointment does not necessarily mean a termination of the contract. *AG Dortmund,*

Judgement, Az. 125 C 5112/92; AG Bad Homburg, Judgement from 25.6.1994, Az. 2 C 3838/93 (MedR 94.487: 94.888 MDR) states that "In case of an unexcused absence, the patient has to pay the usual fee."

15.4 Dental Liability Law

15.4.1 Basics

Dentist and patient frequently meet again in court. This might be caused by juridification spreading in all areas of life, but this development cannot be stopped. The dentist is advised to acquire and adapt the basics of profession-relevant law, especially of tort law. On the other hand, any dentist can be called to assess the work of another dentist in court as an impartial expert.

The term medical malpractice exists neither in the law of the Penal Code nor in the Civil Code. It is defined as improper and damaging behavior by the physician. This means a violation of the general principles of medical science (*BGH, NJW 1953, 257*).

Diagnosis-oriented care, preparation of the oral cavity for holding dentures that need preserving, and periodontal, surgical, orthodontic, and functional therapies to create conditions under which a prosthetic treatment can be successful are components of the treatment contract (Marxkors 1999).

OLG Hamm, Judgement, Az. 3 U 26/94 states that "A dentist had claimed his fee for an extensive crown and bridge restoration in both the upper and the lower jaw, although the entire prosthesis had to be removed a short time after the incorporation due to bad periodontal condition. As a result of faulty planning, there was no doubt that the entire denture was defective and worthless for the patient with the result that the patient was released from paying the fee. It was also noted that the dentist has to bear the cost for removing the prosthesis. The dentist should have omitted the denture or at least he should have done a periodontal treatment and await its results."

OLG Celle, VersR 1987, 591) (Figgener 1993) states that "In cases of doubt, prior to treatment, a consultation with the family doctor or internist is required, his recommendations must be recorded in the treatment register and be guideline for scope and duration of therapeutic measures. Who does not consider these given criteria can be guilty of negligently causing a damage (according to § *276 BGB*)."

Legal liability implications are ruled in a service contract (§ *611ff BGB*), work contract (§ *631ff BGB*), liability for damages caused by an unlawful act (§ *823 BGB*), liability for vicarious agents (§ *831 BGB*), liability for own negligence (§ *276 BGB*), and the fault of the assistant (§ *278 BGB*) (Figgener 1993; Gümpel 1994). Culpably causing damage from a service or work contract can result in both civil and criminal penalties. The Civil law (*BGB*) applies to the (material/immaterial) restitution of damages (§§ *249 ff, 842 ff, 847 BGB*), and the criminal law (*Criminal Code; StGB*) to the penalization of culpable behavior (§§ *223, 230 StGB*).

In civil cases, the applicant shall (in accordance with the rules of evidence) prove whether there is a breach of contractual or legal obligations. In criminal trials, the prosecutor must prove that a criminal accusation is justified. Few allegations against dentists that are the subject of civil proceedings lead to criminal proceedings (Lüer 1948).

In general, in civil law and criminal law, each claimant must demonstrate and prove the facts on which the claim is based. For this reason, two different types of medical malpractice trials are identified (Rohde 1996b):

1. The patient claims compensation for material and nonmaterial damage that resulted from faulty treatment.
2. The physician proceeds against the patient because of unpaid treatment cost. Each party claims compensation for its damages caused by the counterparty.

In both processes, the crucial question is whether medical malpractice exists and whether it can be proven. Because of this burden of proof for patients, the legislation has developed a counterweight. Before any medical treatment, the patient must be informed about the risks of the upcoming surgery. After proper education, the patient shall give consent. Treatment without the patient's consent is an unlawful and culpable assault. The consent must be documented in written form.

Whether an incorrect treatment can be proven and whether the patient has consented to the treatment are decisive for medical liability cases (Rohde 1996b):

1. In case of an incorrect treatment, the dentist must pay compensation for material damage and for pain and suffering.
2. If an incorrect treatment cannot be proven, the patient's complaint is dismissed and the fees are due.
3. If its unclear whether there is an error in treatment and no education was given prior to the treatment, the dentist must pay compensation for damages and for pain and suffering.
4. If it is unclear whether there is an error in treatment, but information was given, the patient's complaint is dismissed and the cost must be paid (Rohde 1996b).

Most medical liability lawsuits end up in a settlement deal; both parties compromise and an agreement can be achieved. Some lawsuits begin with the declared intention not to end up in a settlement. Another factor is that medical liability law is largely unknown and some of its rules are incomprehensible to laypersons.

Thanks to the considerable expertise of the established special courts and senate chambers for medical malpractice, almost all known results from malpractice disputes (settlements or judgments) can be appropriate, knowledgeable, and competent. (Figgener 1997; Rohde 1996b). The large number of settlements suggests that pretrial efforts to resolve the conflict have not been sufficient.

Often, inappropriate behavior of the dentist triggers a conflict. Unfortunately, even simple requests for information are misunderstood as criticism. Patients often have reasonable criticism or wish for more information. It is up to the dentist to solve this conflict by leading a conversation that is more detailed and understandable. This step should never be skipped for time reasons.

A serious and conflict-provoking problem is reckless and careless remarks from the dentist about previous treatments in order to promote the dentist's own knowledge and skills. Remarks such as "who has been doing this" or statements that are even more explicit can lead to the patient's immediate displeasure (Rohde 1996b).

German physician or dentist liability law is not codified as such. It follows the general rules of tort law. Meanwhile, many Senate chambers have established a so-called judicial advanced education to cope with the increasing number of medical liability lawsuits. Legal liability claims by a patient against his dentist because of incorrect treatment can be contractual and/or tort. The Civil Code (BGB) distinguishes two types of contract, the service contract (§§ *611 ff BGB*) and the work contract (§§ *631 ff BGB*). The main difference is that, in the work contract, success is clearly defined, such as a figurative or descriptive work product. In the service contract, the covenanter owes taking action with regard for an object but without guaranteeing its success, such as in the work contract. Further differences are the various warranties and warranty periods. The work contract obliges that the work be free of defects and, in case of defects, removal within a reasonable time.

This strict warranty ends within the period of 6 months after the acceptance of the work (§ *638 para 1 BGB*). In the service contract, a liability occurs only with damages caused by culpability (the warranty period is 30 years). If no culpable behavior is detected, the covenanter is not liable but keeps their wage claim (§ *195 BGB*).

There was a long and intensive dispute regarding the nature of dental contracts. In 1974, the Federal High Court made a landmark decision that dental work, including dental prosthetic activity, underlies the Service Contract. The Federal High Court explains *inter alia*:

"The treatment contract is basically a service contract. A physician/dentist promises only the proper treatment of the patient, but cannot guarantee the desired result: the healing of the disease …

The warranty of the work contract is also valid for the technical production of prostheses. In contrast, the extraction of teeth is a treatment and thus not part of the work contract.

It is true that the technical production of a dental prosthesis is not a medical procedure. It is rather a work as defined in §§ *631ff BGB*, which is often not conducted by the dentist himself, but by a dental technician …

All other tasks related with dental prosthetic in particular the inclusion of the prosthesis in the mouth, are treatments. The success of these treatments depends not only on the skills of the physician/dentist, but also on non-influenceable circumstances."

With this ruling, which contains a comprehensive overview of literature and case law, the Supreme High Court clarified that the dentist is obliged to observe due care in the treatment. The dentist is not liable for circumstances the dentist cannot control, especially for damages as a result of the physical or mental condition of the patient.

15.4.2 Duties from Liability Law

The scope of services for public health patients is governed by the Social Code Book V. The applicable restrictions in the context of dental care are not valid for Private patients. One question regards the scope of services for dental treatments covered by Private Health Insurance (PKV). According to § *27 para 1 sentence 2*, § *28 para 2*, §§ *29*, *30 SGB V*, medical treatment includes the dental treatment and also dentures. This supplying of dentures must be adequate, appropriate, and necessary (§ *12 para 1 sentence 1*, § *70 para 1 sentence 2 SGB V*). A number of typical rights and duties for both sides result from the treatment contract. Obligations of one side reflect the rights of the other side with regard to the cost.

The most significant duties of a dentist from liability law are:

- Medical care
- Obligation for advanced training
- Duty to inform
- Confidentiality
- Duty of documentation (of all important treatment-related facts)

Of course, this list is not exhaustive in detail—the responsibilities can result in many other aspects—but this list is the most common starting point for tort law consequences.

For a liability from the contract, the following conditions must be present:

- Effectively accomplished treatment contract
- Breach of a contractual obligation by the dentist
- Culpability of the dentist
- Damage to the patient
- Causation by breach of duty

In addition to the liability from the contract, there may be legal liability. "Anyone who intentionally or negligently injures the life, body or health of another, is obliged to compensate the damage" (*liability for damages*; § *823 para 1 BGB*).

15.4.3 Compensation for Nonmaterial Damage

The injured person can claim a fair compensation in money (§ *847 BGB – compensation*). Thus, the medical measurability of a surgery and the medical evidence of an impairment are essential features of body and health impairment.

15.4.4 Compensation for Material Damage

The tort claim for compensation of material damage is independent from the contract.

Compensation for damage can only be claimed once.

It may seem surprising at first glance that there is a contractual and tortious liability for the damage. This is, however, in the scheme of our Civil Code, and has good sense and practical importance. The BGB is geared that not only legally connected persons (contractual partners), are liable to careful observance of contractual obligations, but also that parties who meet each other without any contract have the established legal duty not to harm each other.

15.4.5 Content and Scope of Compensation

There must be adequate compensation for damage caused by improper treatment. This includes the full treatment and technology cost of removing the damage (possibly the cost of retreatment and a new preparation of irregular tooth replacement). Furthermore, additional cost for a more extensive treatment must be accepted if the causes are found to be in violation of the original contract (*LG Köln, Judgement of 24.11.1988, Az. 25 O 95/88*).

Court decisions in connection with dental prosthetic treatments demand the following facts (assembled by Rohde 1999). The following conditions must exist for a liability of the dentist (tort liability):

- Unlawful injury to life, body, or health
- Culpability of the dentist
- Damage to the patient
- Causality for the damage

Comparing the conditions of contractual and tortious liability, there must be a contractual breach and an injury to life, limb, or health. Because the obligation of the treatment contract substantially is the positive influence of life and limb, the consequences of a breach of this duty are the constituent elements of tortious liability. Because the other tort law requirements are similar, it should be allowed, to avoid complicated jurisprudence, for the contractual and tortious liability to be set as equal. However, important differences arise in the burden of proof with regard to the scope of the claims, the behavior of the auxiliary personnel, and the statute of limitations.

15.4.6 Limitations

The claim for compensation of a tort damage expires after 3 years, starting after the aggrieved party becomes aware of the damage, even if this is 30 years after the damage occurred (*limitation*; *§ 852 para 1 BGB*). The careful consideration of all of the identified requirements cannot protect the dentist from disputes with his patients. In addition to the financial, time, and emotional stress that a controversy brings for both sides, the dentist and patient should try to agree amicably. If this fails, either party can apply to the insurance company, which usually calls a consultant. If this does not lead to an agreement, a legal argument will be inevitable.

The literature on medical law and medical liability, addressed to all involved parties, is hardly manageable even for lawyers. The publications partly provide advice to patients who believe they have been wronged, partly provide advice to the doctor or dentist to better protect themselves, and also serve as a legal guide for the management of the medical liability process and for the experts.

Despite this detailed literature, case law is always valid for medical liability practice. The jurisdiction in the literature cannot be used as a rigid grid for all cases. The relevant criteria and principles are reassessed for each specific case. We are dealing with not just consolidated, time rigid, rules across time, but with a constantly evolving so-called judge-made law. The following discussion is based, where possible, on individual areas of dental medicine (Figgener 1996).

15.4.7 The Duty of Care

Dentists are obliged to provide comprehensive care for their patients. "The physician/dentist commits a culpable breach of duty, if he negligently disregards the required care" (*§ 276, BGB*). The dentist is obligated to a treatment equivalent of an objective standard of care. Standard of care is the current status of dental knowledge and skills (Figgener 1997).

15.4.8 Obligation to Advanced Education

The physician must not ignore new insights and methods because of convenience, stubbornness, or arrogance. In dentistry, as in general medicine, advanced education is a requirement. The freedom of the doctor to choose a method ends if the superiority of another method is obvious. To have the current state of scientific knowledge as a standard of care of their work, dentists must expand their knowledge and skills constantly and according to the dynamics of progress "to the limit of what is reasonable" (*BGH VersR 1977, 546*; *VersR 1968, 276*). The duty of education, which results from the duty of care, is given in all professional conducts. The fulfillment of the duty of training applies to the due diligence that the physician/dentist has complied with their work (*§ 276 BGB*).

It is obvious, however, that it has become impossible for individuals to understand all of the enormous developments and the immense growth of knowledge in the entire field of dentistry while areas that are even more specialized arise. Because progress only makes sense if the patient benefits from it, dentists have to be able to keep their patients informed about the latest diagnostic and therapeutic possibilities, even if the dentist cannot practice them and has to refer the patient to another doctor. The dentist must be judged on the current state of dentistry. Areas the dentist can no longer master must be excluded from the dentist's activities. Specializations can be found in all areas of work. Those who ignore this development and do not have the required skills for the treatment might be confronted with the so-called accusation of take-over (Figgener 1996).

15.4.9 The Duty to Inform

Another important and highly legally relevant obligation of the dentist is the duty to inform. Its purpose is to ensure the freedom of choice of the patient. Its origin is the principle of the free development of personality and is founded on the self-determination of the patient's body (*derived from the constitutionally enshrined general right under Article 2, Section 1 in conjunction with Article 1 para 1 GG*). Regardless of legal liability standards, the *Professional Code (BO)* in *§ 1a* obliges the doctor to provide information. Without providing adequate and thorough information to the patient, consent cannot be obtained. This may result in medical malpractice consequences.

Only information about the proposed treatment that is proper, individual, and aligned to the intellectual abilities of each individual patient leads to a consent ("informed consent"). The education of patients has been given a concrete form by a variety of judgments (Ankermann and Kullmann 1995). Since the 1950s, information provided before medical and dental procedures has been the subject of disputes in countless court decisions and of an extensive medical–legal literature (Figgener 1996; Rohde 1995b, 1996a).

15.4.10 Principles of the Information

The physician/dentist must personally lead the information of a patient.

1. This cannot be replaced by handing the patient an information sheet.
2. The given information must be comprehensible to the patient, it must be appropriate to the intellectual level of the patient.
3. The given information must include all typical risks of the treatment, regardless of the percentage of instances per 1,000 people.
4. The giving of information must be completed early enough so that patients are able to discuss the information with their family or to seek the advice of another doctor/dentist, or just to think over what was heard (and not right before the surgery or even after premedication).
5. At the time of information, the patient must not yet be premedicated.
6. There are substantial exceptions for information for minor or older patients.
7. For information provided to non-German-speaking persons, an interpreter should be present or another person who has mastered both languages.
8. Before operations with debilitating risks, there should be a sworn interpreter (*OLG München, Judgement of 23.6.1994, Az. 1 U 7286/93*) for patients who do not speak German.

9. The greater the risk of the treatment, the more intense must be the information:
   - If the treatment is controversial within the medical profession
   - If more than typical numbers of treatment alternatives exist
   - If the treatment is more elective (as for aesthetic plastic surgery; *BGH, Judgement, Az. VI ZR 8 / 90, NJW 1991, 2349, BGH, Judgement of 22.11.1995, Az. VI ZR 329 / 94*).

It is generally assumed that the patient must be informed about diagnosis and prognosis, therapy, objective, scope, necessity and urgency, the nature and course of the examination and the treatment course, the involved risks and the relationship between risk and therapeutic benefit, and the cost of the treatment and treatment alternatives (the so-called economic information). The scope of information substantially depends on the circumstances of each case. The range goes from point-like decay up to the dismal tumor of the dental bite to life-threatening illness.

If the patient refuses necessary treatment because they are unable to understand, it is up to the doctor to convince the patient otherwise. If a patient wishes, because of medically nonsensical ideas, to have all of their teeth extracted, the dentist must convince the patient of the absurdity of this treatment. Consent to such a non-indicated treatment was declared invalid by the highest court (Figgener 1997).

The illustrative list of information-relevant factors is far from being complete, because of the singularity of each case. However, the dentist must find the right balance in each case, and the duty of information should not be taken easily, especially from the standpoint that, in case of dispute, the doctor has to prove that proper information was given and informed consent was obtained.

1. The more urgent and imperative the surgery, the less may be the scope of information.
2. The riskier the planned intervention, and the more serious the accompanying risks, the more weighty and substantial must be the information (Laufs 1996a; Muschallik 1998).
3. The more questionable an indication is, the more stringent are the requirements with regard to the informed consent.

According to *OLG Koblenz, Judgement, Az. 7 U 520/94*, "If a doctor wants to apply an outsider method, he is obliged to inform the patient about the fact that this method is not recognized by orthodox medicine, in particular, that there is no sufficient scientific evidence of its suitability."

For the violation of the therapeutic education requirement as a treatment error, the rules of evidence are valid, because the patient is charged with providing evidence for their claim that they had not been sufficiently informed. After evaluation of numerous details from court decisions, it is highly recommended that the date, time, and scope of the information be recorded (Rohde 1996a). In the prevailing case law and medical–legal literature, the biggest conformity exists in the statement that the information must be conveyed personally by a doctor/dentist in a conversation (Deutsch 1991; Ehlers 1987; Giesen 1990; Kern and Laufs 1993; Laufs and Uhlenbruck 1992).

15.4.11 Types of Information

(a) *Self-determined information* ensures that patients can decide, on the basis of diagnosis and findings, if and in which way they agree to the surgery.

(b) *Course information* gives information about the nature and the extent of the surgery, the procedure, and the proposed medication, and also about complications and their control possibilities.

(c) *Risk and complication awareness* informs the patient about the possible permanent or temporary side-effects of a medical procedure that cannot be excluded even under proper performance.

(d) *Information by levels* is divided into:
   1. A written part formalized by information brochures.
   2. An oral part, which is the actual information conveyed in conversation.

(e) *Therapeutic education* is part of medical treatment itself, ranging up to the therapeutic privilege of the physician to withhold certain information, even completely, if the patient's condition so requires. If a medical procedure is urgent and life essential, the information may remain unconveyed if the patient's consent is assumed.

(f) *Omission education* is education about the "consequences of non-treatment" at the initial refusal of consent to the necessary treatment.

(g) *Awareness of treatment alternatives* (e.g., instead of root extraction, various forms of construction of dentures, their advantages and disadvantages, and materials for restorative therapy).

(h) The physician/dentist must also inform the patient about how they should behave after the surgery; if the dentist skips this important part of the information, the dentist may be liable (*OLG Stuttgart Higher Regional Court, judgement of 18.05.1995, Az. 14 U 49/94*).

(i) *Economic information* on the cost of treatment and treatment alternatives must be conveyed. The patient has to be informed about the measures not covered by the public health insurance (*LG Stuttgart, Judgement, Az. 27 O 578/92*; *OLG Stuttgart Higher Regional Court, Judgement, Az. 14 U 41/94*).

Information means weighing, for example, whether a continuation of the treatment (after demolition of instruments or of roots, e.g., by levers, rose drills, blades, or milling) may possibly lead to a greater harm. The referring dentist can convey the information, but the liability is with the surgeon/dentist. For instance, in an orthodontic–surgical treatment combination, if the orthodontist gives an incorrect order regarding which teeth to extract, and the performing dentist extracts the teeth without prior consultation; if the orthodontist insists on his instructions for the extraction, the performing dentist has met their duty of care and is only liable for the proper extraction, not for the indication (Vogel 1980a). The performing dentist is not obligated to perform the extraction if they do not see the need for it.

According to *OLG Oldenburg, Judgement, Az. 5 U 186/94*, "A doctor who does not perform the surgery, but gives information to the patient and also about possible risks, is liable if the given information was insufficient. He is also liable if he does not perform but recommend the surgery."

Rohde (1995b) has investigated how thoroughly patients apprehend the information provided. The result was that more than half of the patients did not retain the information given about the risks of an impending surgery. Only 40 % of the patients could remember the content of information. In another study, the effectiveness of education levels was investigated, with the result that, immediately after the information, only 5 % of all patients could remember at least one of the various risks.

Before an extraction of several teeth, and after sufficient information is given, no further education is required before each extraction (Figgener 1997).

15.4.12 Information About Alternative Therapies

According to judicial case law, the physician shall inform the patient about alternative treatments (*BGH, NJW 1978, S.587*). If the patient insists that the dentist did not inform them about alternative treatments, the patient has the burden of proof that an appropriate treatment-alternative is available and practicable (Scholich 1997).

According to *AG Köln, Judgement, Az. 131 C 83/81*, "If an alternative treatment option (e.g. tooth preserving treatment instead of extraction) is doable in accordance with the rules of medical science, the physician must inform about this alternative."

Pictorial presentation, expressed by leaflets for education, may be an appropriate method of information, according to the Professional Association of German Doctors of Oral and Maxillofacial Surgery.

In a clinical study (survey of 156 ambulatory treated patients, questioned regarding the nature, extent, and clarity of the used leaflets and educational conversation), Aderhold and Frenkel

(1985) came to the conclusion that safe treatment episodes and general complications were only recalled by 57.1 % of the patients (on the day of the surgery) and special complications were recalled only by 64.7 % of the surveyed patients on the day of surgery. The detectable memory gap or misunderstanding of nearly 30 % can lead to the burden proof of the physician/dentist.

15.4.13 Consent to Treatment

All medical and dental treatments require the consent of the patient to be legal. Otherwise, the accusation for bodily injury is justified, even if the treatment was indicated and performed *lege artis*. The patient's consent is the result of proper education by the dentist about the cause, scope, risk, consequences, and possible side effects of the planned intervention (informed consent).

It is a special feature of the medical malpractice trial that the performing physician or dentist has to prove that proper education was given (Figgener 1997; Rohde 1995b, 1996a). This fact might encourage unsatisfied patients to claim this against the physician and move the burden of proof toward the physician. Therefore, every physician and dentist should keep a record of the information (Figgener 1997).

Performing innovative or outsider treatments requires that much more intensive information than with standard methods be conveyed. The patient must be able to think over their decision; to have enough time prior to their consent or to talk it over with a third person (*BGH, NJW 12, 1959, 852*).

Special care is required with patients who are burdened with extraordinary preexisting conditions, such as immunocompromised patients (Schmidt-Westhausen and Strietzel 1997), cancer patients in general, patients with irradiated jaw tumors (Kielbassa and Schilli 1997), noncooperative eligible patients with severe disabilities, patients with anxiety disorders, HIV-positive patients, and AIDS patients (Ratka-Krüger et al. 1997; Cichon and Bader 1997).

Minors under the age of 7 years, because of their legal incapacity (§§ *104, 105 BGB*), are not able to conclude a contract, this must be performed by their legal representatives (usually the parents). There is a limited legal capacity from the ages of 7 to 18 years (§ *106 BGB*). The consent of parents or guardians must be proven (Köhler 1970). Minors younger than 14 years (*limit of criminal culpability of the child*, § *19 StGB*) usually are not able to give a legal consent. The consent can be given by the parents or legal representatives.

The capacity to consent between the ages of 14 and 18 years depends on individual circumstances, scope, and risks of the surgery and also on the intellectual and moral maturity of the minor (so-called natural ability to understand) (Rohde 1997; Uhlenbrock 1976). A treatment contract with a minor is only effective with the consent of the legal representatives, given either before or after the surgery.

If the child is accompanied by his legal representatives, the contract is usually completed by them. The same applies if only one parent is with the child. Before serious treatment with significant risks, however, the dentist should also assure the consent of the other parent to avoid any misunderstandings and to preserve evidence in the case of a dispute. If the child appears alone for the treatment, the contract must still be conducted by the legal representatives.

Another important aspect is the question of who is the addressee for the information. Unlike with the conclusion of the treatment contract, this question is not answered on the basis of specific legal provisions on legal capacity.

15.4.14 Lack of Consent

The dentist is liable if they perform a treatment without the patient's consent. This may lead to the accusation of an assault and represents a factual check and unlawful assault. This is true even if the measure has led to a cure but the patient has not given consent. Liability also arises from improper consent of the patient, i.e., in the absence of or an insufficient ability to reason or insufficient discernment of the patient (*LG Hannover, NJW 1981, 1321*).

The presence of third parties (e.g., as a spectator) during the treatment of a patient without their consent violates medical confidentiality and medical ethics. This ruling of the Court of Appeal is comparable to the judgments, which do not allow the presence of the defendant doctor or dentist at the expert's examination during a trial (Figgener 1999).

15.4.15 Confidentiality

Another important professional duty is medical secrecy. It is ruled in the Professional Code (*§ 3 para 1 MuBerO*), in the Code of Civil Procedure (*§ 383 para 6 ZPO*), and the Criminal Code (*§ 203 para 1 StGB*; *Violation of the personal life and secret area*). All facts that become known to a dentist in their capacity as a trusted professional are covered by the medical confidentiality (also toward family members). This includes not only medical facts, health status, and treatment of patients, but also personal messages and insights into the personal relationships of the patient, either of social, economic, or other nature (*§ 3 para 1 MuBerO*).

The dentist is obligated to teach their staff in written order about the duties of confidentiality (*§ 3 para 2 MuBerO*). The dentist is entitled to disclosure when they were released from the confidentiality or if the disclosure is necessary to protect the legal interests of a higher legally protected right (*§ 3 para 3 MuBerO*).

One particular aspect is applicable in everyday practice. If the dentist gives data to an external billing institution, it is necessary that the patient has given consent in written form before the start of the treatment.

The question of provability in disputes leads to the next important duty in connection with the treatment of a patient, the documentation obligation (Figgener 1998).

15.4.16 Documentation Obligation

As in general medicine, the dentist is obliged to keep careful documentation of all essential details, especially all uncommon features. The documentation requirement is part of the medical education requirement (*BGH, 27.06.1978 – VI ZR 183/76 – JW 1972, 1520; 1; 1978, 2337* (Laufs 1996a; Tiemann 1982).

According to *OLG Saarland (Higher Regional Court), Judgement, Az. 1 U 290/97*, "If the dentist does not perform a proper documentation, this failure may result in a burden of proof." For example, *BGH, Judgement of 9.11.1993, Az. VI ZR 248/92* (*VersR.94, 682*), stated "A patient with severe toothache came to the practice of the holiday representative of his family dentist. After taking an X-ray the doctor extracted the lower left wisdom tooth at the same day. It was more difficult than expected and lasted several hours. After the surgery the patient had a painful nerve damage (facial and oral) and also a persistent osteomyelitis, which could only be mastered by a series of re-operations." The Regional Court (LG) partially accepted the patient's claim. The dentist's appeal at the Higher Regional Court (OLG) led to a complete rejection of the claim. The patient's appeal at the Federal Supreme Court (BGH) resulted in the abolition of the decision, whereby a dentist is not liable for nerve damages and osteomyelitis.

The decisive factors were that "The court noted that no negligent treatment of dental defects could be detected. Based on the expert's statement during the trial, it is clear that an indication for the removal of the wisdom tooth was given. According to both the documentation of the dentist and the presentation by the expert, marks for an acute inflammation stage were not detectable. According to the findings of the expert, the unusually long duration of the surgery cannot be considered as a proof for incorrect treatment."

15.4.17 Documentation

Documentation means collecting, organizing, developing, and saving documents, data, findings, treatments courses, and facts. It is a proactive and retrospective source of information (Wagner and Schneider 1998). Documentation of the treatment is a compulsory exercise that many dentists are reluctant to undergo.

15.4.18 Content and Scope of Documentation

Content and scope of documentation are ruled by § *5 para 1 fixed* of the professional code (*Model Professional Code – MuBerO*). Thus, separate findings for each patient and treatment must be recorded immediately, continuously, and without interruption to put the dentist in the state to give the necessary information upon request and to explain the treatment, e.g., to test instances (§ *20 para 4 BMV-Z*).

The term dental documentation includes any treatment of a patient, such as index cards, medical reports, X-rays, casts, models, calculations, etc. (Ratajczak 1994). It usually consists of the date of treatment, the history, the findings, the diagnosis, the dental formula, the coefficient of performance with further explanations, and last but not least the informed consent discussion/consultation with a short summary.

15.4.19 Anamnesis (Previous History)

Features such as allergies, predispositions for certain diseases, risks from preexisting conditions or accidents; information about the medical condition of the patient (i.e., reactions to treatment, e.g., bleeding, gag reflex, psychosis) should be recorded. Specifically:

- Clinical findings (documentation of findings)
- Medical technical and laboratory findings
- X-ray images
- Diagnoses
- Therapeutic measures (treatment documentation)
- Materials used
- Prescription drugs
- Advice and recommendations to the patient
- Treatment alternatives (e.g., instead of root extraction, various forms of restorations of dentures, their advantages and disadvantages, and materials for restorative therapy)
- Evidence of services rendered to payer (documentation of cost)
- Notes about the informed consent discussion and the consent of the patient

These should all be present in the patient's file in ranked order, so that the timing of the treatment and its results are visible. It is quite common and legally acceptable to use abbreviations, as long as they are understandable without error. Subsequent modifications should be avoided, because they are hard to justify in case of a dispute (Figgener 1995a–d).

A carefully documented treatment means that the dentist has recorded all treatments (that were charged for) and all findings under consideration of current rules. However, this rule also has a downside. It suggests that nondocumented findings are not established and nondocumented treatments have not been performed and the required education was not given (Otto 1998).

The medical/dental records have functions as:

- The personal reminder of the practitioner
- A reference point for information to the patient
- A guide for their own reports and assessments
- A performance record for billing
- To avoid gaps in evidence in court
- A clinical documentation for long-term self-control
- A short-term treatment control (Stratmann 1995)

Such a carefully performed documentation without any contradictions takes time and effort, but is very useful in case of a dispute to protect the dentist from unauthorized claims, because judges usually believe a proper and neat documentation to be true. Inadequate documentation means that the burden of proof is on the dentist, because the dentist must prove that nondocumented treatments have been performed (Figgener 1996). For example, a tooth extraction is not provable if the file card does not include any information about the clinical diagnosis or an X-ray image concerning this tooth.

Deficiencies in the documentation lead to the suspicion that nondocumented treatments or findings have not been performed at all (*OLG Karlsruhe, Judgement, Az. 7 U 29/88*). For example, in *OLG Köln, Judgement* (*MDR 94.994*), "The axial inclination and depth of dental implants was not radiographically checked. Since the documentation of the periodontal condition was not available, it was assumed that this X-ray has not been taken." The X-ray control was missing in the documentation; thus, the court weighed the lack of documentation against the dentist (Deutsch 1998).

The documentation obligation has forensic significance in medical liability processes and especially in law of evidence. Each party has to prove their claim. In cases of doubt, the party that carries the burden of proof will be rejected.

Retention periods for dental records are:

1. Medical records (index cards) "at least 3 years after completion of treatment" (BMV Z-1978 § *5 (2) EC Treaty* § *4.2*); as well 10 years after § *11 para 2 BOÄ*
2. Diagnostic records, including records in orthodontic and periodontal treatment, "at least 3 years after completion of treatment" (BMV-Z § *5 (2) EC Treaty* § *4,2*)
3. Dentures (planning models): 2 years after insertion, SGB V § *135 para 4*
4. X-ray images and X-ray records are required to be stored for much longer periods (§ 28 *X-Ray: X-ray Ordinance – X-Ray, valid in the version from 25.07.1996* (BGBl I, 1172; RöV § *28.4/1*)
   4.1 Records of X-ray treatments: 30 years after the last treatment (*X-ray Ordinance* § *28,4/1*)
   4.2 For X-ray images: 10 years after the last scan (RöV § *28,4/2*)
   The images may be provided upon request (*X-ray Ordinance* § *28,4/2*, § *29,4; from 03.01.1973, valid in the version from 01.08.1987 BGBl I*)
   4.3 Records of the semi-annual teaching of staff: 5 years (*X-ray Ordinance* § *29*) (Andreasen 1988)

15.4.20 Access and Issuance to Dental Records

Another procedural relief for the patient, the right to access and issuance to medical records, not only in case of claim, is of evidentiary significance. According to *AG Essen, Judgement, Az. 12 C 13/97*, "It is necessary that the documents are understandable, especially readable, and comprehensible." Doctors are frequently faced with the problem that the patient wants to have an overview of his medical records as a copy. Doctors often charge too much for this service. The Frankfurt District Court rejected this practice as inadmissible. A patient requested her medical records as copies, the doctor charged her 165,56 € for copying 56 pages, based on the fact that she took 2 h for copying and writing a conclusion. The court awarded the doctor 30,60 €. According to *AG Frankfurt, Judgement, Az. 30 C 1340/98-47*, "The doctor/dentist is obligated to leave records upon request as copies. He is allowed to charge in the following way: 0,50 € per copy and 2,50 € for mailing."

The practitioner has to ensure that all treatment records are accessible at any time. The practitioner is also responsible for the whereabouts of all records, even if they are handed out to a third party, the practitioner must ensure they are sent back (*BGH VI ZR 341/94*).

15.5 Contract Law Between Dentist and Dental Technician

15.5.1 Legal Nature

Regardless of whether the dentist treats a private or public health patient, the relationship between dentist and technician is based on civil law(§ *368 para 6 RVO*) (Tiemann 1982). The dental services for the planning and fitting of metal fillings, bridges, crowns, and/or prostheses are based on service agreements (see Sect. 15.3.1), while the dentist and dental technician have a dental work or work delivery contract.

The legislation provides (regardless of culpability) a limitation period of 6 months for defects in work (short limitation period) (§ *638 BGB*), compared with a 30-year limitation period (general statute of limitations) for culpable violations of the employment contract (§ *195 BGB*) (Figgener 1993; Hempfing 1994).

Obligations from the contract for work/work delivery contract include that the technician owes the contractual and defect-free dental work to the dentist. The dentist in turn owes the agreed remuneration to the dental technician. If the remuneration is not specified, it is based on tax compensation; in the absence of tax, it is based on a usual fee agreement (§ *632 para 2 BGB*). The limit of such agreement is the adequacy of service and return service as well as general principles of law, e.g., good faith or the usury act (§§ *242*, *138 BGB*).

15.5.2 Due Date for Payment

Payment is due with the adoption of the work by the dentist (§ *641 BGB*).

15.5.3 Adoption of the Work

For a tightly fitted crown and bridge restoration, the adoption happens latest with the firm and final cementation. For removable dentures, the adoption is given when the patient and dentist have agreed after a probational period (e.g., 14 days). The short limitation period begins with the acceptance of the work. The risk of accidental loss or accidental deterioration of the work (work risk) moves from the dental technician to the dentist or the patient (§ *644 para 1 BGB*). If the dentist wants to claim a defect in the work, the burden of proof is up to the dentist.

15.5.4 Special Contractual Arrangements

The parties (dentist/dental technician) can frame their contractual relations by agreeing to specific conditions. These must be separately and explicitly agreed and, for evidentiary reasons, must be in written form. This also applies to the so-called terms and conditions (AGB). The terms and conditions are mentioned in the AGB-Act (AGBG) from 9.2.1976 (*BGBl I, p. 3317*).

Examples of terms of technician AGB in violation of the AGB-Act:

- Penalty for nonacceptance by the dentist (§ *11 para 7 AGBG*)
- Liability only for gross negligence by the dental technician (§ *11 para 7 AGBG*)
- Exclusion of liability for promised features (§ *11 para 11 AGBG*)
- Shortening warranty periods (§ *11 para 10 f AGBG*)
- Withholding of correction of faults (§ *11 para 10 d AGBG*)

15.5.5 Warranty for Faults

The dentist has the right to claim defects in dental work, regardless of the technician's fault:

1. Repair/defect removal (§ *633 para 2 BGB*): The exact description of the defect by the dentist is necessary (*BGHZ 61, 42*).
2. Cost of repair in case of a defect must be borne by the dental technician, in particular the transport, travel, labor, and material cost. In return, there is a claim for restitution of the disputed piece of dentures (*BGHZ 63, 306, 309*).
3. Repair by third parties: If the technician is unable to perform the repair, either a third party or a representative may be assigned (§ *633 para 3 BGB*). If the dentist did accept the replacement pieces, the dentist has no right to withdraw from the contract. However, there may be a demand compensation as a result of delayed repair.
4. Change or reduction (§ *634 para 1 BGB*): If the requested repair was not successful, the dentist may request the termination of the contract or reduction of the remuneration.
5. Damages for nonperformance (§ *635 BGB*): The dentist has to prove those damages.

15.5.6 Limitation of Warranty for Defects

The claims of the dentist expire 6 months after acceptance of the dental prosthetic piece (§ *638 para 1 BGB*), while the dentist underlies, in accordance with the provisions of the *SGB V* (§ *135*), a 2-year warranty period. The renewal of dentures (including crowns) can be demanded only if the dentist's fault is proven.

15.5.7 Extension of the Warranty Period

Through contractual agreement, it is possible to extend the warranty period (§ *638 para 2 BGB*). It should not be less than 2 years.

15.5.8 Liability of the Dental Technician to the Patient

According to LG Münster (NJW 1985, 683), "The patient has no contractual claims towards the dental technician, because there is no contractual relation. The contract between dentist and dental technician (work contract) has no protective effect for the benefit of the patient."

15.6 The Medical Devices Act

Based on the European Directive 93/42/EEC, the German Medical Devices Act (MPG) from 1 January 1995 requires a declaration of conformity for all equipment for the preparation of tooth structure (class IIa), based on clinical examination and scientific documentation, in order to make CE-marking mandatory. The purpose of the act (§ *1 MPG*) is to ensure the handling of medical devices for the safety, suitability, and performance of medical devices and health and to protect patients, users, and third parties. (Schorr 1998).

15.6.1 The Medical Devices Act—Implementation in the Dental Practice Lab

Dental practices with their own dental laboratory (practice lab) are manufacturers in terms of the Medical Devices Act. The person in charge of the practice lab (§ *7 MPG*) is the dentist. Both commercial laboratories and practice laboratories are subject to the same safety requirements. In case of doubt, the law requires a continuous recording of the used materials to ensure they meet the current rules.

In general, such information can be derived from the medical record or from the laboratory documents, so that a precise, single case-related documentation is not necessary for each product. However, it is recommended that there be a purchase book in which the batch numbers of all materials are reported. An additional warrant is required, which may be phrased as "It is assured that the designated product meets the requirements according to Annex 1 of Directive 93/42/EEC."

The applications for the Medical Devices Act are accepted by (§ *25 MPG – General Obligation*) the District Dental Association (Chart 15.1). Janda and Kappert (1996) have listed relevant procedures of the Medical Devices Act (MGP).

Chart 15.1
The following special dental products are to be announced to the competent authority (Medical Devices Act—MGP):

Crowns and fixed dentures	**Orthodontic appliances**
1a Crowns, 1b inlays/ onlays, 1c bridges, 1d prostheses	
2 Veneers	
Removable dentures	**Other custom-made products**
3 Partial, 4 total	5 Splints, 6 epitheses etc.

15.7 Liability Risk from Dental Treatment

Treatment risks are very diverse and may lead to a liability of the practitioner (Gümpel 1994) (Table 15.1).

15.7.1 Preliminary Comments

Anamnesis is of major importance before starting a treatment. The biggest mistake of the practitioner is to neglect the anamnesis, which requires not only general basic knowledge, but also some special expertise. This can lead to serious malpractice, as often shown in psychosomatic consultation, especially with patients with orofacial somatization disorders.

Marxkors (1999) describes a treatment that ended as a total failure. An otorhinolaryngologist referred (via telephone) a patient with a trigeminal neuralgia to his dental colleague. After hearing about the patient's discomfort, the dentist immediately started an occlusal treatment in the right upper jaw. The treatment with four crowns in the mandible and a five-unit bridge in the maxilla was a failure. The bridge in the left upper jaw was renewed and the second copy, together with three crowns

Table 15.1 Treatment risks (risk factors, patients at risk (Gümpel 1994))

Category 1	Category 2	Category 3
Somatization disorders	Dialysis patients	Hemophilia of various genesis
AIDS	Endocarditis hazard	Warfarin therapy
Blood disease	Endocrine disorders	
Diabetes mellitus	Cardiovascular problems	
Radiotherapy	Organ transplants	
Cytostatic therapy	Pregnancy	

on the right, had to be removed and replaced by temporaries. During the treatment period, which extended over 9 months, the complaints were sometimes less, sometimes even unbearable.

If the dentist had read the medical history more carefully, he would have seen that the patient had more than 70 appointments during the last 2 years and a 10-year odyssey from specialists of internal medicine to holistic medicine. The patient himself described his discomfort in a previous medical history as "pain in various areas, depression and anxiety…" Gathering a complaint history is the first step and essential for all treatment sequences.

In view of the previous medical history, there was no chance to achieve success solely by dental treatment (Marxkors 1995; Marxkors and Wolowski 1999). Because no medical history was collected, there were no therapeutic–diagnostic investigations, no investigation of the quality of pain, no anesthesia test, no provocation test, no resilience test of the TMJ, and no instrumental functional analysis. This is forensically classified as culpable negligence, because basic knowledge of psychosomatic medicine is required. The statement that the complaints could not be reconciled with the findings raised in line would have led to the suspicion of an orofacial somatization disorder (Bräutigam et al. 1992).

15.8 Dental Procedures and Endocarditis—Prophylaxis

Patients with congenital heart defects are the main risk group for infectious endocarditis (Chart 15.2). Endocarditis prophylaxis is still insufficiently implemented in dental practice (Knirsch et al. 1999). Because of the pathogenesis of infective endocarditis (IE), the possibility of preventive measures in dental surgeries is given. To avoid any failure, dentists must be made aware of this while they are in training.

Bacteremia caused by dental procedures can lead to microbial colonization (given predisposing endocarditis damage) (Horstkotte et al. 1997).

Chart 15.2
Graduation of the endocardium risk (Knirsch et al. 1999)

No increased risk:
- Mitral valve prolapse without insufficiency noise
- Condition after:
  - Coronary bypass operation
  - Pacemaker or defibrillator
  - Implantation of ventriculoperitoneal or ventriculoatrial shunts
  - Closure of *ductus arteriosus* (*ductus Botalli*)
  - Operated heart defects without residual findings (after the first year after surgery)
  - Isolated aortic isthmus stenosis
  - Atrial septal defect of secundum type (ASD II)

Increased risk:
- Congenital heart defects (except atrial septal defect of secundum type (ASD II))
- Acquired valvular heart disease
- Postreeration heart defects with residual findings (without residual findings: only for 1 year)
- Mitral valve prolapse with insufficiency noise without any distinctive myxomatous degeneration

High risk:
- Heart valve replacement using mechanical or biological prostheses
- Condition caused by microbial endocarditis
- Congenital (complex) heart defects with cyanosis

Table 15.2 Orally applicable prophylaxis at dental surgeries (Horstkotte et al. 1997)

	Child	Adult
Without penicillin allergy	50 mg/kg amoxicillin p.o. 60 min before surgery	2 g (<70 kg) to 3 g (=70 kg) amoxicillin p.o. 60 min before surgery
With penicillin allergy	15 mg/kg clindamycin p.o. 60 min before surgery	600 mg clindamycin p.o. 60 min before surgery

After dental–surgical procedures with risk of bleeding, severe bacteremia often occurs, especially with dental extractions, intraligamentous anesthesia, dental cleanings, and in periodontal surgery, root canal treatment, and other dental surgical interventions. Because the oral cavity, under physiological conditions, is populated with more than 200 different species of bacteria and, in particular, the dental sulcus has a particularly high density of bacteria, a high quantity of bacteria reaches the predilection site, compared with other medical procedures (Knirsch et al. 1999).

Bacteremia after dental procedures usually does not last longer than 15 min after the causal surgery. Therefore, a single dose of an antibiotic is prophylactically sufficient. The proposed prophylaxis regimes are adequately tested in animal studies (Glauser and Bernhard 1983; Horstkotte 1985; 1995; Malinverni et al. 1988; Pippert et al. 1991). In the presence of a penicillin allergy, clindamycin provides an equivalent alternative (Table 15.2) in dental practice. This is in line with the recommendation of the American Heart Association (AHA) for high-risk patients. Amoxicillin *per os* (60 min before the planned operation) ensures a sufficiently high serum level to prevent the attachment of bacteria to the vegetation (Dajani et al. 1994).

Martin et al. (1997) evaluated 53 cases of endocarditis that ended in court proceedings. In 48 of the 53 cases, no antibiotic was administered, in 2 cases it was either ineffective or administered at the wrong time. Only in one case was the antibiotic correctly administered. In a German Heart Centre Berlin (DHZB) retrospective analysis over a period of 10 years, endocarditis occurred with dental surgery as the supposed trigger in 4 of 22 patients with congenital heart disease (Knirsch et al. 1999).

15.9 Tooth Restoration Before and After Organ Transplantation

Dental, oral, and maxillofacial surgery is included into the preoperative and postoperative requirements, which ensure a lifelong immunosuppression to maintain the function of the transplant (Otten 1999). Patients with organ transplants have a higher risk for local or hematogenous and transmitted bacterial infection in the oral cavity because of the vital and lasting immunosuppressive medication.

The oral cavity has diverse bacterial colonizations under the predominance of a protective physiological streptococcal flora. In the majority of adult patients, pathogenic bacteria are also potentially present; they have their main location in the periodontium of the teeth. In addition to specific streptococcal species, there are mainly gram-negative anaerobic bacteria. Quality and quantity of the resident flora are not individually assessable, nor is the concrete pathogenic potency. Because of the resident flora of the mouth, the tooth can be an entry point of bacterial infections, manifested as an abscess or osteomyelitis.

The hematogenous spread of the potentially pathogenic agent mixture (known in endocarditis as oral streptococci) may lead to a focal dental infection (secondary bacterial infection). In immunosuppressed organ recipients, anaerobic pathogens (detectable in blood) also have a pathogenic significance.

Before transplantation, this difficulty requires:

1. Clinical and radiographic (panoramic radiograph) investigation and documentation
2. Hygiene instruction and professional tooth cleaning
3. Conservative restoration (endodontics)
4. Surgical rehabilitation
5. Immediate prosthetic supply
6. Reporting of completed dental restoration

Radical restoration treatments are not justified according to current knowledge. Every procedure must take into account the underlying disease and must be performed in consultation with the treating physician (in case of kidney dialysis before the transplantation, heart insufficiency before the heart transplantation, coagulation disorder before liver transplantation, diabetes before the pancreas transplantation, etc.). In individual cases, because of the risk of general complications, the limit of the outpatient treatment options can be exceeded. The fully completed dental restoration (including controlled wound healing) must be documented and reported. This communication is a prerequisite for the approval for the planned on-demand organ transplants.

Analogous to the current recommendations of the American Heart Association (Dajani et al. 1994), the following treatments have an increased risk for endocarditis:

1. Tooth extraction
2. Surgical removal of teeth
3. Apicoectomy
4. Periodontal treatment
5. Periodontology (PAR) examination with probing or PAR surgery
6. Tooth or implant cleaning with local bleeding
7. Dental implant placement and reimplantation
8. Endodontics with preparation
9. Intraligamentous injection (local anesthesia)

All dental treatment measures with bacteremia risks are contraindicated in the first 3 months after transplantation (Otten 1998; Smit et al. 1996).

15.10 Dental Treatment of Patients with Pacemakers

Patient must be asked whether they have a pacemaker. Patients with pacemakers are in possession of a pass that contains all relevant data about the pacemaker type and function, the pacing rate, the electrode type, etc. The pacemaker patient must not be seen as a "problem patient." Routine questioning for medical history usually includes the reference of a pacemaker or implanted defibrillator (ICD).

15.11 Dental Surgery and Diabetes

In the Federal Republic of Germany, more than eight million people suffer from diabetes mellitus. Long-existing and inadequately controlled diabetes mellitus leads to microangiopathy and macroangiopathy, manifested as retinopathy, glomerular sclerosis, neuropathy, and premature arteriosclerosis. This results in an increased incidence of myocardial infarctions, strokes, kidney failure, etc.

In addition to the medical consequences of dental surgery, the general susceptibility to infections and for the oral area in particular are:

- Accumulated periodontal abscesses
- Defective wound healing after extractions
- Persistent ulcerations
- Gingival hyperplasia

If metabolic control is unclear, if the insulin dosage and administration are ambiguous, and before long-term operations, communication with the treating physician is necessary. It should be noted that stress (even the stress of a surgery) can affect the stability of the diabetic state, as well as local infections, trismus, and any fasting. Therefore, a quick change in the insulin dosage and continuous glucose monitoring by both doctor and patient may be necessary. (Wahl 1996). Caution: Children and young people are affected by type II diabetes (formerly named adult-onset diabetes) with increasing frequency. Blood sugar problems are possible, especially in overweight children, and if diabetes runs in the family (Vetter 1999).

15.12 Dental – Surgical Treatment of Patients Taking Warfarin

In the Federal Republic of Germany, approximately 150,000 patients use anticoagulants. Therefore, the treatment guidelines for patients who are taking warfarin should be known to each practitioner (Lechler and Pape 1996). For the prevention of thrombosis and embolism, patients at risk are treated with long-term anticoagulants. The indirect-acting anticoagulants are coumarin derivatives. They alter vitamin K metabolism. By

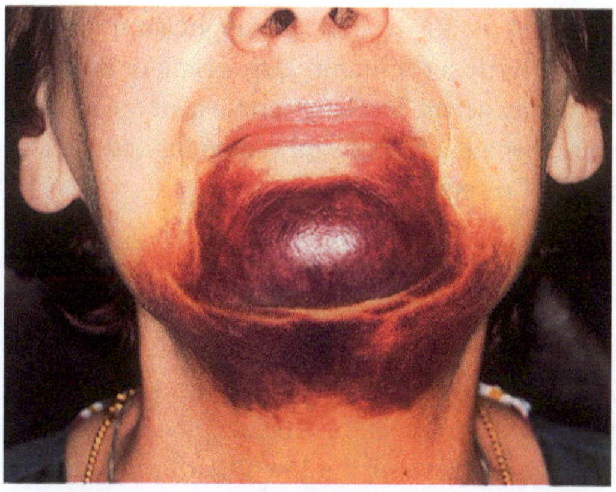

Fig. 15.1 Warfarin-treated patient. The interforaminal implantation was performed without taking into account the increased bleeding tendency

reducing the active form of vitamin K, the synthesis of the coagulation factors II, VII, IX, and X as well as the inhibitors of protein C and protein S are reduced in the liver. Common compounds are warfarin, Falithrom (warfarin), and Coumadin (warfarin). In Germany, phenprocoumon is mainly used. Indications for anticoagulant therapy include vein thrombosis, pulmonary embolism, heart attack, atrial fibrillation, heart valve replacement, and certain heart valve defects.

Before dental–surgical procedures of patients who are taking warfarin, the dentist must be aware of the increased risk of bleeding (Fig. 15.1). The dimension of anticoagulation and thus the risk of bleeding is indicated by the prothrombin time (Quick) or variations such as the thrombotic test. The regular value for both tests is 100 %, with a normal range of about ±25 %. The therapeutic range, i.e., the range of the desired anticoagulation for the Quick test is between 15 and 25 %.

At extensive dental operations or dental restorations with insufficient possibility to stop local bleeding, a temporary increase of the Quick value to 30–40 % is suggested; from 1.6 to 1.9 INR (International Normalized Ratio). In cases of doubt, patients should be stationarily treated to reduce the risks of anticoagulants. In these cases, a syringe pump-controlled dose of heparin can eliminate the risk of thrombosis as well as short-term barriers to control the supply of heparin, intraoperative bleeding, or acute postoperative bleeding.

15.13 Treatment During Pregnancy

Pregnancy requires consideration of specific medical and legal concerns to avoid danger or damage to the unborn child. In addition, the physical and psychological characteristics of pregnant women should be kept in mind (Maeglin 1981).

15.14 Protection Against Radiation

The regulation of protection against damage caused by X-rays (§§ *22, 25, and 28*) contains the specifics of ionizing radiation in women of childbearing age and during pregnancy. Although it is proven that prenatal exposure, depending on the dose and the gestational age, can result in death of the fetus, malformations, growth failure, malignant diseases, and genetic mutations, the radiation risk of dental X-ray images, in consideration of the optimal radiation protection, is extremely low. For shots of the mouth and jaw area, the radiation exposure for the uterus is estimated to be 0.1–1 GY.

However, X-ray examinations during pregnancy should only be performed if strictly indicated, in particular during the first period of gestation. To keep the radiation exposure as low as possible, highly sensitive films, rectangular tubes, and multiple X-ray protections are suggested. The number of shots must be kept to a minimum.

15.15 Toxicity of Amalgam Fillings

The Federal Institute for Drugs and Medical Devices currently recognizes no reasonable suspicion for embryotoxic or fetotoxic mercury risks from amalgam fillings during pregnancy, but recommends not to conduct further amalgam therapy during pregnancy and in women of childbearing age, because experimental, clinical, and epidemiological studies have shown that mercury is transplacentally transferred to the fetus.

The transfer of mercury from amalgam fillings by breast milk to infants has been demonstrated.

A Swedish study of 30 mothers 6 weeks after delivery showed that there is a transfer of inorganic mercury from the blood into the milk, the mercury level in the milk was about half of that set by the WHO as the acceptable daily intake for adults (Oskarsson et al. 1996).

15.16 Prescription of Drugs

Even if prescription drug effects on the mother are known, the risk assessment of drug effects to the fetus is difficult. The nature of the fetal damage depends on the intrauterine development. The treating dentist is responsible for any drug therapy in pregnancy.

15.16.1 Antibiotics

Penicillin, cephalosporin, and macrolide antibiotics have no embryotoxic effects.

15.16.2 Analgesics

Taking into account some special features, the aniline derivative of paracetamol and antipyrine or propyphenazone is suitable for the use in pregnancy. Evidence of teratogenic effects are not available. Paracetamol crosses the placenta, therefore, high doses (for a longer time) should be avoided to prevent liver damage.

Aspirin (acetylsalicylic acid) inhibits prostaglandin synthesis and should therefore not be prescribed in the last month of pregnancy in order to prevent birth delay. Aspirin should not be given during pregnancy, because bleeding in pregnant women and fetuses were observed (aspirin may also lead to premature closure of the *ductus arteriosus Botalli*).

In special situations of pain with severe swelling, the use of derivatives of weak acids (nonsteroidal anti-inflammatory drugs) may be considered, such as arylacetic acids and arylpropionic acids; the best known are diclofenac and ibuprofen.

In special cases, the use of opiates and opioid analgesics, which are subject to narcotics regulation, is necessary. Evidence of a malformation potential is not found. In application shortly before birth, a respiratory depression of the newborn may occur. The long-term use of opiates can cause neonatal withdrawal symptoms and impairment of responsiveness.

15.16.3 Sedatives and Hypnotics

Anxiolytics may be prescribed for a short duration. The group of benzodiazepines is recommended because of the low rate of side effects. Diazepam is the most studied compound out of this group.

15.16.4 Local Anesthetics

Local anesthetics have a high lipid solubility and can therefore easily pass the placenta. The sooner the transition from maternal to fetal blood, the less the local anesthetic is bound to plasma proteins. Therefore, the local anesthetics with the highest protein binding rates are preferred. There are no reports of harmful effects to the fetus by local anesthetics during dental treatment.

Adrenaline as a vasoconstrictor additive is dosed as low as possible (1:200,000). On behalf of gynecologists, there are no objections to adrenaline derivatives, those substances are used as tocolytics (ache-inhibiting drugs). Intravascular administration must be avoided, because systemically resorbed adrenaline may lead to a constriction of the uterine vessels.

Norepinephrine and felypressin are contraindicated. Articaine, bupivacaine, and etidocaine may be used during pregnancy. The amides prilocaine and mepivacaine are to be considered more critically.

15.17 Damages Caused by Incorrect Treatment from the Perspective of Malpractice Assessments

Vogel presented (1982) a review of 584 claims, whereupon 42 % of dental damages were caused by surgical treatment (Tables 15.3 and

15.4), 32.4 % were caused by prosthetic measures (Table 15.5), and 16.6 % were caused by conservative treatments. Similar cases often resulted in widely divergent court decisions (Vogel 1982). Of medical liability lawsuits, 4 % are against dentists (Dajani et al. 1994).

Table 15.3 Main complaints of 584 patients after dental treatment (Vogel 1982)

Damage caused by	*n*	Percent	From dental treatment	Percent
Surgery	246	42.1	10	4.0
Prosthetics	189	32.4	13	6.9
Conservative treatment	97	16.6	3	3.1
Local anesthesia	33	5.6	2	6.1
Orthodontics	15	2.6	1	6.7
General disease	3	0.5	1	33.3
General anesthesia	1	0.2	–	–
Total	584	100	30	5.1

There is a comprehensive collection of judgments by Oehler (1999) concerning dental treatments and a list of information about various court judgments (*BGH – Supreme Court, OLG – Court of Appeals, LG*). Note also that the behavior after the occurrence of the damage will be assessed. A proper medical history, diagnosis, and treatment or referral to the appropriate further medical treatment is not only a medical duty but also a duty according to the insurance contract.

15.18 Dental Surgery

Klaus Rötzscher and Rolf Singer

Each oral surgical treatment bears complications that are either predictable or unpredictable (Egyedi 1998). Damages by surgical treatment measures are the most common complaints; nerve damage is the most common cause for liability claims (Vogel 1980a, 1982).

Table 15.4 Liability claims after dental surgery (Vogel 1980a)

Caused by	Main accusation	Additional accusation	Justified	Compensation rejected	Unknown
Sensory disturbance	46	–	22	3	21
Untreated root residues	43	7	15	1	27
Broken jaw	33	–	12	4	17
Mouth–antrum contacts	24	–	6	7	11
Tooth damage	20	2	9	2	9
Confusion in extraction	19	–	11	1	7
Root fragments in the maxillary sinus	12	1	5	1	11
Untreated debris	12	1	5	1	6
Temporomandibular joint (TMJ) damage	7	–	0	1	6
Osteomyelitis, caused or incorrect treatment	6	3	2	2	2
Soft tissue injury	5	–	3	0	2
Incorrect diagnosis	4	–	1	2	1
Soft tissue infection, caused or incorrect treatment	3	–	0	3	0
Side confusion in operation	3		2	0	0
Lack of consent	3	–	2	0	1
Non-indicated extraction	3	–	0	2	1
Error in root tip resection	2	3	0	1	1
Preprosthetic surgery	1	–	0	1	0
Total	246	17	92	31	123

Table 15.5 Liability claims after conservative treatment (Vogel 1980b)

Caused by	Main accusation	Additional accusation	Justified	Compensation rejected	Unknown
Swallowing of root canal instruments	27	–	16	–	11
Soft tissue injuries	23	–	10	–	–
Broken root canal instruments	20	1	7	4	9
Via falsa	8	1	3	–	5
Damage after root canal treatment	6	–	1	2	1
Chemical burns caused by drugs	4	–	4	–	–
Incomplete root filling	3	–	–	2	1
Swallowing of filling parts	2	–	–	–	2
Inhaling of root canal instruments	2	–	2	–	–
TMJ dislocation	1	–	–	1	–
Secondary caries and pulp damage	1	3	–	–	1
Total	97	5	43	9	45

15.18.1 General and Local Anesthesia

If general anesthesia is performed by an anesthesiologist in dental practice (outpatient), the dentist is responsible for the indication of the anesthesia, but not for the implementation. The anesthesiologist is responsible for the method of anesthesia (Günther 1966).

Differentiated local anesthesia has been established as a fundamental form of analgesia in dental treatment of children as well as in adults. If, in certain situations, a treatment under local anesthesia is not considered possible by the dentist, or on the recommendation of the attending physician (GP/Internist), dental treatment may be carried out under general anesthesia. This may occur, for example, in acute diseases (e.g., inflammatory processes or trauma) and/or as a result of general medical risks or medical history (such as physical, mental, and psychological disabilities) or behavioral disorders. If the dentist comes to the conclusion that a further and adequate treatment under local anesthesia is not possible, e.g., unwilling children, this can also be seen as an indication for the implementation of a general anesthesia.

General anesthesia should only be performed by a doctor with the academic title "Doctor of Anesthesiology." "The anesthesiologist is in charge for the anesthesia procedure and for monitoring of vital functions during and after surgery. This includes the management of complications and the incident involved therapy during and after anesthesia. After an outpatient's anesthesia, monitoring to stabilize the vital signs is particularly important. The determination of timing and modalities of the home travel is one of the most responsible duties of care for anesthesia physicians" (*Opinion of the German Association of Anaesthetists – In: Anesthesiology and Intensive Care Medicine 2/89*).

In the decision between a nasal or oral intubation, the specific requirements of dental treatment are to be considered. With the invention of the intraligamental anesthesia procedure, the problem of reuse of opened cartridges arose, because this form of anesthesia often requires very little anesthetic and therefore (motivated by economy), one carpule is reused (with different needles) in other patients.

15.18.2 Risk of Infectiousness

Risk of even 1 % or less in view of the negligent transmission of infectious diseases is too high. The most important example is the risk of negligent transmission of hepatitis B (and HI) virus. Not only the injection needle but also the carpule must be replaced after each patient, even if anesthesia fluid is lost (Maeglin 1981). Disregarding this is a grossly negligent act, with all of the consequences of culpable behavior. "During injections of local anesthesia it may come to cardiac, central nervous and general reactions and side effects of the vasoconstrictive additives (especially in overdose, inadvertent intravascular injection and non-regarding of predisposing diseases, but also during local anesthesia performed lege artis). This may become acutely life-threatening and requires instant countermeasures" (Frenkel 1978).

Even a properly applied adjuvant (adrenaline) has a significant absorption rate in healthy patients (Lipp et al. 1988). Therefore, it is obvious that general intoxication can occur in correctly administered, and even more dramatically in accidentally administered, intravascular administration of catecholamines. Local anesthetics, accidentally injected intravenously with addition of a vasoconstrictor, have a significantly higher toxicity (Niesel and Kaiser 1991). Failure of aspiration followed by intravascular injection may lead to the accusation of breach of duty, similar to the accusation of disregarding previous illness or exceeding the maximum amount of supplementary injection.

It is a culpable act to leave (after local anesthetic) a pale and dizzy patient unattended. Less known are symptomatic psychoses in the sense of ordered semi-consciousness, presumably often misinterpreted because of their volatility, so the patient is not able to drive a motor vehicle for the next 24 h.

15.18.3 Infiltration Anesthesia and Fitness to Drive

A causal connection between infiltration anesthesia and a disturbance of consciousness (causing an accident) is often denied because of the low concentration of active ingredients and temporal relation. Both, however, can be explained by pharmacokinetics of the combination of local anesthetic and vasoconstrictive substance. The vasoconstrictive addition is intended to prevent a rapid absorption of local anesthetic at the target site and to prolong and deepen the effect. If the vasoconstrictive effect fades after 1–3 h, the vasodilatory effect of the local anesthetic in the well-vascularized mucosa starts. This can lead to increased washout and a short-term influx of the drug into the bloodstream. Local anesthetics are not metabolized at the site of action, but in the liver, some already partially in the blood. An effect similar to that of a relative overdose would be possible.

The absolute level of an active ingredient is less significant than the increase of concentration. In this context, it should be noted that clouding of consciousness, according to the severity classifications, can already be observed after a mild intoxication (Hempel et al. 1982).

Vasoconstrictors are added to local anesthetics to improve the local effect and to lower the blood levels, which are reduced after the absorption of local anesthetic as an expression of distribution of the substance in the body. The correctly administered local anesthetic in addition to a vasoconstrictor seems more compatible as a possibly vasoconstrictor-free substance. If the vasoconstrictor is injected intravenously by mistake, this increases not only the local anesthetic effect, but also the vasoconstriction (Niesel and Kaiser 1991).

There is a considerable link between oral infiltration anesthesia and the ability to drive. Conductive anesthesia must not be given if it is known that the patient will drive a motor vehicle after treatment. A limitation of driving ability may already arise from stress caused by dental surgery and must be part of the education. In addition, a duty of education also arises from relevant warnings by manufacturers of the anesthetics. According to current Supreme Court jurisprudence (BGH), the physician must inform the patient about all possible risks that cannot be excluded with certainty (Haffner and Graw 1995).

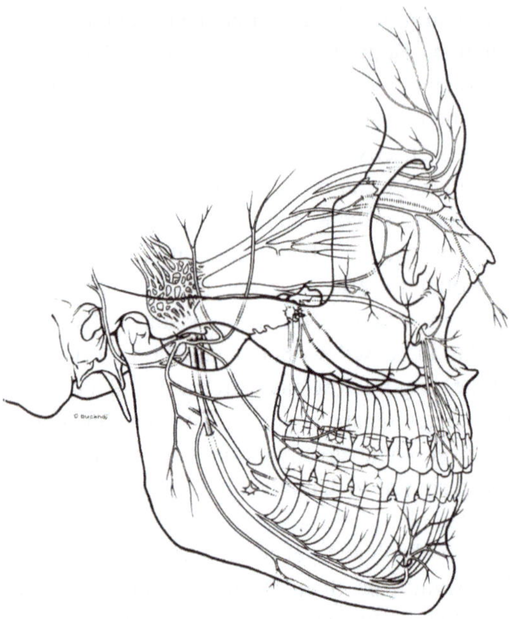

Fig. 15.2 *N. mandibularis*, side view (Evers 1983)

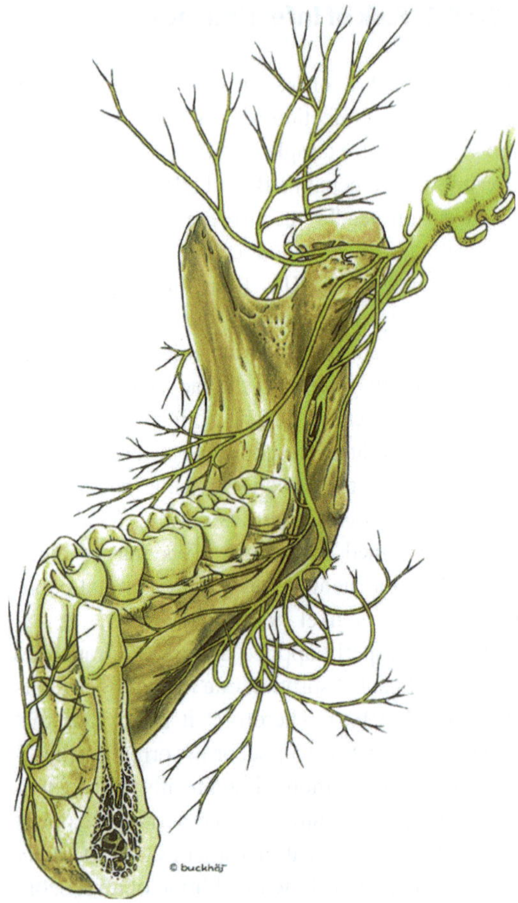

Fig. 15.3 *N. mandibularis*, frontal view (Evers 1983)

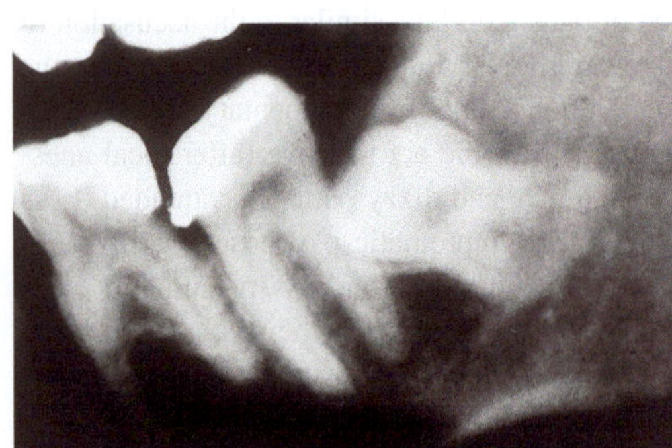

Fig. 15.4 *N. mandibularis*, X-ray before extraction (operation)

15.18.4 Postoperative Sensory Disturbances

Irreversible sensory loss after dental treatment (mainly after tooth extractions and surgical procedures, less after anesthesia) has significantly increased in recent years (Vogel 1980a, b). Contact of the root tip to the mandibular canal or a direct trauma by instruments or dislocated roots can result in irreversible damage to the *N. alveolaris inferior*.

The *N. mandibularis* (Figs. 15.2 and 15.3) is a mixed but predominantly sensory nerve. It reaches the infratemporal spatium through the foramen ovale. The locomotor units of the chewing muscles leave the nerve trunk in the infratemporal fossa. Afterwards, the bifurcation distributes in sensory branches (Evers 1983). Prior to each extraction, an X-ray image should be taken. In order to detect rare anatomical variations, the dentist must be oriented to the anatomic conditions in the root zone in order to identify the nerve course (Figs. 15.4, 15.5 and 15.6). The *N. lingualis* is usually injured by slipping instruments in the floor of the mouth or by conductive anesthesia at the wrong place. Scoring the periosteum with the needle tip during injection must be strictly avoided (Fig. 15.7).

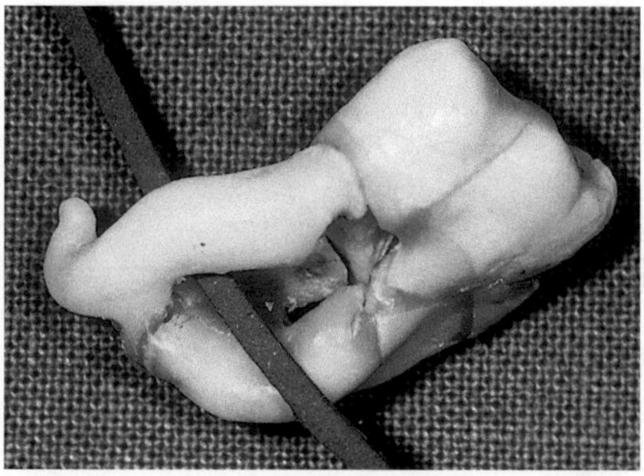

Fig. 15.5 *N. mandibularis*, presentation of the nerve course

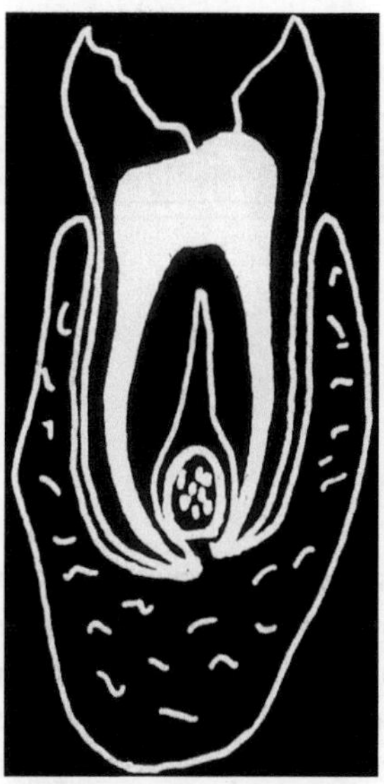

Fig. 15.6 *N. mandibularis*, presentation of the course of the nerve (drawing)

15.18.4.1 Types of Nerve Lesions/ Complications

Injury to nerves, arteries, or veins during the local/conductive anesthesia may be caused by:

- The surgical procedure itself
- Contaminated needles with subsequent infection
- Quick injection with subsequent postoperative pain by ripping the tissue or necrosis
- Large injection volume (do not use more local anesthetic than necessary) or injection into infected area
- Trismus (usually caused by injection into the *M. pterygoid internus*)
- Bleeding at the site of injection (using solutions with low-dosed vasoconstrictor additives)
- Facial paralysis (injection at the posterior border of the ascending ramus) with atony of the lower lip (hanging mouth) (Evers 1983)

15.18.4.2 Consequences of Nerve Lesions

Typical clinical symptoms of nerve injury are:

- Hyperesthesia
- Hypoesthesia
- Paresthesia
- Anesthesia and anesthesia dolorosa

15.18.4.3 Duration of the Nerve Injury

Lesions may be temporary or permanent (>2–3 years after surgery). Injuries of the sensory branches of the *N. trigeminus* are a very painful complication. Most common are impairments of *N. alveolaris inferior*, the *N. mentalis*, and the *N. lingual* (*Opinion DGZMK 6/ 89*). With the increasing awareness of modern microsurgical nerve–surgical options to restore function after nerve lesions, considerable progress has been achieved. Damages to the nerves are no longer accepted as an irreversible fate, because patients are now referred to microsurgical therapy at an early stage.

In cases where there is a close anatomic relationship of *N. lingualis* to the mandible body and *N. alveolaris inferior* to the teeth, there is a risk of damaging those nerves during dental, surgical, and some conservation measures. The most common lesion sites of the *N. lingual* and *alveolaris inferior* are in the range of the mandibular angle, especially in the third molar region.

According to *OLG Munich* (*Higher Regional Court*), *Judgement of 20.11.1996*, *Az. 4810 AHRS*, "Prior to conductive anesthesia, an education about the rare and usually avoidable risk of damaging the *N. Alveolaris* is not required." In contrast, the OLG (Higher Regional Court) of Munich ruled (*Az. 26-O-285/78*) with the tenor that it is a rare (0.1 %) but typical complication. The *N. Mentalis* is mostly injured outside the

Fig. 15.7 The needle tip should never be introduced into the foramen, because the risk of vascular or nerve injury is high and complications such as hematoma and paresthesias (longer lasting) can occur (Evers 1983)

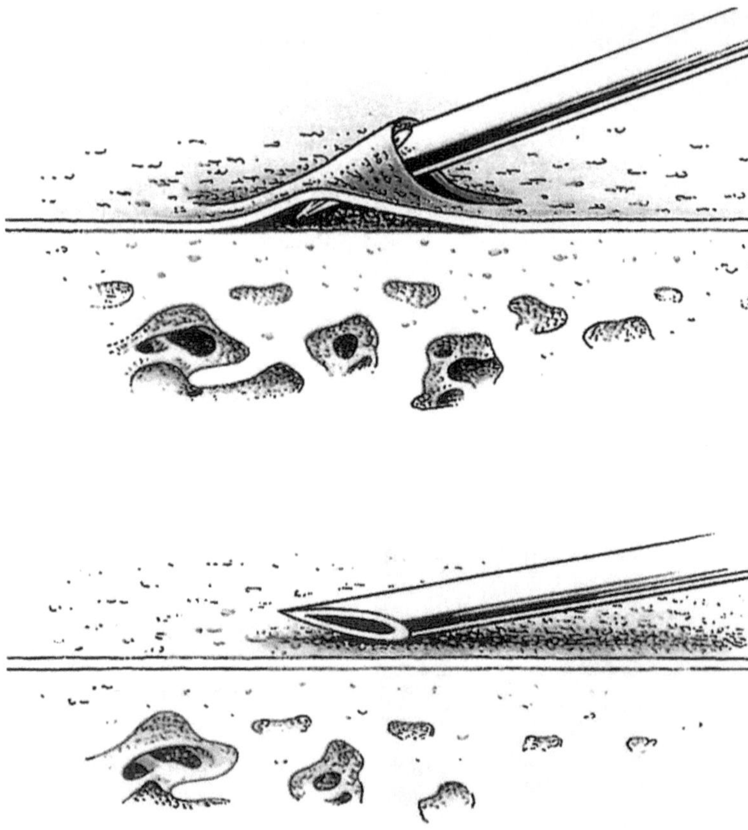

mental foramen (injury of branches of the trigeminal nerve II are very rare). Nerve injuries are usually not noticed during the operation. The often-described symptom of a dull pain occurs only rarely.

15.18.4.4 Symptoms of Nerve Injury During Injection – The Immediate Pain

If the trunk of the *N. lingualis* or *N. mandibularis* is hit during conductive anesthesia, this is accompanied by a flashing defensive movement of the patient or with a shooting pain in the lower lip or tongue. This phenomenon always should be documented in the patient file in order to point to a possibly sensory disturbance.

If, as a result of close anatomical relationship of the root tips to the mandibular canal, the risk was obvious, a claim for compensation may be entitled because of lack of education (lack of preoperative X-ray diagnosis or incomplete image of the root tips in case of damage). A survey (during a legal dispute) showed that a *N. lingualis* injury in a sole anesthetic block may occur only by the pressure rise caused be the anesthetic solution, or more likely caused by hemorrhage and clot formation and subsequent fibrosis in and around the nerve.

15.18.4.5 Injury of the *N. Mandibularis* During Surgery

Prior to the surgery, the dentist must inform the patient about the risk of irritation of the nerve. There is current consensus that, in a nonurgent medical intervention, the rare complication of nerve injury must be explained to the patient (*OLG Köln, Judgement of 22.8.1998, Az. 5 U 232/96*). *LG Dortmund, Judgement of 27.09.1979, Az 2029/79; OLG Hamm, Judgement of 12.02.1980, Az AHRS 4800/1; LG Mannheim, Judgement of 04/30/1986, Ref 9 – O-6/85; OLG Dusseldorf Higher Regional Court, Judgement of*

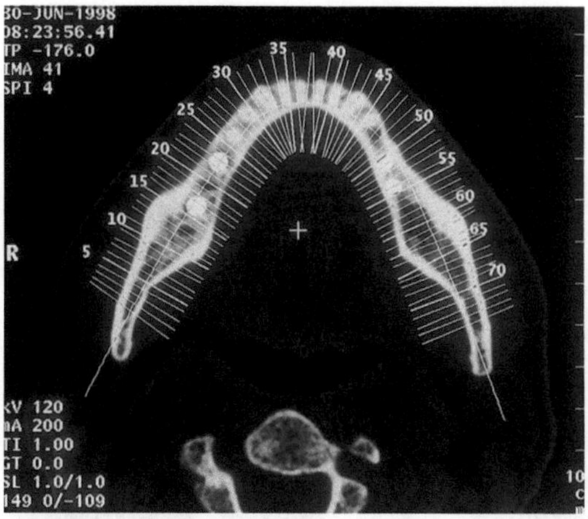

Fig. 15.8 CT scanning

25.07.1991, Az. AHRS 2694/12 states that "Prior to a non-critical extraction/surgical removal of a wisdom tooth, the patient must be educated about the risk of damage to the *N. mandibularis* and its consequences."

Very often the clinician tries to shift the responsibility for an injury of *N. mandibular* to a postoperative tissue swelling or a postoperative bleeding. *OLG Dusseldorf Higher Regional Court, Judgement of 25.07.1991, Az. AHRS 2694/12*, and *OLG Stuttgart Higher Regional Court, Judgement, Az. 12 U 25/95* found that "The postoperative tissue swelling is not such as the nerve (covered by a bony layer) gets damaged. It is also possible that the nerve injury is based on a post-operative bleeding, because bleeding caused by such compression, leads only to temporary neural deficits." The dentist's argument that a scarred structure around the nerves was the cause of the injury was dismissed by court because the sensitivity loss had occurred immediately after surgery but a scar formation takes days or weeks.

Damage to the *N. mandibularis* can also occur during an implantation in the mandible. For example, during the postoperative control after an implantation in the left and right lower jaw, the patient complained about numbness in the *N. mandibularis*. A CT scan was recommended (Figs. 15.8 and 15.9). The family dentist removed the two implants and replaced them by 2-mm-shorter implants. The paresthesia was completely healed within 3 months.

In postoperative lesions/irritations of the *N. mandibularis* after implantation, a three-dimensional image should be taken to discuss the therapeutic alternatives with the patient. Both distal ends (47 and also 46) project themselves into the nerve canal (Fig. 15.10). The radiograph (see Fig. 15.9) (layer 54) shows that the drill hole passes lingually.

A lesion of the *N. mandibularis* may be related to a root filling in the lower posterior teeth by the passage of the root canal in the mandibular canal. For example, the distal implant (coating level 54) is projected above the nerve canal (Fig. 15.11). The X-ray control must be performed immediately after root canal filling to detect the passage of the material into the nerve region in time (Fig. 15.12). Thus, the very different toxicity of the root canal fillings has a significant role. The panoramic display shows the expansion of the overstuffed root filling. Contrary to primary advice, an intraoral neurolysis was conducted to remove the root filling material. This resulted in a rupture of the nerve, which was followed by a nerve transplant and ended up in anesthesia dolorosa.

Chloropercha, e.g., develops relatively low toxic stimuli compared with compounds that include plastic state unpolymerized constituents or iodoform or paraformaldehyde. Additionally, calcium hydroxide preparations are not harmless, because they are highly alkaline and etching. Toxic damage occurs immediately and the material must be removed quickly. Because root canal filling materials (once applied into the mandibular canal) must be removed by microsurgical interventions, it is wrong to extract the tooth (after overstuffing) with the intent that root filling material could be drained.

15.18.4.6 Injury of the *N. lingualis* During Surgery

Nerve injuries of *N. lingualis* can lead to numbness of the affected half of the tongue and/or to a unilateral failure of the taste perception. If only the sensitivity in the branching of *N. Lingualis* is disturbed, this indicates a partial lesion of *N. Lingualis*.

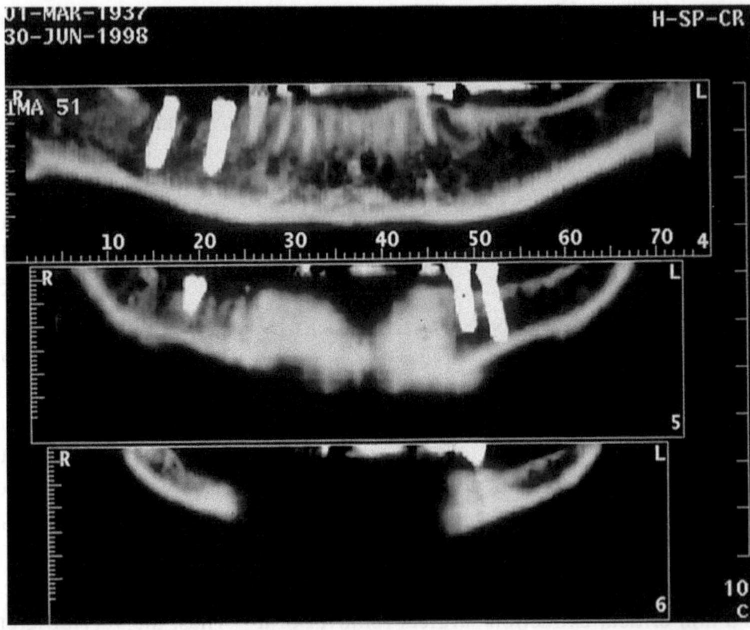

Fig. 15.9 Both implants in the right and left mandible are displayed

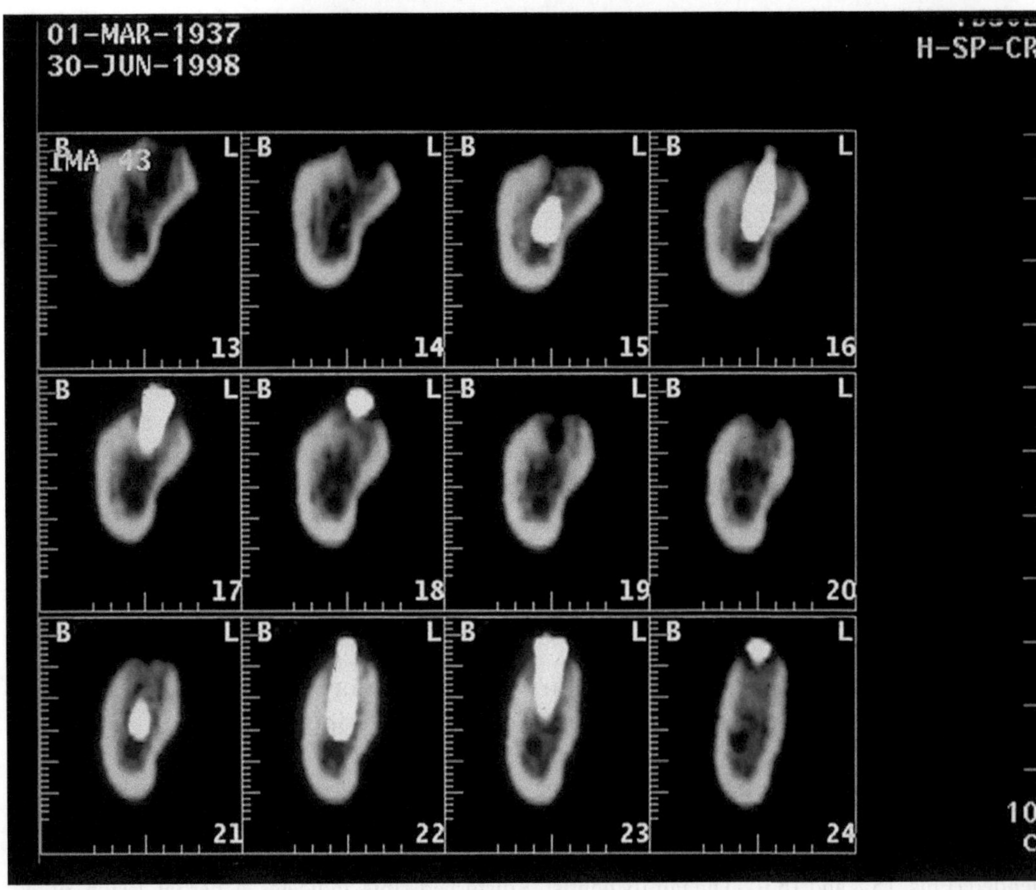

Fig. 15.10 Both distal ends (47 and also 46) project themselves into the nerve canal

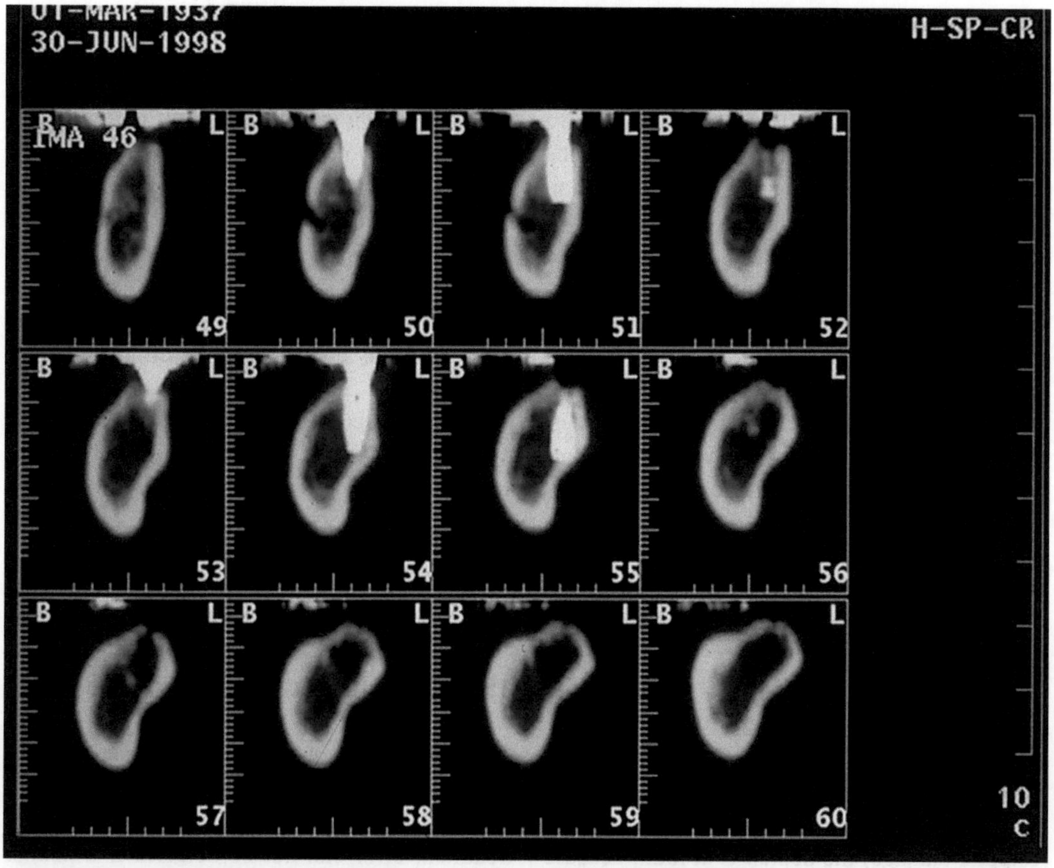

Fig. 15.11 The distal implant (coating level 54) is projected above the nerve canal

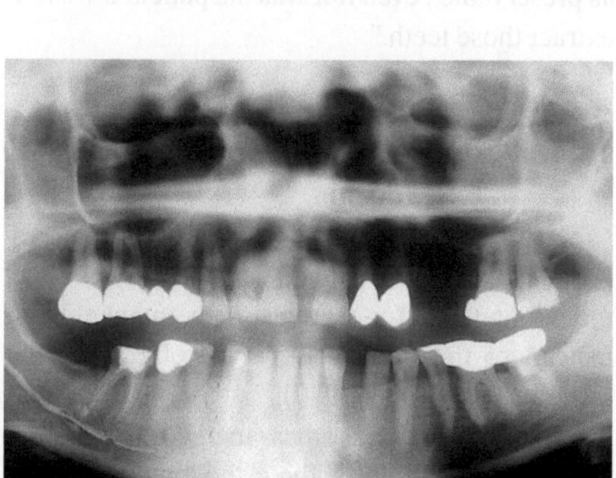

Fig. 15.12 Condition after root treatment of tooth 46 with overstuffed and spread filling material

LG Frankfurt, Judgement of 02/03/1981, File number: *2/16 S 172/80* found that:

1. A nerve injury of the *N. lingualis* with permanent numbness of the left half of the tongue during the surgical removal of the impacted wisdom tooth 38 can not be causing for an infraction during the anesthesia or the surgery itself.
2. In approximately ten million cases of conductive anesthesia per year, only about ten lead to a long-term damage of the *N. lingualis*, so there is no duty to inform.

These findings also apply to the rare complication of *N. Lingualis* damage caused by anesthesia. For instance, *LG Duisburg, Judgement of 15.6.1988, Az. 6 O 34/86* found that "The damage of *N. lingualis* after surgical removal of wisdom tooth 38 may have been caused either by the previous block anesthesia or the surgery itself. This damage is, however, a statistically unusual rare complication and a duty to inform is not given." The damage of *N. Suralis* justified a compensation of 10,000 €, because the loss of the sense of taste (the patient was a butcher) required a reanastomose by inserting a part from the dorsum of the foot.

The rate of nerve injury caused by conductive anesthesia is very low. Local anesthesia has to be injected as closely as possible to the nerve root. The dentist would act culpably by using only a blunt or bent needle tip. The standard needle length should be at least 42 mm (see needle breakage). *OLG Köln, Judgement of 23.4.1999, Az. 5 U 232/96* found that "In case of an urgent surgical measure, there is no duty to inform." It is to be assumed that the claimant would also have undergone the surgery if they had received proper information. The experts have convincingly shown that the procedure was indicated as urgent because there was a difficult displacement of the tooth, but also the wisdom tooth had significant decay and an acute inflammatory process had started.

15.18.5 Needle Breakage

According to the principles of *prima facie* evidence, in case of a needle breakage (and the resulting damage) the dentist is at fault, because the damage is typically caused by incorrect treatment (see *LG Darmstadt, Judgement, Az. 130160/70*). For example, *the Hanseatic Higher Regional Court (OLG), Judgement of 18.06.1953, Az. 6 U 80/53*; *LG Hamburg, Judgement, AZ. 12 0 208/51* found that "The use of a carpule syringe with a very thin needle was not objectionable at the time of the treatment. It is not an incorrect behavior of the dentist if the needle breaks (during an anesthetic injection) and a fragment of 1.5 cm length remains in the tissue, since several causes for the breakage are possible (material defects, sudden movement of the patient)." Because of the known possible complications, anesthesia should not be administered with used and resterilized needles.

In *OLG Frankfurt, Judgement, Az. U-235/71*, "The dentist argued that the patient unexpectedly moved his head during the injection and the needle broke. The patient has the burden of proof that he did not unexpectedly move his head and caused the needle breakage." Since a cannula fracture occurs only at the transition to the cone, it is required that only needles with at least 42 mm length may be used in order to remove the needle fragment in case of a breakage.

In nerve reconstructions by transplantation of an autologous transplant, there is a risk of an amputation neuroma in the area of the sampling nerves. Surveys on our own patients show that this risk is in the lower percentages. For successful reconstruction, however, the advantage at the receiver site is greater than the disadvantage in the donor site. Education is not required due to the rarity of recorded complications in the literature of oral and maxillofacial surgery (Haßfeld 1999).

The fact of nerve damage cannot lead to the suspicion of incorrect treatment, but rather the delayed surgical treatment of the injured nerve.

15.18.6 Nonindicated Extractions

The dentist may not perform any extraction without a clinical diagnosis. *LG Frankfurt, Judgement of 20.09.1954, AZ. 2 O 372/53* stated that "A treatment error can not be detected if a dentist denies the extraction of teeth which he considers as preservable , even if it was the patient's wish to extract those teeth."

15.18.7 Confusion in Tooth Extractions

It is a lack of care if a dentist erroneously extracts the wrong teeth, for example the permanent teeth instead of the milk teeth (after referral by the orthodontist) (Vogel 1979).

If the orthodontist has marked the wrong teeth, the culpability is the orthodontists. Before unusual demands (e.g. the removal of permanent canines or premolars with agenesis of second premolars), the orthodontist should explicitly confirm the instructions.

15.18.7.1 Side Confusion in Surgeries

It is a classic mistake to confuse the left and right side (e.g., impacted wisdom teeth, upper canine teeth) because of inadequate radiology diagnostic or incorrect labeling of the included X-ray images. The surgeon cannot rely on incorrect documentation, because the surgeon is responsible for the correct side localization.

15.18.7.2 Mouth–Antrum Connections

Such defects can occur at extractions or surgical removal of upper premolars and molars because of topographic–maxillary anatomical features. The narrow spatial relationship between the tooth and sinus system may cause, even with appropriate diligence, one of the most common complications in dental surgical treatment.

OLG Oldenburg, Judgement of 29.10.1991, Az. 5 U 50/91 states that "A patient had undergone the extraction of her last three teeth 23, 26 and 27 in mid-November 1984. A week later, a complete denture had been inserted in the upper jaw. Afterwards she was free of symptoms. In early 1988 an inflammatory swelling in region 27/28 was radiologically detected in an oral surgery clinic and a root residue was removed. The result was a mouth-antrum connection that had to be closed in another operation 2 weeks later. Ambulatory treatment was completed in early 1991. The patient claimed the dentist, who had performed the extractions in 1984, for compensation of material damage of 4.050 Euro and 1.500 Euro for pain and suffering." The lawsuit and also the appeal were dismissed. The root residue could not be assigned without doubt to one of the extractions in 1984. The reasoning was provided by experts in a comprehensive discussion, including the structure and migration patterns of roots in the jaw area. The court came to the conclusion there was no context between the inflammation in 1988 and the retained root. The court also denied (in another opinion) the obligation of the dentist to take an X-ray image in order to provide evidence for a possible medical malpractice debate. Because the patient was not able to prove her accusation that the extractions in 1984 were causal for the retained root, the claim was dismissed (Rohde 1995a).

More fatal is the unconscious dislocation of foreign bodies in the antrum, resulting in perforation of the maxillary sinus. A dental assistant had left a cone-shaped hand piece of a root canal instrument in the maxillary sinus (the instrument was wrapped in a swab). The physician is liable for a culpable error of an assistant, because the surgeon has to ensure the correct performance of the surgery (Berg 1966; Bünger 1980). Even implants that are introduced into the upper jaw can cause the dislocation of the implant into the maxillary sinus (Figs. 15.13 and 15.14). It is a culpable negligence if the surgeon does not check (after treatment or operation) the possibility of iatrogenic perforation of the maxillary sinus, which may require a plastic closure.

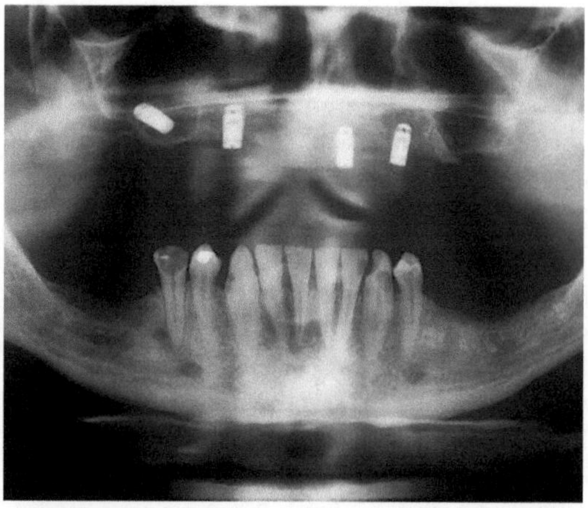

Fig. 15.13 Postoperative control of four implants in the upper jaw

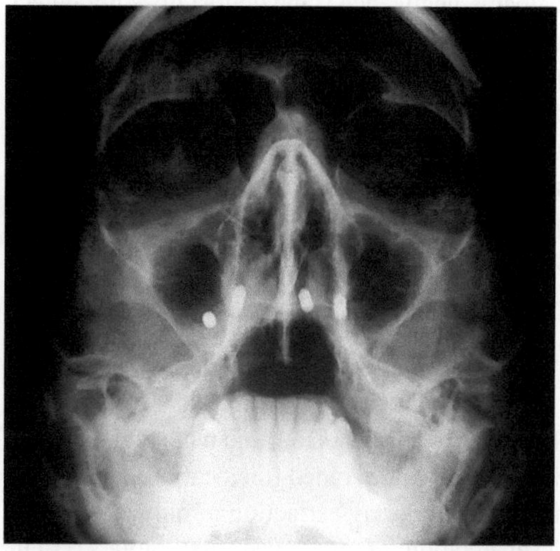

Fig. 15.14 Postoperative X-ray image control of the sinus. The dislocated implant is visible in the maxillary sinus

For example, in *LG Darmstadt, Judgement of 03.02.1981, Az. 13 O 156/77*, "The emergence of a mouth-antrum connection related to the extraction of the tooth 26 is not inevitable. It was a treatment error to treat only 2 out of 3 roots of the tooth 26 and to fix a crown on this tooth at the same day. Together with the damages caused by two bridges in the lower jaw (due to early contacts) a compensation of 3.000 Euro was justified."

15.18.7.3 Dislocated Root Fragments and Foreign Bodies in the Maxillary Sinus

Root fractures or dislocation of roots into the maxillary sinus are complications that are not caused by incorrect treatment. However, it is a culpable negligence if the dentist does not detect a root fracture or if the dentist does not refer the patient to a specialist, if unable to remove the fragments (this also refers to the removal of fractured milling and drilling). The duty of care is met when the patient is informed about the complications that occurred and their consequences and is referred to a dentist for oral surgery or to an oral and maxillofacial surgeon.

15.18.7.4 Damaging of Teeth During Treatment

Damages to adjacent teeth and teeth in the opposing jaw must be avoided (dislocation, removal of tooth germs during extraction of milk teeth). The lever-luxation of destroyed first molars (Bein lever) must be conducted with great care to avoid a peripheral dislocation of the mixed dentition of mesial premolars (Fig. 15.15). The patient should be informed about the possible risk of damages to adjacent filled teeth.

OLG Köln, Judgement of 09.03.1992, Az. 27 U 144/92 stated "A 25-year old junior doctor tried to extract tooth 48 only with a leverage tool. Despite the use of substantial leverage, a significant loosening of the tooth could not be reached until the tooth 47 was fractured and could not be restored. The hospital (as an employer of the dental assistant) was sentenced to compensation of 750 Euro for loss of tooth 47. According to the experts, the leverage (after consideration of the X-ray images) was unlikely to succeed since a

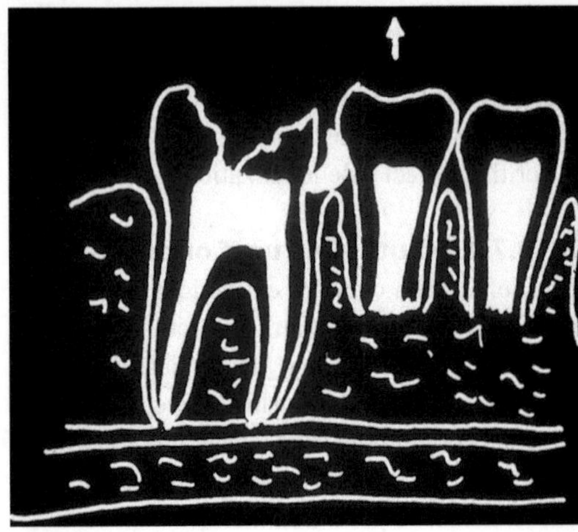

Fig. 15.15 Dislocation of a destroyed molar by using a Bein lever resulted in peripheral dislocation of mesial standing premolars in the mixed dentition

considerable resistance in the bone was given by inclination of the tooth dislocation. In view of the faulty treatment and because of the generally known consequences caused by an increased use of force with a lever tool, the handler should have aborted his attempt at an earlier stage and instead arrange a surgical removal of the tooth 48."

15.18.7.5 Apicoectomies and Hemisection

The apicoectomy, especially in the posterior region, is one of the most difficult procedures of dental surgery, with many possible complications. The apicoectomy, also the root tip amputation together with a hemisection (halving of a multirooted tooth—preferably of mandibular molars—the retention of only one root is also practicable) and intentional replantation are attributed to endodontic surgery. This procedure is a tooth preservation in the final consequence. Prosthetically usable portions of multirooted teeth are protected from loss by a partial resection. Before a surgery, it is advisable to explain that the surgery is an attempt to retain the teeth, but that success cannot be guaranteed.

The prophylactic use of hemisection or root amputation for minor furcation problems or minimal periodontal lesions is contraindicated. Prior to indications for endodontal problems, all conservative treatment options must be exhausted.

Posssible error sources are:

- Inadequate endodontic treatment
- Failure to observe the furcation and root anatomy of molars (periodontal problems)
- Lack of postoperative prosthetic treatment (no fracture prevention, inaccuracies in the adjustment)

15.18.7.6 Mandibular Fractures/ Foreign Bodies in the Lower Jaw

Iatrogenic mandibular fractures by wisdom tooth extractions or surgical removal of wisdom teeth are one of the most unpleasant complications. Gross treatment errors or insufficient information can result in a judicial proceeding. Errors especially occur in wisdom tooth extractions and surgical removal of impacted premolar teeth or in connection with cysts. Late fractures are also possible by lever removal in the full row of teeth.

LG Heidelberg, Judgement of 15.08.1990, Az. 3 O 323/88 states that "A postoperative X-Ray image is necessary to avoid a fracture of the jaw during the removal of an impacted wisdom teeth."

OLG Celle, Judgement, Az. 1 U 31/92 states that "Prior to the insertion of a removable partial denture for a 88-year-old woman, the horizontally impacted wisdom tooth 48 was prophylactically removed and has caused a fracture in the mandible with a significant dislocation, which was detected after 1 week. The fixation of the plate splint in stationary treatment took 4 weeks. The court admitted a compensation of Euro 3.843,00."

"There is substantial evidence that the dentist removed the tooth 48 without sufficient clinical indication, since the patient had no complaints at this time.

The defendant has not expressed the risk of a possible mandibular fracture and in addition the fracture was detected only 1 week later and caused a delay in treatment of 1 week."

OLG Dusseldorf, Judgement of 21.03.1996, Az. 8 U 153/95 states that "A fracture in context with the surgical removal of a wisdom tooth is a proof for faulty treatment. Education about the rare possibility of a jaw fracture during the surgical wisdom tooth removal is not necessary. The court admitted a compensation of 10.000 Euro."

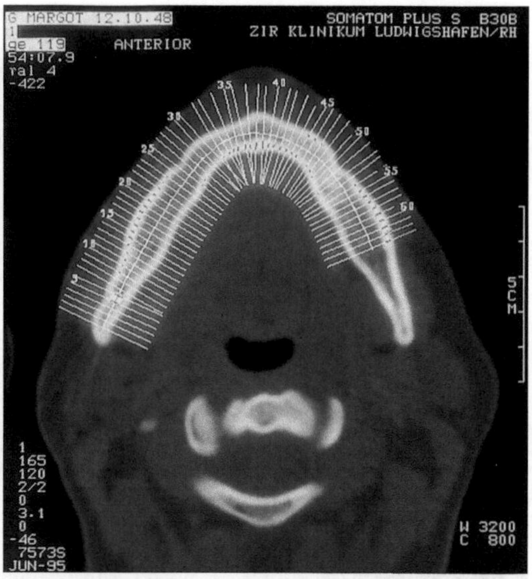

Fig. 15.16 Dental CT scanning of the mandible. Radiopaque foreign body in the layer—Level 5

As part of the backup information, the dentist must inform the patient about the appropriate behavior measures after the surgery. If the Bein lever or other instruments cause a fracture, a three-dimensional X-ray image should be taken prior to any attempt to remove foreign bodies (Fig. 15.16). In Fig. 15.17, the grid of a dental CT of the lower jaw shows a radiopaque foreign body in the layer level five. The foreign body in layer five (Fig. 15.17) had to be removed by an extraoral access.

15.18.7.7 Soft Tissue Injuries

Rotating instruments, scalpels, and periosteal elevators and ligatures are the most common causes for cut, torn, crushed, or strangled nerves. In some cases, extensive soft tissue injuries can cause nerve hemorrhage as well as compression and scarring. Soft tissue may also be injured during the preparation by grinding wheels, turbines, and by milling or during the insertion and the removal of crowns. Injures may also occur during the insertion of gangrenous teeth in bridge constructions, as well as damages of the pulp after crown

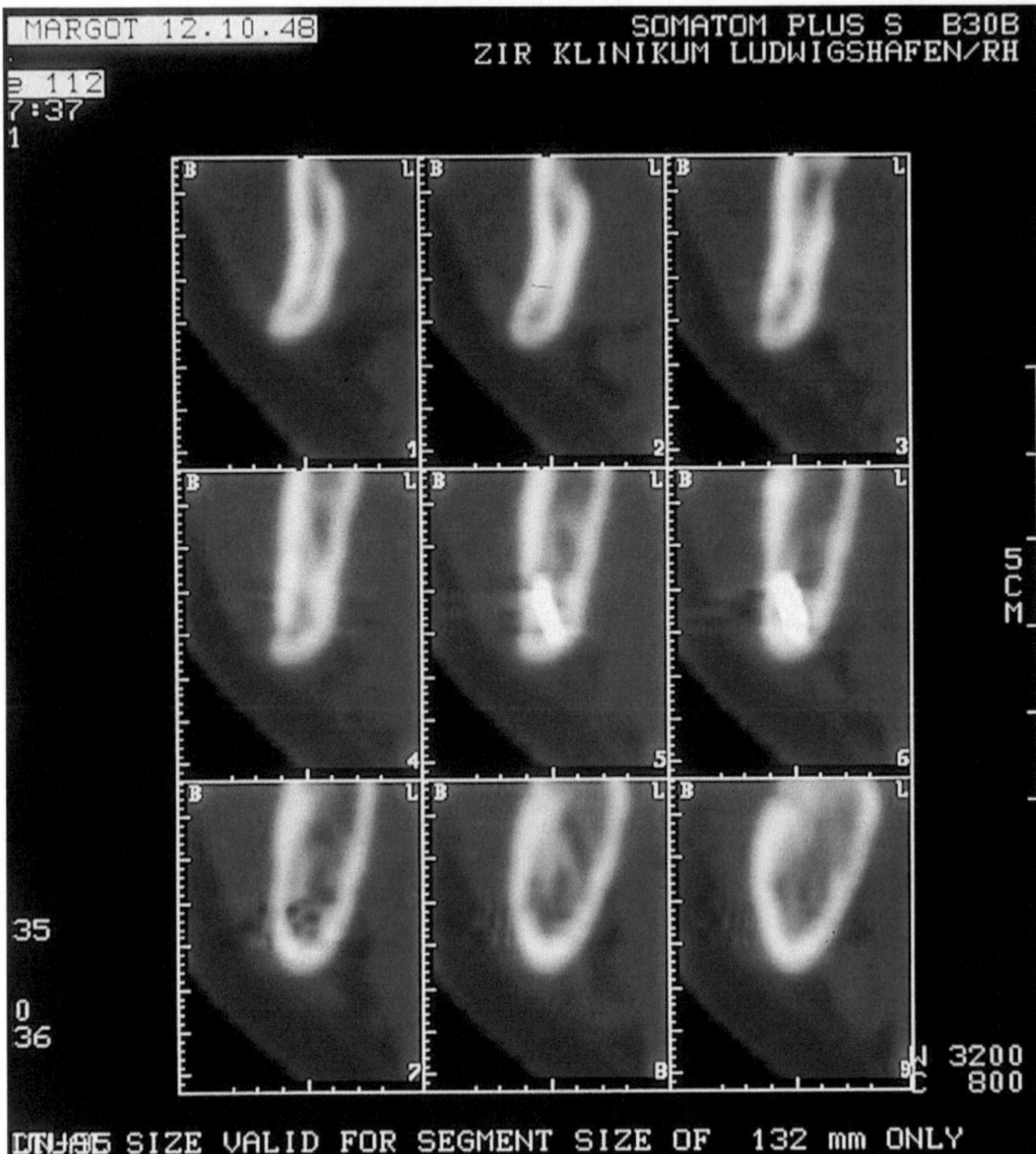

Fig. 15.17 Exact location of a foreign body in the mandible basal edge layer—Level 5

preparation, swallowing and aspiration of crown and bridge parts, improperly crowned teeth, not recognized and left roots (error in radiographic diagnostic) prior to the insertion of bridges and dentures, and damages by faulty fixed and removable dentures. All of these damages will justify compensation if faulty treatment is proven.

Larger injuries or perforation of the oral mucosa, for example by a slipping Bein lever or by bone milling, caused by insufficient bracing (disc protection), suggest a lack of care. For example, *OLG Stuttgart, Judgement, Az. 14 U 34/98* states that "The fact that the dentist left the actual area (during surgical removal of a tooth by using a Rose-head burr and a Lindemann burr) and penetrated the adjacent soft tissue, which caused a nerve injury, leads to the accusation of culpable negligence."

15.18.7.8 Soft Tissue Infections

The dentist is responsible for soft tissue infections/osteomyelitis caused by untreated root residues, unless the patient was given appropriate instructions right after the root fracture. A breach of duty of care is given if extractions in inflamed or decayed areas are performed without previous restoration, if referrals to a specialist are delayed, or antibiotic therapy is not prescribed.

The dentist is not at fault in cases of primary chronic osteomyelitis or inflammatory reactions after correctly performed extractions (performed *lege artis*). Chronic osteomyelitis of the jaw is a rare complication after tooth extractions. Therefore, antibiotic treatment has priority over surgical intervention (Farmand 1984). Even today, in times of increasing antibiotic applications, this clinical diagnosis requires a surgical intervention; 90 % of decortication is relapse-free, compared with only 50 % with curettage (Handschel et al. 1998). All non-vital teeth as well as tooth decay and periodontal disease are classic centers of infection in 80 % of cases of osteomyelitis. Osteomyelitis also may arise from an apical periodontitis.

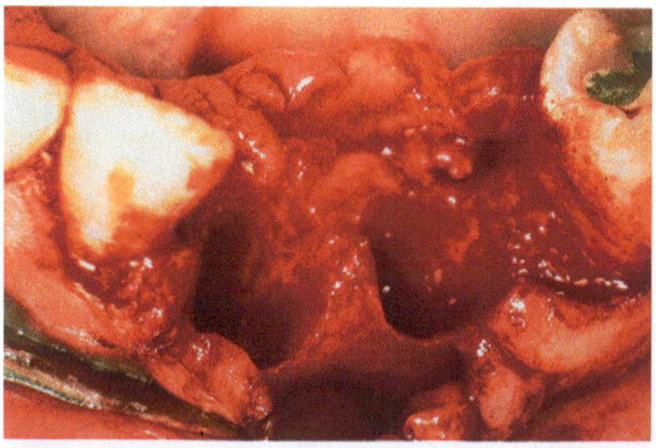

Fig. 15.18 Extraction alveoli of fractured teeth in the mandible

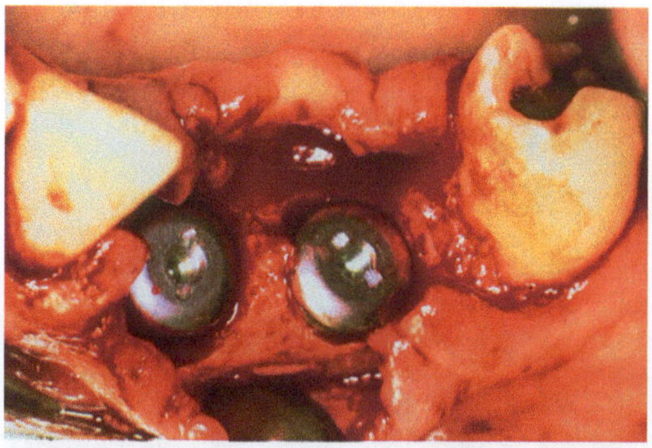

Fig. 15.19 Two FRIALIT-2 implants immediately implanted after trauma (Courtesy of Dr. J. Schiel, Basel)

15.19 Oral Implantology

Initially the placement of implants was in the foreground. Implants have only been placed where the existing bone substance has allowed them to be placed, with compromises regarding the axis direction. Nowadays, techniques for guided bone regeneration in conjunction with simultaneous bone transplantation or replacement materials are used. Bone dehiscences and fenestrations of the implant are accepted and compensated. The long-term prognosis for this procedure is not secured yet, so, in case of doubt, the previous bone transplantation is preferable.

The endosseous implant is the method of choice (safer and more predictable) for the supply of partially edentulous or edentulous jaws (Wolf and Courant 1998). Because of good biocompatibility of pure titanium implants, allergic reactions have not been described thus far (Schiel and Besimo 1997; Spiekermann 1997). The rotationally symmetrical titanium implant allows an osseointegration (Figs. 15.18 and 15.19). The discussion regarding the surface design (smooth surface, titanium plasma-coated sandblasted and etched surface) has not yet been concluded. This does not mean that defects in blade implants would be inherent. The advantage of blade implants is the fact that they even can be used where rotationally symmetrical implants cannot be inserted without extensive augmentation measures. For example, after insertion of disc implants in April 1998 (Fig. 15.20), the extent of vertical bone loss at single disc implants in both the upper and lower jaw was detected after the OPG control in November 1998, caused by insufficient depth of the insertion (Fig. 15.21).

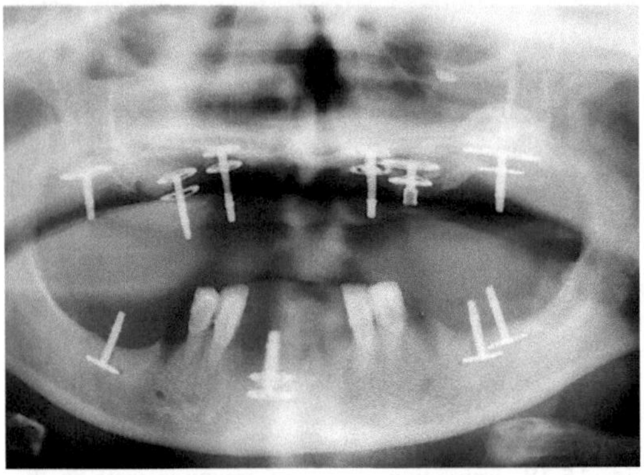

Fig. 15.20 Condition after implantation 4/98 with disc implants

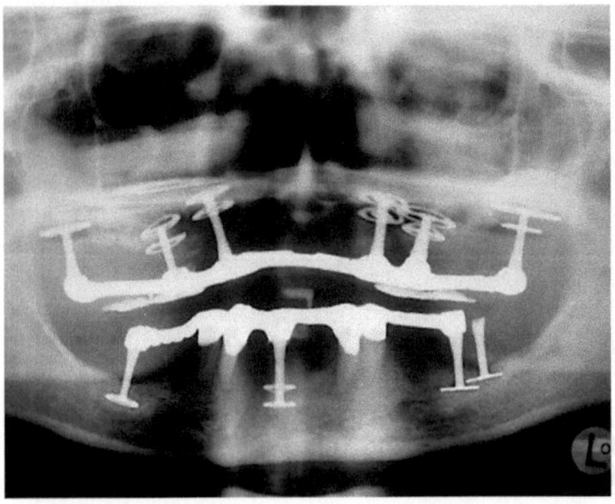

Fig. 15.21 OPG—control 11/98

15.19.1 Preprosthetic Planning

Successful dental implantation is based on precise preoperative findings and diagnoses (Kornas et al. 1998). The assessment of the implant ground by quantity and quality is the most important preoperative decision. Basic parameters are a dental film and/or an orthopantomography with test fixture and plaster models/saw cut, and possibly a mucosal thickness measurement. Preprosthetic planning should always include a clinical and radiological diagnosis and evaluation. The classification of bone quantity and quality is ultimately decisive for a successful implantation.

A topic of discussion is whether open or closed healing has a safer osseointegration and can offer a better connection between the bone and the implant. *OLG Köln, Judgement of the 5th Senate of 25.2.1998, Az. 5 U 157/97* states that "A compensation of Euro 12.5000 was admitted due to a grossly erroneous insertion of a prosthesis (superstructure). In spite of a detectable (X-ray images were taken before the surgery) progressed bone resorption in the edentulous maxilla, the dentist inserted the implants without sufficient bone support."

A lateral skull cephalometric (lateral cephalogram (FRS)) or a so-called mandibular lateral view can be very helpful to estimate the position of the symphysis and the width of the bone tender. Because of the two-dimensional representation of the overlying bone contour and volume, those images are not sufficient to reconstruct an accurate three-dimensional representation (Fuhrmann et al. 1993, 1994).

The computed tomography (CT) diagnosis (so-called dental CT) provides diagnostic information for planning in unprecedented precision and versatility. The metric accuracy of three-dimensional measurement of CT data with the combination Picker CT PQ 2000 with spiral CT option (Picker, Cleveland, Ohio, USA) and ISG Allegro was evaluated (1998) by Kornas et al. to be approximately 0.3 mm for the lower jaw and 0.5 mm for maxillary preparations. The limiting factor is the possibility of intraoperative implementation of diagnostic data.

The main criticisms of CT for use in dental practice (compared with conventional X-ray procedures) are the increased radiation exposure and the greater technical and financial costs (Kornas et al. 1998). Because of the radiation exposure and cost-effectiveness, CT is not a routine investigation and should be limited to marginal indications.

Data from six dental practices (750 patients with a total of 2,346 implants). CT analysis was performed in only 2 % of the cases; of those, a lateral cephalogram was conducted in 5 % and an OPG was conducted in 94 %. Regarding the diagnosis from the prosthetic view, situation models were found only in 35 % of the cases (of which, only 14 % were articulated); surgical guides or wax-ups were made in only 5 % of the cases (Richter 1999).

15.19.2 The Question of Reasonable Medical Necessity of Dental-Implantology Measures

A medical indication is not equivalent to a medically acceptable necessity. A restoration of the functioning of the masticatory system can also be achieved by conventional prosthetic measures. Dental implantology lies between the conflicting priorities of medical needs and medical necessity. Experts for implant-supported dentures are constantly confronted with whether a dental implant treatment is medically indicated or whether necessity has been exceeded.

The use of 14 or more implants in the upper jaw, necessary in many so-called bone-forming measures (within the meaning of sinus lift operations), is justified by the so-called root replacement, where 14–16 teeth per jaw exist in a fully toothed patient. These maximum treatments are justified with regard to the so-called biodynamic beneficial effects, because the implant-supported dentures counteract the physiological bone loss and influence the atrophy of the ridge much better than a mucosa-supported care, for example, in a complete denture.

The most common need for implants is in the atrophic edentulous mandible. The interforamina district provides the most favorable preconditions. The lower jaw (too fine) and several closely spaced implants have a stress-induced fracture risk.

Six, eight, or more implants, together with augmentation measures, may be medically indicated in some patients, but the degree of reasonable medical necessity must be questioned. *LG Wuppertal, Judgement of 23.10.1997, Az. 7-O-492/93* (*Comment*) found that "In the opinion of the court, the health insurance must not bear the cost for an implant treatment of Euro 37.324.-, which is a multiple of the conventional treatment cost."

The following options for the implant supply of an edentulous maxilla or mandible are currently discussed:

- A fixed denture in the maxilla requires up to eight pillars and up to six pillars in the lower jaw
- A removable denture in the upper jaw requires up to six implants and up to four implants in the lower jaw
- The minimum supply of the upper jaw consists of four pillars and two pillars in the lower jaw

Most of the conflicts in view of the number of implants arise during the planning phase. To decide how many pillars at one- or two-sided free-end conditions in the upper and lower jaw are needed, it must be considered that, in each quadrant, six replaced dental units are sufficient for functionality. If teeth 41–43 are existing, two or three implants are sufficient to reach functionality of the 4th quadrant. If tooth 47 and 48 are replaced by implantology, it may exceed the medical necessity, even if medically indicated, due to economic reasons.

15.20 Concerning Private Health Insurance

For reasonableness, the cost is also significant. The cost for implants must not be more than twice as high as for the alternative treatment. To avoid later disputes with the patient and/or the private health insurance, the practitioner must calculate a detailed therapeutic cost schedule prior to treatment.

15.21 Concerning Public Health Insurance

Implant-supported or subsidized supply measures are not covered by the public health insurance. In certain cases, if other generally accepted methods are not available or cannot be used in this particular patient, exemptions may be granted. It should be noted that the treatment contract and the insurance contract are not congruent. The cost of treatment on one hand, and the reimbursement claims after the specifications of the insurance contract, on the other hand, are not congruent. "Prior to an implant treatment the patient must check the scope of his health insurance. It is not the task of the dentist to find out whether the treatment is covered or not."

15.22 Failings and Errors

15.22.1 Failings and Errors in the Planning Phase

Implant planning (interforaminal) in the posterior region of the mandible should always consider the risk of irritation of the *N. mandibularis* or *N. mentalis*. Attention must be paid to the Canalis mandibulae. Basically, there should be a safety distance of 2 mm above the *Canalis mandibulae* because of possible radiographic measurement errors. Furthermore, it should be noted that, in measuring the bone bed/implant bone supporting area, the drill bit goes 0.5- to 1.4-mm deeper than the length of the implant.

The most common errors in planning are made by implanting into areas that are not convenient for prosthesis or the intermaxillary relation was not taken into account, because of lack of model analysis. It should be checked that enough space is existing (in the mesiodistal direction) between the implant and the natural tooth or between the implants. A rule of thumb could be that the smallest gap should be half of the implant diameter. Additionally, a pilot hole can reduce the risk of damaging the adjacent teeth. Contraindications and limitations for surgical procedures must be carefully recorded in the medical history (Wolf and Courant 1998).

15.22.2 System-Specific Causes of Failings

If the expert opinion about the failing has detected system-specific causes, the current state of the art as well as the state of scientific knowledge must be regarded. This applies in particular for the indication of subperiosteal implants, a method used in the 1960s, which can worsen, in case of failing, the situation in the upper or lower jaw.

15.22.3 Indication-Specific Causes of Failings

Endosseous implants are not indicated if, e.g., the implants cannot be inserted in a prosthetic concept. Another indication-specific cause for a failing can be the fact that the available space, both vertically and transversely, is not sufficient for the planned number of endosseous implants. The implants should be completely surrounded by bones (only the periosteal soft tissue is in contact with the implant surface). In forensic disputes concerning fractures in the mandible central region after interforaminal implantation, the discrepancy between the number of implants and the width of the available bone stock was always the cause of the fracture. Five or six holes (to incorporate the appropriate number of endosseous implants) can lead to weakness and inevitable fracture.

15.22.4 Patient-Specific Aspects of Failings

The preparation phase with medical history, indication, selection of patients, and the plans to obtain the best conditions for a successful implantation are essential. If these parameters are not or only partially met, defects and legal consequences are inevitable. Contraindications for endosseous implants are all diseases that also apply to other selective dental, oral, and maxillofacial surgeries. Endosseous implants are contraindicated during immunosuppressive therapy and in insulin-requiring diabetes that is not optimally controlled (values over 200 mg% are a relative contraindication, values above 300 mg% are an absolute contraindication). Another relative contraindication is the lack of motivation for optimal oral hygiene.

15.22.5 Operation-Specific Defects

Because implantology is an elective treatment of plastic and reconstructive surgery, 100 % success is demanded by the patient (Schiel and Besimo 1997). A guarantee for medical success is not possible, but maximum diligence must be granted. The surgeon and the assisting staff must have adequate surgical experience and training, as well as an appropriate infrastructure of the operating room to provide sterile conditions.

Dislocation of implants in the sinus cavity and nerve lesions are the most common causes for forensic arguments. The dislocation of endosseous implants in the sinus cavity during the surgery or within the scope of excavation is always chargeable to the dentist. The dentist is also culpable for leaving dislocated implants or dislocation of teeth or root fragments in the maxillary sinus. A postoperative radiograph is therefore indicated to prove that the implants have been properly inserted. An X-ray prior to the denudation is indicated, because (unnoticed by the patient) implants may drop into the maxillary sinus. The most serious complication in the endosseous implantation is damage to the *N. mandibularis* during the surgery. Usually a faulty treatment, together with errors in planning and implementation, is causal.

In case of malfunction (paresthesia) on the first postoperative day, a dental CT scan is indicated if a panoramic X-ray image is not precise enough. Dental CT diagnosis can be established in three dimensions, whether the implant rises in the *canalis mandibulae* or whether the roof bones of the nerve canal were perforated. The implant must be removed if it has touched the nerve canal (detectable by X-ray image). In this case, a reimplantation or a shorter implant must be discussed. The immediate decompression of the nerve by removing the implant will help to regenerate the nerve. If there is no nerve regeneration within 2 years, a nerve lesion of *N. mandibularis* must be considered (current jurisdiction admits a compensation of 5,000 €). The worst complication after a nerve transplantation is anesthesia dolorosa, with the result that stereotactic operations on the Gasserian ganglion are necessary. In such cases, up to 100,000 € for treatment cost and compensation may be justified.

15.22.6 Behavior After Implant Loss

The patient typically has no claim for reimbursement or reduced treatment cost after the loss of implants. In case of doubt whether the treatment was performed according to the approved rules of implantology, the patient may refer to the arbitration board of the Dental Association (cost-neutral arrangement) or civil jurisdiction.

There are two alternatives in terms of a "goodwill" arrangement:

(a) If the implant is lost within the so-called healing time, most dentists will not charge for the implants or they will reimburse all paid cost. Material cost will either be reimbursed by the manufacturer or must be paid by the patient.
(b) In the few cases of implant loss within healing time, the dentists charge full treatment and material cost, but are willing to perform a reimplantation free of charge.

If there is an implant loss after the prosthetic restoration but a violation against the approved rules of implantology is not provable, the dentist will not be liable for the implant loss.

The most convenient position for implants in the upper jaw is the caninus pillar. In most cases, there is sufficient bone structure for dental implants, often for the first premolars. The residual maxillary sinus is only a thin bony contour, especially with advanced atrophy. For implant restoration supply, the posterior region of the upper jaw still is a problematic area (Hürzeler 1996).

The so-called sinus lift procedure consists of anchoring the lateral implants in a bone graft (bone by bone grafting). This must usually be performed in two stages, because the implant fixation is not stable through the graft in the alveolar bone. The sinus lift procedure involves a risk of sinusitis. Because the alveolar process is not increased, the subsequent prosthetic teeth may be extended. If there is not enough material for jawbone augmentation, the bone graft must be gathered from bone reserves in the body, e.g., from the iliac crest (stationary treatment is necessary). Larger bone removal in the chin area may cause changes in facial profile and disturbances of the innervation of the lips.

The direct functional connection between bone and implant surface is known as osseointegration or ankylosis. At the worst, the foreign body cuts into connective tissue and leads to implant loss. Guided bone regeneration through membranes is currently not scientifically accepted as a treatment method (Strietzel 1998). The interval function of absorbable materials, the complexity and dynamics of the processes occurring in the controlled bone regeneration, the process of resorption of the membrane and its fixing aids, and the osteoconduction in the application of appropriate augmentation and osseointegration have not been evaluated, nor have the prediction for the long-term preservation and long-term viability of regenerated tissue or whether the regenerated bone really offers the possibility of osseointegration of the implants (Strietzel 1998).

The immediate prosthetic structure has been proven with good results but only in the regions of the *mandible interforaminalis* with four splinted implants. The healing time for implants varies, 2–6 months in all regions, 4 months for mandible, and 6 months for upper jaw. For simultaneous sinus floor augmentation with implants, a longer healing time (8–9 months) seems reasonable.

There is no doubt that augmentation measures are complicated and require a high degree of surgical skill. Until today, there has been no long-term prognosis for augmented bone compared with the local bone. Furthermore, it is unclear which augmentation material might be used (beside autologous bone). Recommended materials for bone substitute are hydroxyapatite ceramics and decalcified freeze-dried bone. However, all of these materials are still in the experimental stage.

The implant loss rate with scientifically accepted implant systems during the healing period is under 2 % (Spiekermann 1997). Endosseous implantation for restoration of a fixed single tooth replacement or as a retainer for removable reconstruction in tooth loss has increased in importance. Nevertheless, implants may not be used to stabilize periodontally involved teeth.

During recent years, orthodontic considerations (for edentulous patients) were included in the prosthetic implantology. The complex displacement of teeth usually is not promising, because these gaps do not have a sufficient ground for implants. To prevent defects, these measures should always be performed very defensively and with great expertise. Appropriate alternatives should be discussed (Steinhilber 1997).

15.23 Prosthetics

15.23.1 Crowns and Bridges

The pretreatment for a crown includes surgical, restorative, and periodontal rehabilitation, a sensitivity test, and a radiological control of the abutment teeth. This prognosis should be foreseeable for several years, because (premature) loss of teeth with crowns and bridges always requires replacement. In cases of doubtful prognosis, temporary crown and bridge restorations are indicated. Nonvital, successfully treated teeth should be supplied with a core-build stump to ensure sufficient retention for the crown. In the upper jaw, a 14-membered bridge can be used; in the lower jaw, a 5-membered bridge should not be exceeded because of functional-related deformation.

Each dentin preparation of a vital tooth can traumatize the pulpa (the deeper the preparation, the higher the risk). Another important traumatogenic factor is the heat generation during preparation (depending on speed, contact pressure, nature, and structure of the cutting surfaces and the geometry of the preparation instrument). Rotary instruments may not exceed the maximum speed.

- The amount of cooling water should be greater than 50 ml/min. If rotary instruments have a diameter of 1.8 mm (ISO 018) or a total length of >19 mm, additional water cooling or spray cooling is required. A rule of thumb is that the active instrument parts and preferably also the tooth must be completely wetted by the cooling medium.
- Improper selection and application of preparation instruments (for example roughness, diamond coating (>ISO 524) and/or diameters over 1.4 mm) may result in dentin destruction. Furthermore, excessive roughness (>30 mm) may be produced, enamel rods may be broken, or adjacent teeth may be damaged. By applying oscillating diamond instruments in the contact area, a violation of the neighboring teeth can be avoided:
  - Adjacent teeth must be protected, e.g., by Matrix.

  - All preparation margins must be reworked with smoothing instruments.
  - A rule of thumb for the minimum thickness of dentin (in crowning) is 0.7 mm at narrow tubules and 1.4 mm at wide tubules.
  - The circular stump walls should have a convergence angle of 6–12°, so that crown and bridge anchors have sufficient adhesion and loosening can be avoided.
- The possible size of the marginal gap ranges from 50 μm (in some areas of the crown margin) to 300 μm. The width should not exceed 100 μm. The final crown margin is a key criterion; the wider the marginal gap, the higher the risk of carious lesions and periodontal damage.
- Temporary cementing is recommended to allow subsequent corrections before the partial or total reconstruction of the occlusion (or ceramic parts).
- Full-ceramic parts cannot be provisionally cemented.
- In courses without complications, crowns and bridges may be finally cemented immediately after the trial period (Wichmann 1999).

Manufacturers of work equipment for tooth structure preparation (class IIa) must have a declaration of conformity to ensure clinical examination and scientific documentation (CE marking). Additionally, a risk analysis and a detailed instruction sheet are compulsory (*European Directive 93/42/EEC, based on German medical devices Act of 1 January 1995*).

15.23.1.1 Disinfection of Dental Impressions

Asepsis is of essential importance, not only in view of the HI virus. Many germs can be washed off under running water. Nevertheless, a number of pathogenic bacteria remain viable and fertile, therefore, routine disinfection is mandatory.

15.23.1.2 Dimensional Stability of Disinfected Impressions

There are concerns that disinfection may influence the accuracy or the quality of the impression. Not all disinfection methods are suitable for dental impressions, especially for hydrocolloid impression materials (which have a high water content). However, because alginates are not designed for precision impressions, the accuracy requirements are not as high as for elastomers. Additionally, alginate impressions can be disinfected, even if a swelling leads to larger, but negligible dimensional changes. Solutions of 2 % glutaraldehyde are suitable for all material groups. Alginate impressions should not stay longer than 10 s in 2 % glutaraldehyde solution and no longer than 5 min in a closed vessel (Hygrophor) for rinsing.

15.24 Prosthetics from the View of Medical Malpractice – Assessment

In an evaluation of 121 clinical expert reports about prosthetic treatments that led to legal disputes (from West German Jaw Clinic Center for Dental, Oral and Maxillofacial Surgery, Heinrich-Heine-University Düsseldorf, 1970 to 1992), 18.2 % of the cases were free of defects, in 23.1 %, minor deficiencies were found, and 50.4 % had serious failings. In 15 of 20 cases where medical malpractice was detected, a treatment with fixed dentures had been previously performed (Diedrichs et al. 1990). The analysis of 67 completed liability cases (from District Court Frankfurt/Main from 1990–1995) showed that the focus was on denture treatments.

Possible causes for the increasing number of liability claims against dentists may be the great cost of prosthetic restorative treatments and also the high expectations of the patients as well as the performance of risky treatments without sufficient diligence, e.g., an abrasive trauma with loss of the pulp after the bridge work or by incorrect recording of the bite. The triggering factor on the patient side may be the unintended error that a prosthetic supply must lead to a full compensation of the restrictions because of tooth defects or tooth loss.

The increasing number of such conflicts will lead to growing importance of science-based expert opinion for legal disputes because the judges can hardly solve these cases without the support of the expert (Gümpel 1980).

15.25 Gnathology

The determination of the jaw relation (gnathology) represents a complex of methods to avoid or eliminate so-far tolerated inaccuracies in dental procedures. Risk-prone procedures or single steps of the gnathological analysis must be assessed from the legal point that diagnostic measures may not increase the already inherent "risk propensity."

The clinical and instrumental function analysis is considered as a scientifically valid diagnostic procedure. With its help, the dysfunction of the orofacial system is recorded in order to draw conclusions for the therapeutic function restoration. Without the functional analysis, the diagnosis and treatment of functional disorders and diseases is not possible.

The results (initial and final findings) should be documented on an inquiry (e.g., clinical functional status of German Society for Dental, Oral, and Maxillofacial Surgery (DGZMK)), as well as the functional analysis measures. Furthermore, the articulator-mounted upper and lower jaw models and possibly the movement records should be available (Freesmeyer et al. 1999). *OLG Koblenz, Judgement, Az. 3 U 806/79*; *LG Koblenz, Judgement of 06.01.1981, Az. 10 0 201/77* states that "A compensation of EURO 3,000.- was admitted for the insertion of a faulty bridge, which had no bite function and caused sibilants and articulation problems."

15.26 Orthodontics

Günter Seifert

This section is more detailed than the other sections regarding treatment risks because orthodontics is a very specific area of dentistry, where orthodontists act, but also general dentists act who do have not enough detailed knowledge and do not recognize possible late effects.

In orthodontics, a lack of information about caries susceptibility during a multiband treatment leads to liability claims, as well as errors in diagnosis and therapy (Alfter 1997; Seifert 1997). Compared with regular dental measures, orthodontic treatments seem to be fraught with a very low risk for treatment incidents. In order to capture the incident frequency, a nationwide survey of 1,500 orthodontists was conducted in 1995, and 338 questionnaires were evaluated.

Injuries caused by removable orthodontic devices are negligible. Although they occur in large numbers (in 49.8 % of the 338 cases, which is a total of 268), they mostly cause only minor injuries. Fixed devices have a higher risk of injuries. A total of 282 cases (88.5 %) was observed (22 cases with headgear). Headgear may cause rare but serious injuries of the eyes, one of those cases even led to the loss of the eye.

In 58 % of the 338 practices, allergic reactions during treatment were reported. A suspected nickel allergy in two cases caused acute respiratory distress. Overall, the suspected diagnosis of an allergy must be carefully assessed, because it often leads to eczematous skin lesions.

Suspected inhalation of a foreign body during treatment occurred in 18 cases and outside the treatment in 13 cases. Despite the relatively low frequency of inhaling, this is a serious hazard, especially because of the associated complications and its invasive therapeutic treatment. In 11 cases, the foreign body had to be removed by bronchoscopy. Brackets were inhaled in five cases and pieces of wire in four cases.

Swallowed foreign bodies were reported more frequently (174 during and 75 outside of the treatment). Complications occurred in five cases, in one case, the foreign body had to be endoscopically removed.

Vitality loss of teeth during orthodontic treatment was described in 139 cases, the cause could not clearly be identified, and, therefore, a connection with orthodontic treatment is not proven. Vitality loss in the upper incisors was described in 92 cases; in the lower anterior, in 12 cases. Three cases were reported in the lateral tooth area (both upper and lower jaw).

Thirty-two medical malpractice trials were reported. The main reasons for those disputes were root resorption ($n=6$), periodontal diseases ($n=5$), decalcification or caries ($n=3$), and incorrect extractions ($n=2$). In one case, the treating orthodontist was sued by a patient because the orthodontist had inflicted an iatrogenic injury.

Incidents as part of the orthodontic treatment cannot be excluded. According to the parties, some of the incidents could have been avoided by better protection. Both dentist and patient benefit from a maximum of care during the treatment as well as from an extensive communication between orthodontist and dentist (Alfter 1997).

Errors in orthodontic treatments result in health and financial damages for the patient as well as forensic consequences for the dentist. Most of those errors arise during the following stages of treatment (Seifert 1997):

1. Preventive orthodontics
   (a) Education about oral hygiene, nutrition, fluoridation
   (b) Conservation of deciduous teeth
   (c) Relief of dysfunctions
   (d) Setting the correct breathing
   (e) Inserting placeholders
   (f) Interceptive orthodontics
   (g) Control of the dentition
   (h) Transfer of cross-bite
   (i) Trauma prevention
   (j) Myofunctional treatment
2. Corrective orthodontics
   (a) Introductory treatment – correction or improvement of skeletal abnormalities
   (b) Main treatment – fine tuning of occlusion and articulation
3. Retention treatment
4. Relapse treatment

ad 1. Many preventable dental deformities occur in the first phase of treatment of early loss of deciduous teeth, if no placeholder is used. The problem occurs especially during premature loss of deciduous teeth in a limited space of the permanent teeth. Crowding of the permanent teeth dissolves into the vacated space, leading to tooth misalignment, which can only be corrected with great effort.

Worst are the following consequences of premature loss of deciduous teeth:

1. At the loss of the second deciduous molars, the first permanent molars migrate mesially to the upper jaw, where they tilt and rotate (Figs. 15.22 and 15.23). In addition to this displacement of the molars, there is an intermaxillar mistoothing and retention of the second premolar (Fig. 15.24).

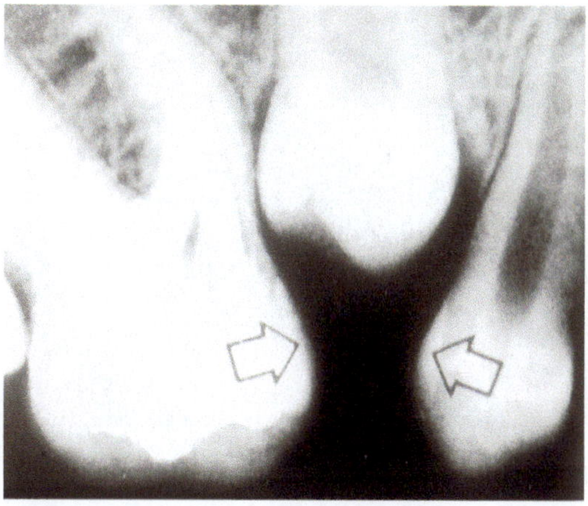

Fig. 15.22 Loss of tooth 55 (X-ray image). Episodes: leading 16, retention 15

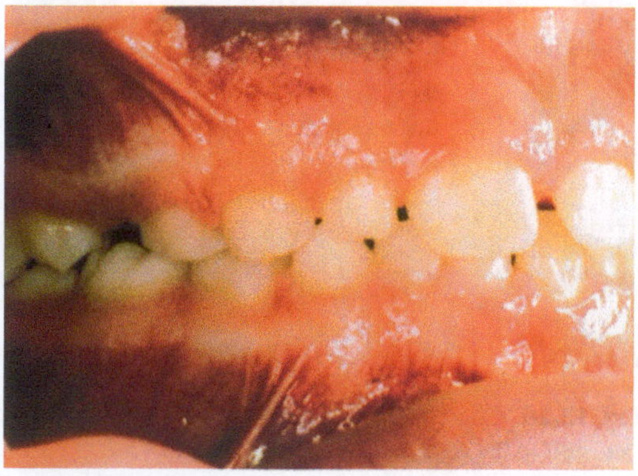

Fig. 15.23 Distal occlusion of teeth 16 and 46

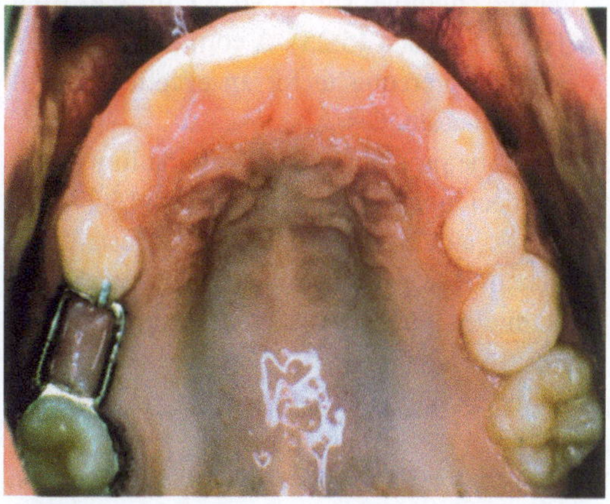

Fig. 15.24 Placeholder for tooth 15, gap opening

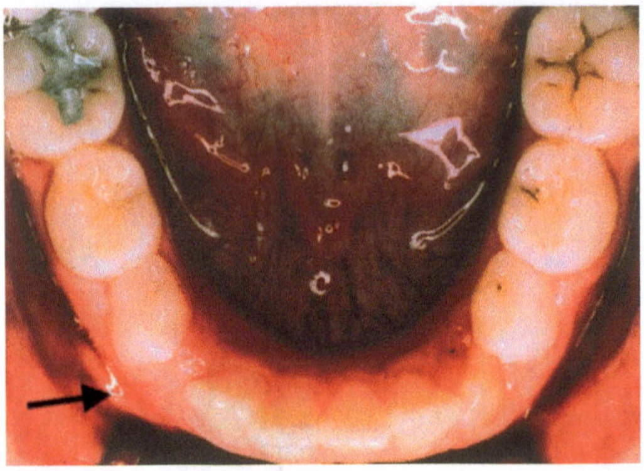

Fig. 15.25 Early loss of tooth 83 (*arrow*)

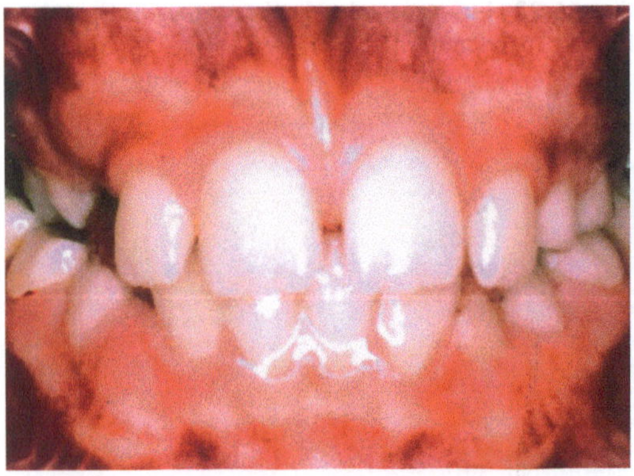

Fig. 15.26 Consequences of early loss of tooth 83: midline shift to the right, loss of space for tooth 43

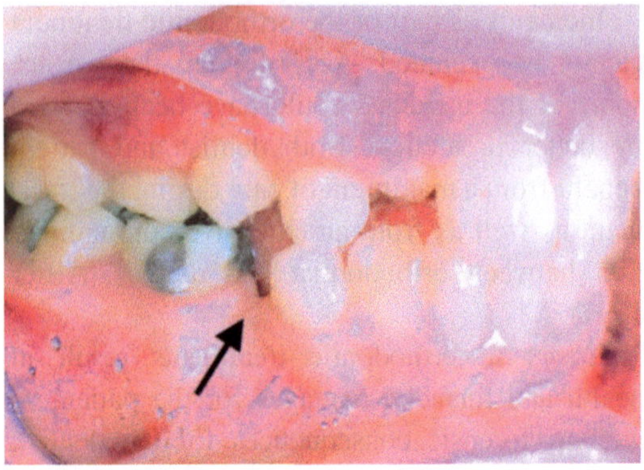

Fig. 15.27 Early loss of tooth 84 with crowding in the lower anterior region (*arrow*)

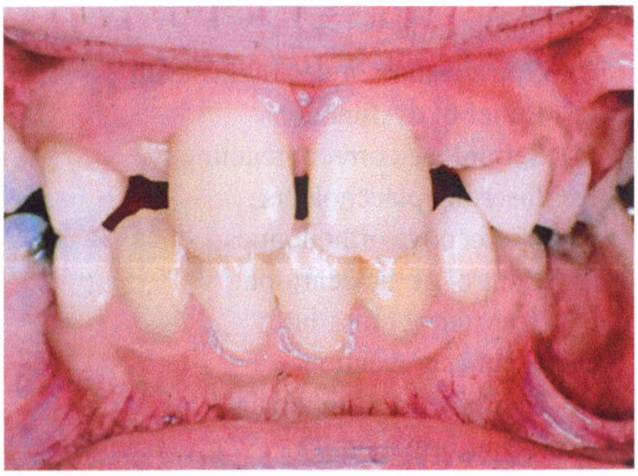

Fig. 15.28 Consequences of early loss of tooth 84: distal migration of tooth 83, gap narrowing of tooth 44, retention of tooth 44, and midline shift of the front

2. At the loss of the deciduous canine, there is a marked midline shift (MLV) of the front (Figs. 15.24 and 15.25). A correct center is an essential prerequisite for an excellent occlusion and aesthetics.
3. The same problem occurs with the loss of the first deciduous molar (Figs. 15.26, 15.27, and 15.28), although it might be suggested that such a vigorous deciduous tooth is preventing the midline shift toward the resulting gap.

ad 2. During the interception phase, errors are primarily committed in the dentition, i.e., lacking intervention at the change of teeth:

1. Persistent deciduous teeth and root remain and are not removed in time and lead to the retention or faulty eruption of the permanent teeth.
2. Often, the planned exchange of space between the permanent canine and second premolar (especially in the upper jaw) is absent and must be performed by dentist in order to prevent difficult correctable deformities (Figs. 15.29 and 15.30):

   The upper molar moves mesially in a distal occlusion and takes the space that is provided for the permanent canine (Fig. 15.31).

   The canine breaks (rotating because of lack of space or labial or palatal deformity (Fig. 15.32).

   Because of lack of space, a retention and relocation of the canine occurs with the risk of cyst formation and root resorption of the lateral incisor.
3. Eruption barriers such as cysts, odontoma, and supernumerary tooth germs are not detected and removed in a timely manner, leading to the retention of the permanent teeth (Figs. 15.33 and 15.34).

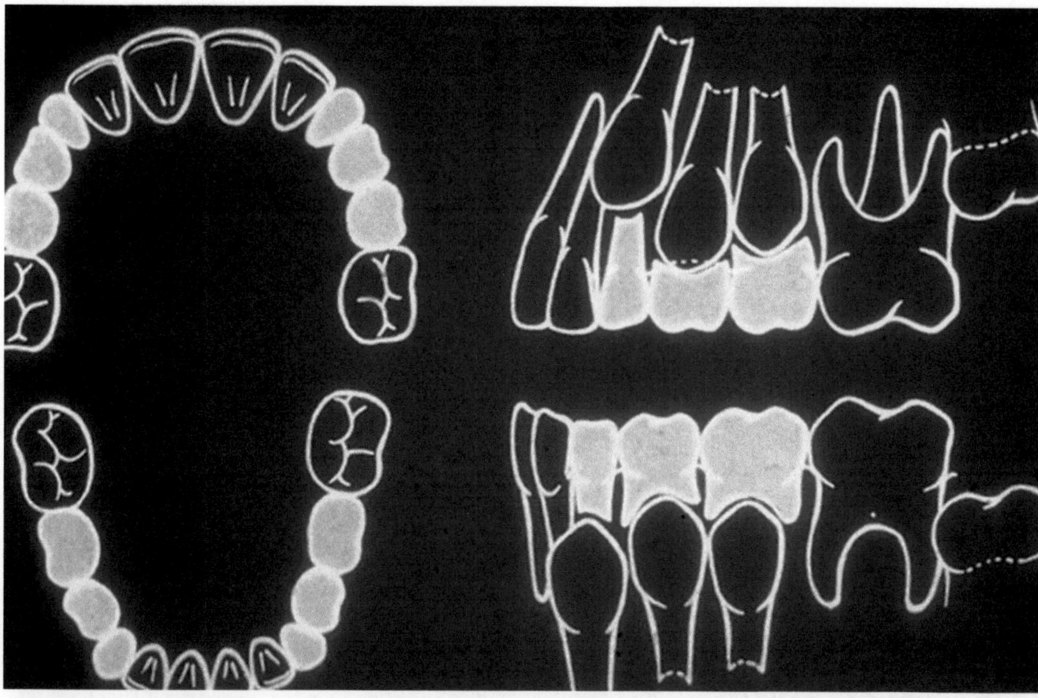

Fig. 15.29 The control of tooth loss in the dental side area is of great significance for correct occlusion

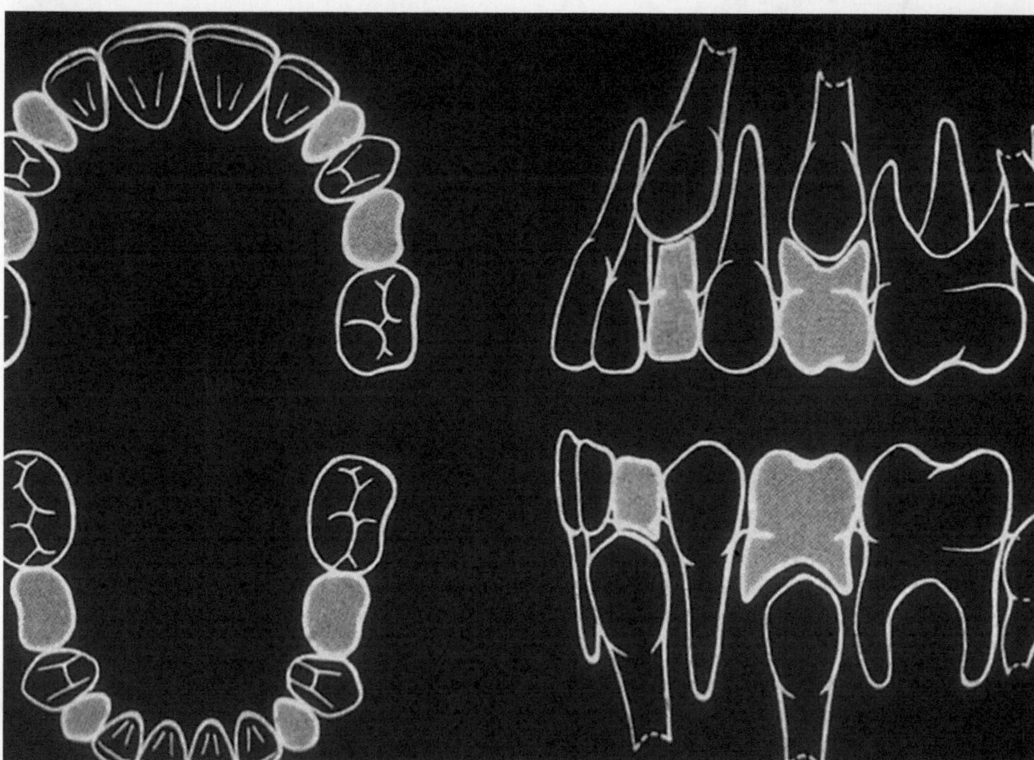

Fig. 15.30 The space is not replaceable. The canine erupts in the wrong position

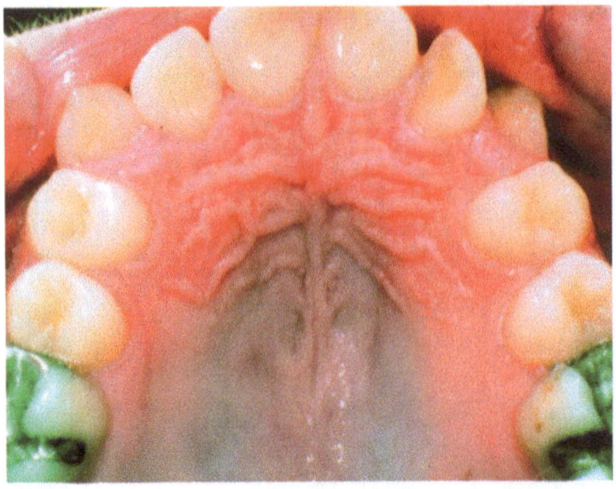

Fig. 15.31 Forward line of left and right posterior region cause by an early loss of teeth 55 and 65

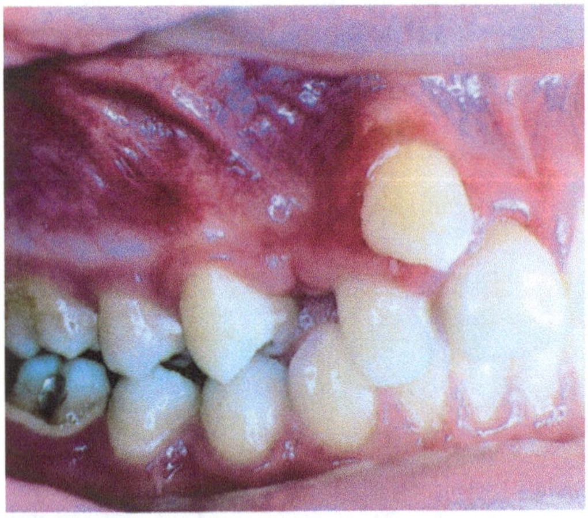

Fig. 15.32 Lack of space for teeth 13 and 23 with buccal cutting as a result of the forward line in the posterior region

4. Ankylotic milk teeth, mostly the first or second molars, are not recognized as a danger and, therefore, not removed (Fig. 15.35).

   The permanent teeth cannot cut. The neighboring teeth grow together over the ankylotic milk teeth in the wrong position (Fig. 15.36).
5. Cross-bites are usually detected and corrected in an early stage. However, in this case, a time delay causes no significant damage. An exception is a cross-bite overloaded compulsive lower front tooth that can react with a labial gingival recession and cause corresponding bone loss.

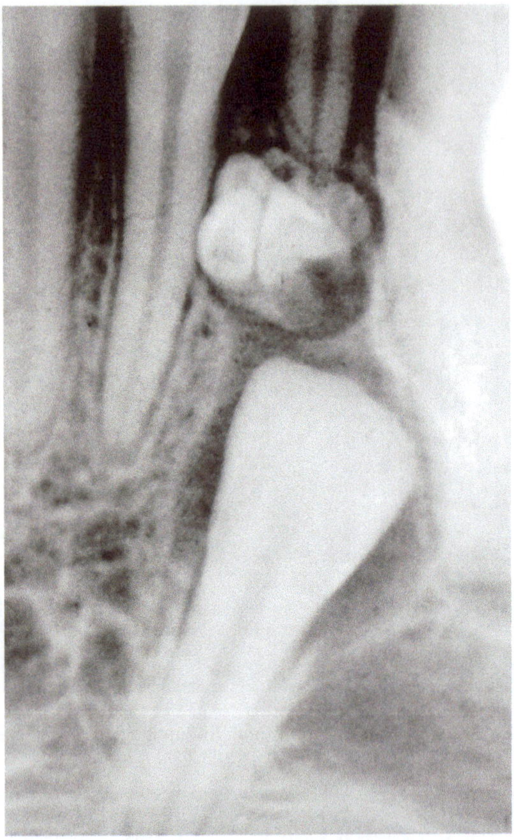

Fig. 15.33 Odontoma prevents the eruption of tooth 32

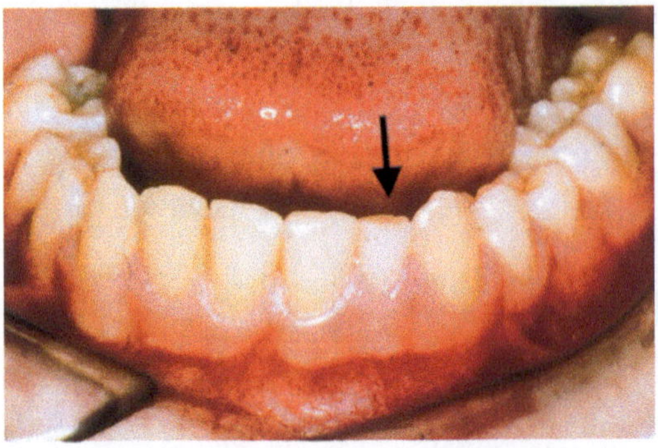

Fig. 15.34 Because of the size difference between tooth 72 (*arrow*) and tooth 32, it is difficult to identify tooth 32 in the classified row

This misconduct causes the following damages:

(a) In eugnathic dentures without actually need of any treatment, malocclusions occur that require a complex and costly treatment.

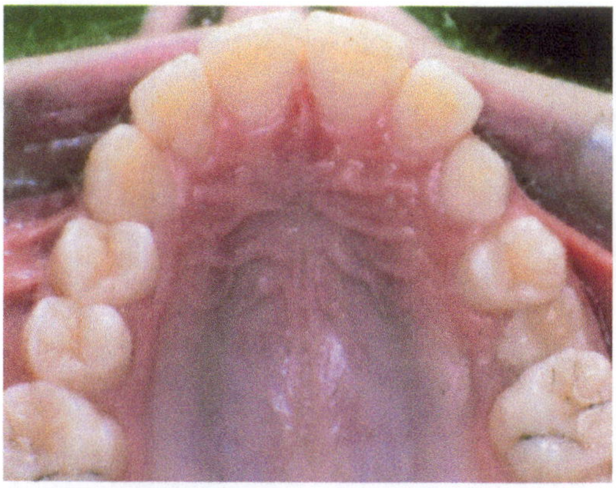

Fig. 15.35 Ankylosis of tooth 65. Because of delayed removal, teeth 24 and 26 grow together in deformity over tooth 65

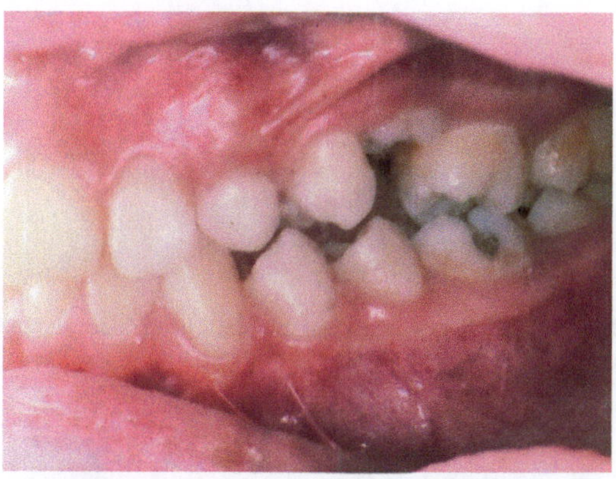

Fig. 15.36 Misalignment of tooth and retention of tooth 25 as a result of a not timely removal of tooth 65

(b) In patients with tooth and jaw misalignment, additional dislocations occur that complicate and prolong the correction of the initial anomaly.

Mistakes made in these two phases of treatment are based less on special orthodontic expertise than in dental–orthodontic action, as in the following context:

1. During training, the significance of this simple but crucial necessity of treatment is neglected.
2. The treatment options are not taken seriously because the dentist is not aware of the consequences and thinks they can be corrected at a later time without major problems.

The consequences for the patient are iatrogenic dental malocclusion. It must be clarified in what way this might have forensic consequences.

15.26.1 Errors in the Initial Treatment

The most common abnormality in orthodontics is malocclusion (distal bites), the so-called Angle $Kl.II_1$ and $Kl.II_2$. This distal occlusion describes a false toothing in the sagittal plane, which can be combined with different basal anomalies. For many orthodontists, the correction of malocclusion is in the foreground. Because they do not observe any other skeletal variations, growth direction, and growth potential, this leads to inappropriate treatment that fails in the orthodontic goal of ideal function and aesthetics.

The distal occlusion can be combined in the sagittal plane with a distal, neutral, or low mesial and in the vertical plane with a deep, neutral, or open jaw relationship. These anomaly types can have large, low, or no growth potential and be combined with a favorable or unfavorable growth direction of the upper and lower jaw. The treatment depends on the combination form of these anomalies.

The most common and important treatment errors are:

1. The distal occlusion is associated with a large skeletal deviation in the sagittal plane (ANB angle >6°) with low or no growth potential. In this case, functional (orthodontic device (KFO)) equipment (as commonly used for correction of malocclusion) is contraindicated.This fault mostly arises from the fact that the patient is referred too late after the main growth phase. In girls, this may already be the age of 12–13 years (Figs. 15.37, 15.38 and 15.39). After this date, the anomaly should be orthodontically/orthognathically treated. Nevertheless, there are dental attempts to compensate this jaw deformity that lead to the following disadvantages:

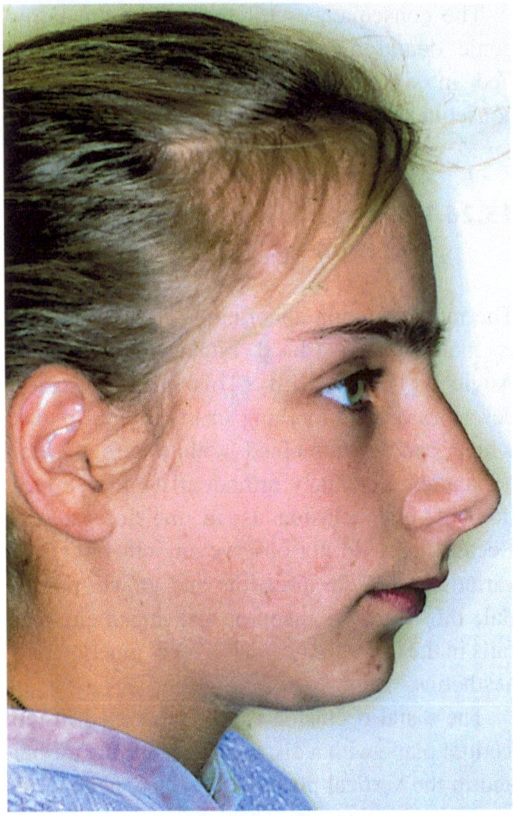

Fig. 15.37 Fourteen-year-old girl with severe retrognathic position of the mandible

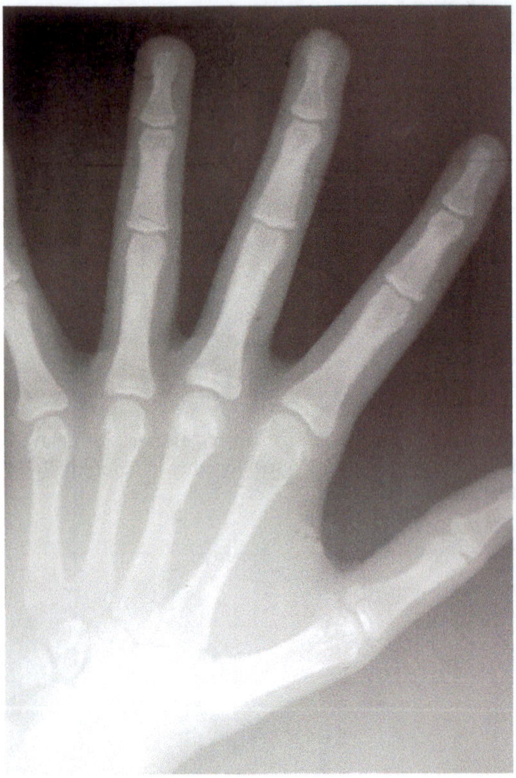

Fig. 15.38 X-ray image of the left hand side shows closed growth

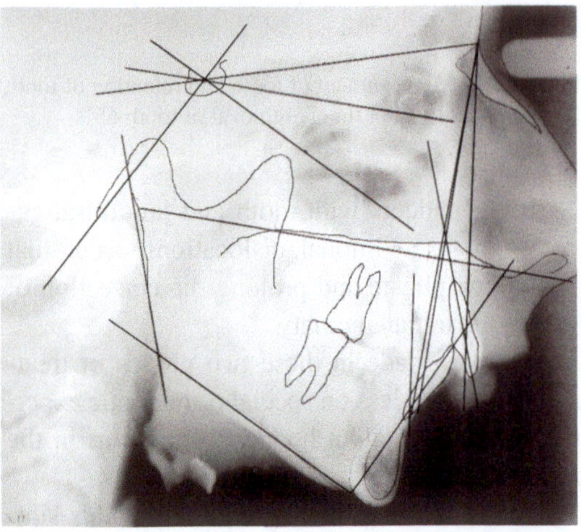

Fig. 15.39 Lateral cephalogram for cephalometric analysis

- No skeletal improvement
- Too steep upper jaw front
- Large nasolabial angle
- Large nose profile
- Excessively protruded lower jaw; front improper frontal load
- Risk of relapse

2. The distal occlusion is associated with a tendency for mesial (progenic) (Class III) jaw relationship (ANB angle <1°). At the same time, there is a large potential for growth of the mandible in front with a positive growth direction.In this case, the insertion of a functional orthopedic appliance for the correction of malocclusion (distal bite) can have serious consequences, developed by a mandibular prognathism, which must be surgically corrected after the completion of growth.
3. The distal occlusion is associated with an open jaw relation, which is compensated by a normal anterior overbite. Moderate growth in an unfavorable direction of growth is connected with a large growth potential. The

insertion of an orthodontic device (KFO) or of a cervical headgear for the correction of distal occlusion leads to unwanted extrusion of the posterior region. Combined with unfavorable growth direction, this results in the posterior rotation of the mandible, deterioration of the open basal relation, and the emergence of an anterior open bite. This deterioration of function and aesthetics requires difficult and expensive treatment.
4. A lateral cross-bite is associated with a narrow frontal overbite, an open jaw relationship, and an unfavorable direction of growth.

If a normal maxillary expansion plate without side jig and without occipital headgear is used, it leads (caused by the buccal tip of the side teeth) to hanging palatal cusps of the molars. This leads, in addition, to dysfunction in the posterior region, to an open front bite.

In addition to the Class III malocclusion, this represents a particular problem, because the growth potential of the lower jaw is not predictable and also not able to be inhibited. In patients with a poor prognosis (poor previous medical history, predental compensated front teeth, relatively large skeletal deviation), lengthy treatments must not be performed.

In no case is the extraction of teeth in the lower jaw without space problems allowed with the intent to inhibit the mandibular growth or to transfer the lower front of the cross-bite. Another presurgical treatment (for decompensation with gap opening) and a surgical correction of the anomaly after the completion of growth would be the inevitable consequence.

15.26.2 Errors and Complications in the Main Treatment

The main treatment, i.e., the fine adjustment of occlusion and articulation using the multiband treatment, is extremely error prone, whereby these technical errors are easily detectable and correctable. Worse are the complications such as damage to the tooth structure and to the periodontium with inadequate dental care, especially the root resorption to the upper front teeth and the

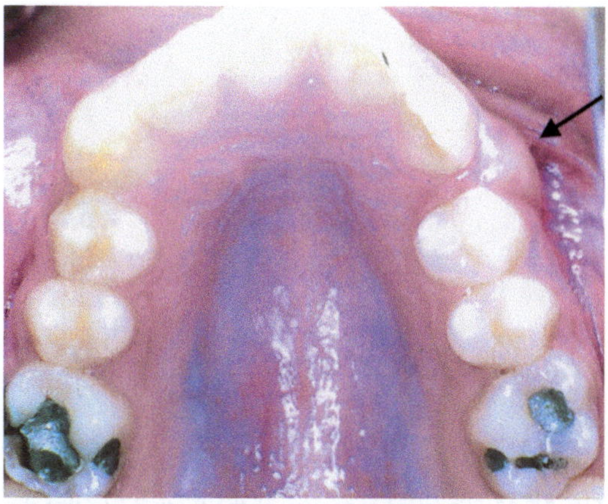

Fig. 15.40 Consequences from late referral: complete lack of space for tooth 23 (*arrow*) with retention of the left posterior region by the midline shift to the left

anchorage loss after tooth extractions in case of inadequate anchorage. Forensic consequences may result if the orthodontist cannot prove the fulfillment of appropriate information.

15.26.3 Errors in Treatment of Special Cases

15.26.3.1 Errors in the Setting of the Canine Tooth

Beside the first molars, the canine is the most important tooth in human dentition. As a solid pillar on the transition from the front to the posterior region, it has a crucial functional role as well as a significant role for facial aesthetics in the nasolabial fold. The canine problem is a prime example of prophylactic thinking and acting. Because of its long eruption path (so-called "eye tooth") and the greater diversity between the milk and permanent canine, appropriate intervention is absolutely indicated. Unfortunately, orthodontic treatment often starts too late, because dentists await the eruption of all teeth; however, by this time, 2–3 mm space for the canine may already be missing (Fig. 15.40). This late referral may have legal consequences. To what extent failure of a dentist can be concluded in this unique technical consulting situation must be proven.

The entire posterior area must be distalized to open the gap for the canine. This task can only be

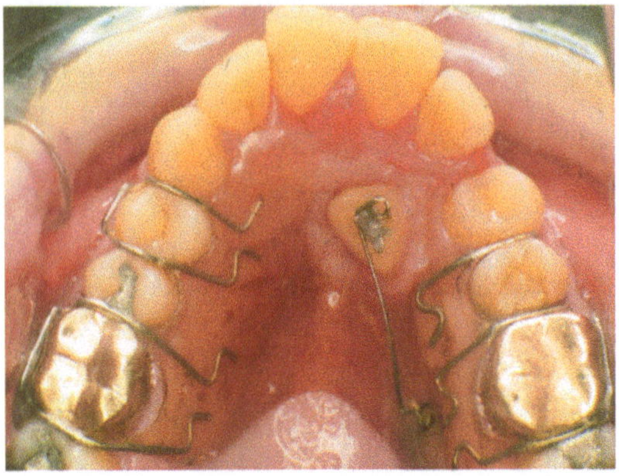

Fig. 15.41 Surgical exposure of the tooth 23 to test the mobility

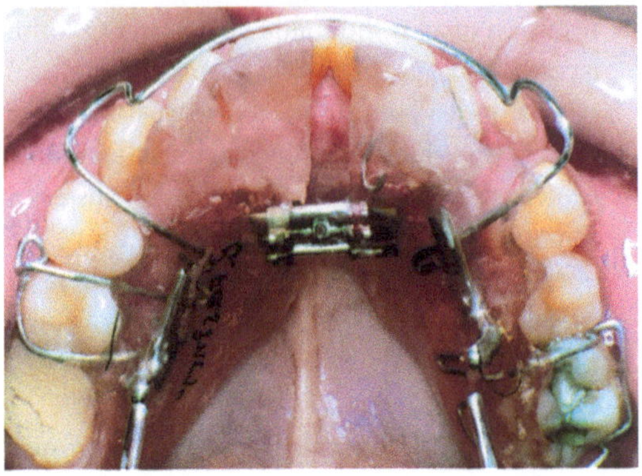

Fig. 15.42 A maxillary expansion plate is contraindicated for the complete opening of the canines, as well as in the position of a lateral cross-bite in open bite

solved by a maximum of cooperation of the patient and by help of the headgear, eventually by extraction of two or four premolars and a complete multiband treatment. During surgical exposure, errors may occur because of lack of cooperation between orthodontists and oral surgeons. Too much attached gingiva that is necessary for a good periodontal closure of the canine may be excised. The same applies for removal of too much of the alveolar bone. The neck region of the canine tooth may be damaged. The roots of adjacent teeth may be injured. Since the introduction of the bonding technique, the latter complication can be minimized, in contrast to the technique of circumferential wiring. It is an obvious gross negligence if the bracket is glued to the apex of the tooth instead of to the crown.

Especially in treatment of adults, whether the tooth can be adjusted or whether it is ankylosed must be checked (after surgical exposure) before starting a costly orthodontic treatment (Fig. 15.41). A seemingly correct treatment can also cause substantial damage, as in this example. The upper canine shows a residual tendency. The gap is closed and cannot be orthodontically opened. For this reason, the first premolar is usually extracted to set the impacted canine. One fatal disastrous might be that the canine deviates from its eruption path and absorbs the root of the lateral incisor. Thus, the patient loses two healthy teeth.

The gap that was created by the extraction of the first premolar is closed by the mesial migration of the first molar and second premolar. Again, the extraction was in vain. The premolar may only be extracted if it is assured that the canine is adjustable and was pulled from the root area of the lateral incisor to avoid root resorption. The gap created by the extraction of the first premolar must be kept open using a placeholder or at least must be frequently controlled.

Another serious error may arise from opening the gap for the canine, which is a sagittal, and not, as often mistakenly assumed, a transversal problem. A gap for the canine must therefore be opened by mesially and distally moving adjacent teeth. This cannot be achieved by using a transversely acting expansion plate (Fig. 15.42).

15.27 Errors in Extractions and Nonindicated Extractions

1. Indicated extraction: If an extraction is indicated, but the dentist tries to solve this problem without performing an extraction, the result is usually a bimaxillary protrusion of the front teeth with an unaesthetic lip profile, adverse loads of the front teeth, and a gingival recession with a high relapse rate (Figs. 15.43 and 15.44).
2. Nonindicated extraction: If an extraction is conducted but not indicated, or at hypodontia, the gaps are closed without lack of space, they can reopen. The result is a so-called grandmother profile with receding lips

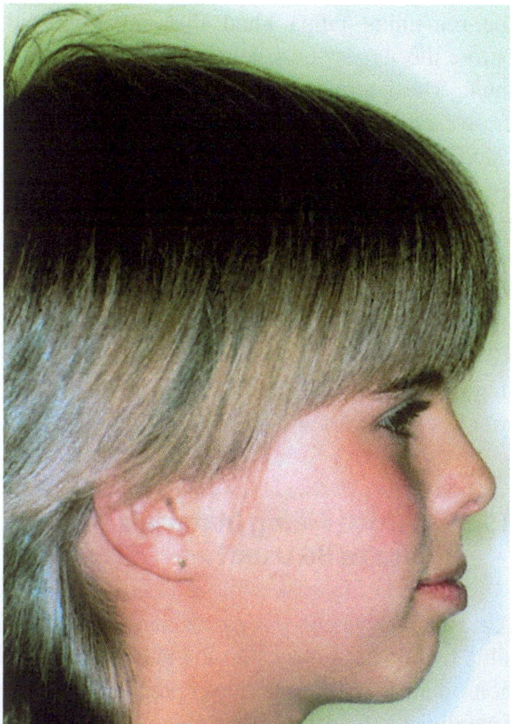

Fig. 15.43 Extraction case treated as non-extraction

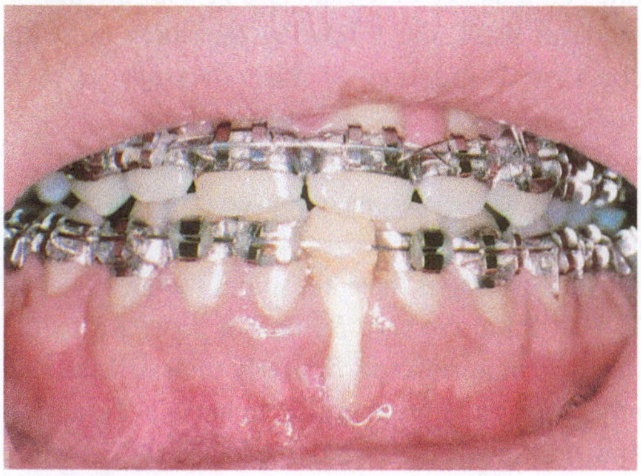

Fig. 15.44 Gingiva recession as a result of non-extraction

(Fig. 15.45). In few cases, the gaps must be reopened and fitted with a prosthesis.

3. Indicated extractions: Often the gaps in the upper jaw are partially closed from the wrong side, which leads to an anchorage loss. Consequently, the space problem is not solved. The sagittal step remains and the teeth are unfailingly extracted (Figs. 15.46 and 15.47).

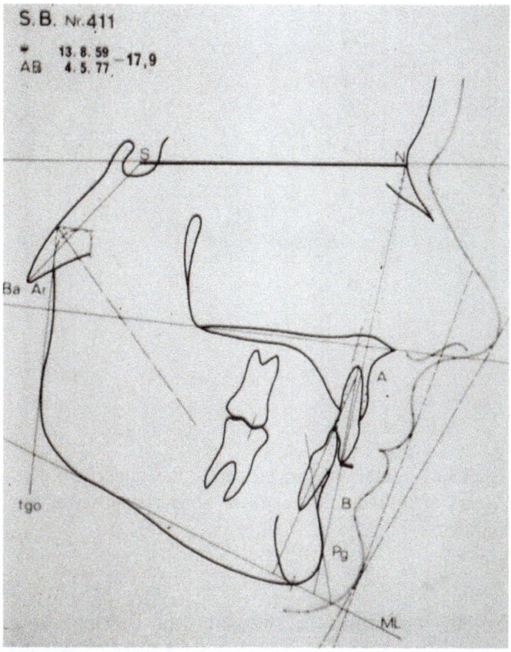

Fig. 15.45 Non-extraction case was treated as an extraction case with the consequence of a retruded front (concave lip profile)

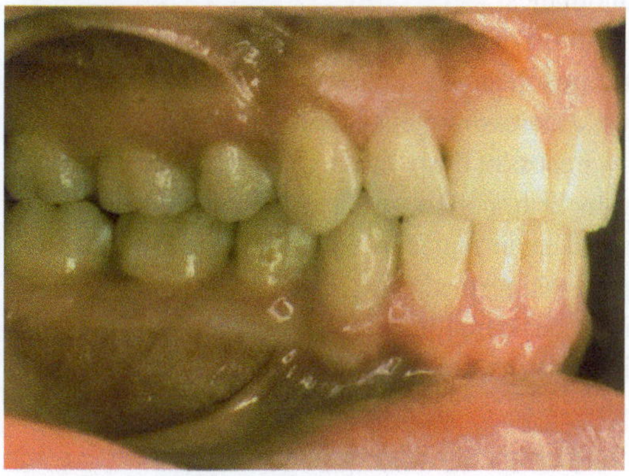

Fig. 15.46 Retruded front in a non-extraction case, treated as extraction case (concave lip profile)

In these three cases, a claim for compensation is justified (Seifert 1997).

15.28 Combination of Orthodontic and Surgical Treatment

Orthodontic surgery has now reached a high level and become an essential part of the orthodontic treatment in adult patients. From a certain size of

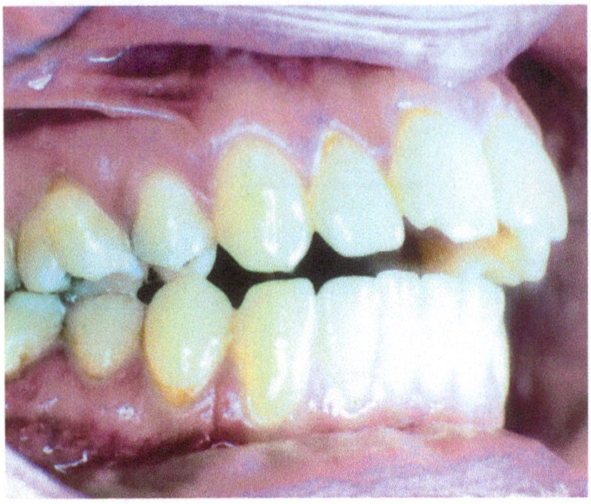

Fig. 15.47 Total anchorage loss in the upper jaw after 3 years of orthodontic treatment with extraction of two premolars

skeletal deviation in the sagittal, vertical, and transverse planes, a reasonable dental treatment is not possible. The object of orthodontic treatment—optimal in function and aesthetics—cannot be reached without the correction of skeletal anomalies.

Court disputes concerning failures in orthodontic treatment are rather the exception. However, with increasing copayment and increasing health awareness of the patients, the forensic problem will gain in importance. It can be concluded that, to avoid errors and legal disputes, a precise treatment plan taking medical, technical, and time options into consideration, as well as properly documented information, is mandatory (Seifert 1997).

15.29 Conservative Dentistry

As measured by the number of liability cases with only 18 % error the rate, of the main subject of dentistry is almost negligible. Damage-causing errors are made during diagnosis and treatment planning; in cavity preparation and restorative treatment; during root canal treatment because of omission, lack of preparation, and incorrect interpretation of radiographs; in superficial caries diagnostics and by ignoring occlusal defects (Günther and Heifer 1984).

In "vital amputation," the most common cause for failure of pulpotomy is a bacterial infection of the remaining pulpa blunt that either existed before the surgery or developed during the treatment. The internal absorption and other degenerative changes in the dental pulp, such as the calcification and the pathological reactions cause by the iatrogenic, mechanical, and chemical trauma, are significant. For early detection of such problems, regular clinical checks (sensitivity test) and radiographs are required, in order to initiate an immediate root canal treatment to avoid serious complications, such as the formation of a periapical lesion or a perforation of the root by an internal absorption.

15.30 Which Filling Materials Are to Be Used?

A reasonable benefit–risk assessment is only possible by taking into account the individual situation (dental status, allergies, pregnancy, etc.). Sometimes the final decision regarding the materials can only be made during a surgery (after removal of a filling or caries). It should be noted that none of the known filling materials constitutes an unacceptable risk. Along with the filling material itself, the following measures must be considered (*Supreme Court decision II StR 397/97*):

- Radiation exposure by X-ray images
- Allergic reactions caused by drainage materials
- Side effects of local anesthetics, etc.

For definitive restorations in posterior teeth, metallic materials (particularly metal alloys and amalgams) and nonmetallic materials (ceramics and composite resins) are available. Other materials (such as dental cements) can only be classified as temporary or semipermanent fillings.

15.31 What Side Effects May Occur?

The risk of undesired systemic and local side effects of correctly used filling materials is very low, but cannot be excluded, as in all drugs and medical products.

15.32 Allergies

Dissatisfied patients may try to claim compensation for alleged or actual complaints with the accusation that harmful materials have been used (Figgener 1996). *OLG Köln, Judgement, Az. 5 U 212/94*; *OLG Hamm, Judgement, Az. 3 U 19/98* states that "If no concrete clues for an allergy are existing, the dentist is not obliged to conduct an allergy testing." Except for rare hypersensitivity reactions (allergies, lichenoid changes), there is no substantiated evidence that adequately prepared gold, amalgam, composite, or ceramic restorations can cause health problems.

15.33 Risks of Filling Materials

All filling materials continuously release substances in tiny amounts. Preferably, the number of different metal alloys should be kept small.

15.33.1 Amalgam Fillings

Patients with amalgam fillings have (depending on the number of fillings) a higher level of mercury in body organs and fluids than amalgam-free patients. A clinically significant toxicity is, according to current knowledge, not to be expected. The removal of existing intact fillings because of alleged "detoxification" is scientifically not indicated. According to *OLG Koblenz, Judgement of 16.06.1999, Az. 3 U 328/87*, "Dental amalgam fillings are generally not associated with a health risk. Although amalgam fillings lead to an increased mercury levels, a toxicological risk is not proven."

A study (Rowland et al. 1992) showed that dental personnel are exposed to a higher risk for reduced fertility and increased abortion rate by inhaling mercury vapor. This leads to a storage of mercury in the pituitary gland, ovaries, and adrenal glands (Nylander et al. 1987; Störtebecker 1989). Under increased mercury levels, prolactin is frequently elevated, the concentration of progesterone is reduced, and the frequency of normal ovulation is reduced to approximately half, and the adrenaline hormones, cortisol and dehydroepiandrosterone, are decreased.

15.34 Protective Measures

Neglecting safeguards, for example, measures against swallowing or inhaling of small instruments or other objects, is a "culpable malpractice." Treatments with small instruments (such as nerve needles) always bear the risk that these instruments might enter the throat by swallowing or inhaling. This risk can be reduced by appropriate protective measures. Neglecting of these measures may have legal consequences (accusation of negligence). According to *OLG Nürnberg, Judgement of 19.10.1953, Az. 2 U 22/52*, (*MDR 53, 483*; *AHRS 6410/5*), "If the patients swallows a nerve needle which was not secured, the dentist is liable for any damage."

Swallowing objects is less dangerous than inhaling objects. In most cases, swallowing ends with natural excretion, and intestinal complications are the exception; however, barbed objects (including root canal instruments, drills, and nerve and injection needles) may cause severe damage (perforation of the stomach and intestinal wall, peritonitis). Inhaling usually has serious consequences, and the legal assessment also depends on whether appropriate measures (such as the immediate referral to the hospital) were taken. *OLG Dusseldorf, Judgement, Az. 8 U 127/91* states that "If there are no appropriate safeguarding measures available e.g. for fitting a primary telescopic crown, the dentist is not liable for damages caused by inhaling."

In all cases of complications, the patient must immediately be informed about the incident and possible damages (Gaisbauer 1998). There are internationally accepted standards (ISO 25, ISO 35) for root canal instruments concerning the breakage, warping, and bending strengths. Only instruments that meet these quality criteria should be used and must be checked prior to each introduction into the oral cavity.

15.35 Periodontology

About 95 % of Germans between the age of 35 and 54 years suffer from gingival disease. About 20 % are severe cases that lead to irreversible degradation of the jaw bone and tooth loss (Meyle 1999).

15.35.1 Microbiological Diagnosis of Marginal Periodontal Disease

The progression of marginal periodontitis is determined by the virulence and bacterial count of periodontal bacteria in the periodontal pocket as well as predisposing systemic and exogenous factors. Periodontal therapy is only successful if the number of periodontal bacteria in the oral cavity is reduced. A microbiological analysis (diagnosis) of subgingival plaque is only indicated, based on current knowledge and under consideration of a low cost–benefit ratio, in the following "aggressive" marginal periodontitis:

- Periodontitis in early years (prepubertal, juvenile, rapidly progressive)
- Severe generalized periodontitis in adults (>50 % alveolar bone loss in >14 teeth)
- Refractory periodontitis
- Severe marginal periodontitis with systemic diseases (especially diabetes mellitus, HIV infection with CD4 <200/mm^3)

Except for refractory periodontitis, all other forms require microbiological diagnosis before beginning a treatment. Microbiological methods with maximum positive and negative predictive values are recommended. For correct interpretation of the results, detailed knowledge about the validity of the methods is essential. In chronic gingivitis and mild-to-moderate adult periodontitis, a conventional periodontal therapy with (supragingival and subgingival scaling and possibly flap surgery) antibiotics has no additional benefit. According to current knowledge, a microbiological diagnosis is not indicated (Flemmig et al. 1998).

15.35.2 Adjuvant Antibiotics in Marginal Periodontal Diseases

A therapy exclusively with antibiotics is only slightly effective, because the biofilm structure of plaque inhibits the antibiotic effect. A therapy with antibiotics as support is indicated in aggressive marginal periodontitis and additionally in:

- Periodontal abscesses with a tendency to spread into the adjacent boxes, fever, and/or severe lymphadenopathy
- Necrotizing ulcerative gingivitis or periodontal disease with fever and/or significant lymphadenopathy

By systemic administration of antibiotics, all periodontal pockets and other niches of the oral cavity can be reached. General contraindications for antibiotics and their interactions with other drugs must be considered (Flemmig and Karch 1998).

15.35.3 Hormonal Contraceptives and Marginal Periodontium

Approximately one-third of women of childbearing age in Germany currently use hormonal contraceptives (most common are products containing ethinyl estradiol and progestin). If the plaque control is not sufficient, hormonal contraceptives may deteriorate the clinical symptoms of gingivitis. Patients should be advised that hormonal contraceptives may lead to an increased gingivitis reaction to the bacterial plaque.

15.35.4 Bone and Bone Substitutes for Periodontal Regeneration

The histological result of periodontal regeneration (development of the alveolar bone, root cementum, and functionally oriented periodontal ligament) corresponds to a clinical attachment gain and a reduction of the probing depth. To promote the periodontal regeneration, bone grafts, implants, and bone substitute materials are used.

Allogenic bone implants are usually made from the long bones of multiorgan donors. Frozen or freeze-dried bone implants have a considerable risk of pathogen transmission and sensitization. This risk can be reduced by a combination of demineralization and freeze-drying of allogenic bone. After the implantation of demineralized freeze-dried bone allograft (demineralized freeze-dried bone allograft (DFDBA)), sensitization was not observed (in quantities needed for regenerative periodontal surgery). The transmission risk of pathogens during correct processing of DFDBA is extremely low, but not completely excluded. The estimated risk for HIV infection is $1{:}8 \times 10^6$.

The risk of prion transmission has not yet been evaluated. Patients should always be informed about the potential risks associated with the implantation of DFDBA, and the consent should be documented in written form (Ehmke and Flemmig 1998).

15.36 Radiology

The X-ray image is used for clinical diagnosis for which the dentist is responsible. The dentist should always choose the technology that provides the best information value for diagnosis, even if this method bears a risk of higher radiation exposure. In general, an X-ray image is necessary if the clinical examination is not sufficient for a diagnosis. The X-ray image is also essential for the planning of treatment steps, monitoring, correction (if necessary), and documenting of treatment results. The significance of the X-ray image as documentation must be especially pointed out (RöV § *28, 2*).

The use of X-ray images for diagnostic purposes is subject to the "*Regulation for protection against damage caused by X rays*" (*dated 8.1.1987*). Whether and in what way X-ray images will be used is up to the dentist, who must have acquired sufficient appropriate knowledge. Radiation exposure must be limited as much as is compatible with the requirements of medical science. During pregnancy, all options for reducing the X-ray radiation of the fetus must be considered. Unnecessary images must be avoided (*RöV* § *24,3*, and § *25,1*).

The value of the panoramic X-ray radiography is undisputed, because it is almost indispensable for orthodontic and surgical diagnoses. The more circumscribed the area to be examined, the more subtle must be the radiography. Intraoral dental film is unsurpassed in display of details. Several shots must be taken if necessary for a precise diagnosis.

15.37 Complementary Methods

The classification of a theory as unscientific does not necessarily mean that this method is wrong, because human judgments do not have absolute certainty. Certain elements of classic naturopathy and possibly also medical systems of other cultures may be integrated into dental education and training, if their effectiveness is proven and related to dental, oral, and maxillofacial surgery. The term complementary methods contains many different procedures with ratings from recognized to questionable and even absurd. Medical procedures find scientific recognition if they are useful or effective as measured by scientific criteria (verifiability, repeatability, significance) as being useful and/or effective. Anyone who champions a medical procedure has to prove the alleged capability.

A precise distinction between paramedical procedures and unconventional methods is difficult. Paramedical procedures are characterized by the fact that they do not have any value for rational diagnostic and therapeutic procedures (e.g., diagnosis with the involvement of divining pendulum, mind healing and long-distance healing). Unconventional procedures are often seen as largely ineffective, but also harmless. However, at least some of these processes serve as a diagnostic basis for highly invasive procedures (unnecessary replacement of restoration materials and extraction of teeth, or even milling on the jawbone). Such nonindicated invasive measures are to be refused.

15.38 Lasers in Dentistry

A multipurpose laser for dental treatments does not exist, because there are many different application areas for various types of lasers. The advantages of laser welding (in a dental lab) of metallic dentures with a powerful pulsed Nd:YAG laser ($\lambda = 1{,}064$ µm) are scientifically proven. Compared with soldering, laser welding offers significant advantages in manufacture and repair of metallic prosthesis parts. The resilience of the welds is high and different materials can be directly welded even in close vicinity to veneers or prosthetic teeth.

In oral surgery, a cw-Nd:YAG laser (λ=1,064 μm) is approved for coagulation in patients with hemorrhagic diathesis or platelet function defects. There is an advantageous use of cw-CO_2 lasers (λ=9,600 μm; 10,600 μm) in the local treatment of various oral lesions for the ablation of leukoplakia. The uses of other lasers for different indications in oral and maxillofacial surgery are currently being investigated in experimental and clinical trials.

The application of CO_2 lasers for selected indications of soft tissue surgery is regarded as a profound alternative, but has no larger advantages over established techniques (scalpel or radiofrequency surgery) in removal of carious changes in dental hard tissues with the water-cooled Er:YAG laser. In the field of dental surgery, there are no absolute indications.

A precise preparation of healthy tooth structure with laser systems for cast fillings, crowns, or bridges still is not possible. A variety of different laser types is discussed for this purpose. For the treatment of dental hard tissues, only laser radiation works well because its interaction with the tooth structure is not of only a thermal nature. The Er:YAG-laser (λ=2.940 μm) is used for painless cavity preparation, but has a higher time requirement compared with conventional therapy with rotary instruments. The Excimer laser (λ=193–351 μm) is also discussed for these applications but is not yet in use because of technical reasons. Excimer lasers for channel processing or apical surgery with CO_2 and Er:YAG lasers are being investigated in the basic research stage. All other methods (especially in periodontology) are still in experimental testing and are discussed very controversially. Nd:YAG lasers, no matter what kind, cannot be used for treatment of hard tissue.

Up to now, there is no scientific evidence for a possible enamel conditioning with a laser to receive adhesive restorative materials. The suitability of other laser types for the selective removal of caries is still in the experimental stage. Removing of old fillings (amalgam, composites, cements) may produce hazardous fumes or vapors; therefore, additional fundamental research is required.

Before using a laser for any treatment, the dentist and staff must undergo an appropriate training, and the strict observance of safety guidelines is mandatory. Because of the potential danger of coherent and monochromatic laser radiation (VBG 93), protective measures (MedGV, VBG 93) for the patient, practitioner, and the staff must be strictly followed. Using a laser without protective goggles is irresponsible and may have legal consequences. Contrary to some optimistic opinions, the widespread use of lasers in dentistry is not imminent. However, basic research is useful and necessary (Visser 1997).

15.39 Behavior in Case of Damage

In case of damage, the professional liability insurance carrier must be informed immediately, even if the patient has not yet made any claims. In case of an incident, the patient is to be informed in an appropriate way (in the presence of the assistant) and all necessary steps to eliminate or alleviate the consequences must be taken. This is not only medical duty, but also corresponds to the harm reduction clause of the insurance contract. In addition to the oral information about the possible complications of the surgical intervention, alternative methods should be mentioned.

15.40 Trauma

Avulsion trauma (total luxations) and severe dislocation trauma of the anterior teeth (which reach their "age peak" in milk teeth around the age of 2 years (Garcia-Godoy and Garcia-Godoy 1987; Andreasen 1988), especially the milk incisors of the upper jaw, occur more and more frequently (Fillipi et al. 1998). The dentist (in practice and clinic) must be prepared for immediate reimplantation and replantation of the extraoral root-filled primary tooth (Frenkel et al. 1989; Will 1983). Cytotoxic manipulations, such as the use of oxidizing substrates (e.g., H_2O_2) may not be conducted. Early loss of milk teeth leads to an unfavorable development of the dental arch (Rinderer 1981; Frenkel et al. 1989; Filippi et al. 1998).

15.41 Teeth, Jaw, and Soft Tissue Injuries After Child Abuse

In approximately 2.9 million cases of child abuse per year in the USA, more than 50 % of the injuries are on the face or head (soft tissue injury) and neck region. Nevertheless, in Illinois, only 9 % of the cases were reported by dentists. This low percentage is explicable more by ignorance than by neglect, because dentists are required to report any suspect of child abuse to the Department of Child and Family Services (DCFS) (Becker et al. 1978).

In Norway, Switzerland, and Spain, the obligation to notify authorities has priority over medical confidentiality. In Norway, an estimated 85 out of 1,000,000 children per year are maltreated and an estimated 3–4 children die from such injuries (with a population of 4.4 million).

Dentists freely admit that they often do not know what to look for during the examination in suspected child abuse and how to confront the parents when abuse is suspected. In case of suspected sexual child abuse, an immediate physical examination is required. Documentation and an interdisciplinary approach (pediatrician, surgeon, gynecologist, forensic physician) is beneficial (Brinkmann and Banaschak 1997).

Although the apparent findings, such as extensive bruises, marks by objects, cuts and strangulation marks, multiple fractures, burns, frostbites, and bite marks are obvious and easy to interpret; in contrast, the legal assessment may be difficult (Trube-Becker 1973, 1974, 1977, 1982; Kenney and Spencer 1995).

A maximum of attention is indicated because the statistics are shocking. Oral injuries include damage of the inside lip, torn labial frenulum, or tooth damage. Children under 3 years old are mainly affected. Fifty percent of all cases of child abuse are cases of recurrence (Laskin 1973).

References

Aderhold L, Frenkel G (1985) Preoperative information to the patient before maxillary surgery interventions based on a standardized procedure. Fortschr Kiefer Gesichtschir 30:15–18

Alfter G (1997) Mögliche Zwischenfälle während einer kieferorthopädischen Behandlung – Ergebnisse einer bundesweiten Befragung. AKFOS Newsl Jg 4(3): 52–53

Andreasen JO (1988) Traumatologie der Zähne. Schlütersche Verlagsanstalt, Hannover

Ankermann E, Kullmann J (1995) Arztpflicht-Rechtsprechung. Ergänzbare Rechtsprechungs-sammlung zur gesamten Arzthaftpflicht. E. Schmidt, Berlin 1987, p 51. Lieferung

Becker DB, Needleman HL, Kotelchuk M (1978) Child abuse & Dentistry; Orofacial Trauma and its Recognition by Dentists. JADA 97(1978):24–28

Berg SP (1966) Gerichtliche Medizin. 7.verb.Aufl. Rudolph Müller & Steinicke, München

Bräutigam W, Christian P, Von Rad M (1992) Psychosoamtische Medizin. Thieme, Stuttgart

Brinkmann B, Banaschak S (1997) Sexueller Kindesmißbrauch. Editorial. Rechtsmedizin 8(1):1

Bünger B (1980) Zahnärztliche Sorgfaltspflichtverletzung – ein kasuistischer Beitrag. ZWR 89(2):54–58

Cichon P, Bader J (1997) Die zahnärztliche Behandlung in Intubationsnarkose. In: Fortbildungsteil 2/97, Zahnärztl Mitt 87 Nr.21,1.11.97: 74–80

Dajani AS, Bawdon RE, Berry MC (1994) Oral amoxicillin as prophylaxis for endocarditis: what is the optimal dose? Clin Infect Dis 18:157–160

Deutsch E (1991) Arztrecht und Arzneimittelrecht. 2.Aufl. A. Springer, Berlin, p 64

Deutsch E (1998) Die Beweiskraft der EDV-Dokumentation bei zahnärztlicher Behandlung. AKFOS Newsl Jg 5(1):3–11

Diedrichs G, Schikowski V, Bötger H (1990) Entwicklung der Sachverständigentätigkeit in der zahnärztlichen Prothetik. Zahnarztl Mitt 80:1479

Egyedi P (1998) Komplikationen bei oralchirurgischen Eingriffen. In: Linn EW, Eijkman MA (eds) Mißerfolge bei der zahnärztlichen Behandlung. Kap.13. Deutscher Ärzte-Verlag, Köln, pp 226–243

Ehlers APF (1987) Die ärztliche Aufklärung vor medizinischen Eingriffen. Heymann, Köln

Ehmke B, Flemmig TF (1998) Knochen und Knochenersatzmaterialien zur parodontalen Regeneration. Gemeinsame Stellungnahme der Deutschen Gesellschaft für Parodontologie (DGP) und der Deutschen Gesellschaft für Zahn-, Mund- und Kieferkrankheiten (DGZMK), 8/98. Dtsch Zahnärtl Z 54(3):141–142

Evers H (1983) Technik der regionalen Anästhesie in der Zahnheilkunde, In: Evers H, Haegerstam G (Hrsg) Lokalanästhesie in der Zahnheilkunde. Springer, Berlin/Heidelberg/New York, S 74, 203–205

Farmand M (1984) Bedeutung der Knochenbiopsie bei besonderer Verlaufsform der Osteomyelitis des Unterkiefers zur mikrobiologischen und histologischen Untersuchung. In: Pfeifer G, Schwenzer N (eds) Fortschr Kiefer Gesichtschir Bd.XXIX. G. Thieme, Stuttgart/New York

Figgener L (1993) Die Rechtsverhältnisse zwischen Patient, Zahnarzt und Zahntechniker. ZMK 9.Jg. April, 3:36–38

Figgener L (1995a) Die Pflicht zur Dokumentation. Stellungnahme der DGZMK 10/94, Stand 30.11.1994; Diese Fassung ersetzt die frühere Stellungnahme 3/84. Dtsch Zahnarztl Z 50(3):175

Figgener L (1995b) Zahnarzt und Recht – Unterlassene Endokarditisprophylaxe – Ein Behandlungsfehler. AKFOS Newsl Jg 2(2):39

Figgener L (1995c) Zahnarzt und Recht – Vorbehandlung vor prothetischer Versorgung – Ein häufiger Streitpunkt. AKFOS Newsl Jg 2(2):40

Figgener L (1995d) Zahnarzt und Recht – Aspirationsprophylaxe in der zahnärztlichen Praxis – Ein altbekanntes und doch immer aktuelles forensisches Thema. AKFOS Newsl Jg 2(2):41–42

Figgener L (1996) Neue Rechtsprechung zum Haftpflichtrecht. Zahnärztl Nachr Sachsen-Anhalt 8:1–4

Figgener L (1997) Neue Rechtsprechung zum Haftpflichtrecht. Zahnärztl Nachr Sachsen-Anhalt 8:1–8

Figgener L (1998) Neue Rechtsprechung zum Haftpflichtrecht. Zahnärztl Nachr Sachsen-Anhalt 9: 1–8

Figgener L (1999) Aktuelle Rechtsprechung zum zahnärztlichen Haftpflichtrecht. Rhein Zahnärztebl 5: 17–27

Filippi A, Kirschner H, Kraus U, Pohl Y, Robert F, Tekin U (1998) Avulsionstrauma der Frontzähne. Der Freie Zahnarzt 3:48–54

Flemmig TF, Karch H (1998) Adjuvante Antibiotika bei der Therapie marginaler Parontopathien. Gemeinsame Stellungnahme 9/98 der DGP und der DGZMK, Stand Juni 1998. Mitt DGZMK 4/98. Dtsch Zahnärztl Z 53(12):824

Flemmig TF, Christgau M, Karch H (1998) Mikrobiologische Diagnostik bei marginalern Parodontopathien. Gemeinsame Stellungnahme 10/98 der DGP und der DGZMK, Stand Juni 1998. Mitt DGZMK 4/98. Dtsch Zahnärztl Z 53(12):825–826

Freesmeyer WB, Koeck B, Reber T (1999) Funktionsanalytische Maßnahmen. Stellungnahme der DGZMK. Dtsch Zahnarztl Z 54(8):471

Frenkel G (1978) Die Schmerzausschaltung. In: Haunfelder et al. Praxis der Zahnheilkunde, Ergänzung B1. Urban & Schwarzenberg, München

Frenkel G, Aderholt L, Leilich G, Raetzke P (1989) Die ambulante Chirurgie des Zahnarztes. C. Hanser, München/Wien

Fuhrmann R, Wehrbein HM, Diedrich P (1993) Dreidimensionale computertomographische Darstellung des bezahnten Alveolarkamms. Ein radiologisch-histologischer Vergleich. Fortschr Kieferorthop 54:91

Fuhrmann R, Langen HJ, Günther R, Diedrich P (1994) Radiologische Diagnostik artifizieller intraalveoläreer Knochendefekte. Dtsch Zahnarztl Z 49:336

Gaisbauer G (1998) Verschlucken und Einatmen von Fremdkörpern in der zahnärztlichen Praxis aus haftungsrechtlicher Sicht. VersR 7:279–285

Garcia-Godoy F, Garcia-Godoy FM (1987) Primary teeth traumatic injuries at a private pediatric dental center. Endodont Dent Traumatol 3:126

Giesen D (1990) Arzthaftungsrecht. Gieseking, Bielefeld

Glauser M, Bernard B (1983) Successful single-dose amoxicillin prophylaxis against experimental streptococcal endocarditis. Evidence of two mechanisms of protection. J Infect Dis 147:568

Gümpel G (1980) Vorgerichtliche Begutachtung. Dtsch Zahnarztl Z 35:369

Gümpel G (1994) Rechtliche Bedeutung prophylaktischer Maßnahmen und Haftungsrisiko des Zahnarztes. AKFOS Newsl Jg 1(1):13

Günther H (1966) Indikationsstellung, fachliche und rechtliche Probleme der Allgemeinanästhesie in der zahnärztlichen Praxis. Dtsch Zahnarztl Z 21: 1167

Günther H, Heifer U (1984) Rechtsmedizin und Begutachtung in der zahnärztlichen Praxis. G. Thieme, Stuttgart/New York, pp 113–121

Haffner TH, Graw M (1995) Zur Bewertung der Fahrtauglichkeit nach zahnärztlicher Infiltrationsanästhesie aus rechtsmedizinischer Sicht. AKFOS Newsl Jg 2(3):67–68

Handschel J, Kleinheinz J, Ahrberg W (1998) Chronische Kieferosteomyelitis nach Zahnextraktion. Ist ein chirurgische Vorgehen noch zeitgemäß ? Der Freie Zahnarzt 3:56–60

Haßfeld (1999) Nervus lingualis. Zahnärztl Mitt 89 5/1.3.1999 (470):6

Hempel A, et al. (1982) In: Haffner TH und Graw M (1995) Zur Bewertung der Fahrtauglichkeit nach zahnärztlicher Infiltrationsanästhesie aus rechtsmedizinischer Sicht. AKFOS Newsl Jg 2(3):67–68

Hempfing W (1994) Zahnarztvertrag ist Dienstvertrag. Zahnärztl Praxis 2/1991. AKFOS Newsl Jg 1(2):31

Horstkotte D (1985) Endokarditisprophylaxe bei Zahnärztlichen Eingriffen. Mitt DGZMK 4,85

Horstkotte D (1995) Mikrobiell verursachte Endokarditis: Klinische und tierexperimentelle Untersuchungen. Steinkopff, Darmstadt, S 149

Horstkotte D, Piper C, Schultheiß HP (1997) Prophylaxe und Recidivprophylaxe bakterieller Endokarditiden bei zahnärztlich-chirurgischen Eingriffen. Dtsch Zahnarztl Z 52:650–656

Hürzeler MB (1996) Versorgung der augmentierten Kieferhöhle mit implantatgetragenem Zahnersatz. Quintessenz, Berlin

Janda R, Kappert HF (1996) Medizinproduktegesetz MPG. Quintessenz, Berlin, 11,12,17,19,20,23ff,65

Kenney JP, Spencer DE (1995) Child abuse and neglect. Chapter 6. Human abuse and neglect. In: Bowers CM, Bell GL (eds) Manual of forensic odontology. ASFO, Saratoga Springs, pp 191–199

Kern BR, Laufs A (1993) Die ärztliche Aufklärungspflicht. A. Springer, Berlin, p 193

Kielbassa AM, Schilli K (1997) Betreuung des tumortherapeutisch bestrahlten Patienten aus Sicht der Zahnerhaltung. In: Fortbildungsteil 2/97, Zahnärztl Mitt 87 Nr.21,1.11.97: 58–68

Knirsch W, Finke CH, Adam M, Vogel M, Lange PE (1999) Der Risikopatient. So erkennen und schützen Sie Ihren Endokarditis-Risikopatienten. Zahnärztl Mitt 89 Nr 21:32–37

Köhler JA (1970) Beitrag zur forensischen Zahn-, Mund- und Kieferheilkunde. Zahnärztl Welt/Rdsch 79:892

Kornas M, Haßfeld S, Mende U, Zöller J (1998) Metrische Genauigkeit der CT-Analyse vor enossaler Implantation. Dtsch Zahnarztl Z 52(2):120–126

Laskin DM (1973) The battered-child syndrome. J Oral Surg 31:903

Laufs A (1996a) Die Entwicklung des Arztrechts. NJW 1992: 1529–1539, NJW 1993: 1497–1506, NJW 1994: 1562–1571

Laufs A (1996b) Das Recht des Patienten auf Teilhabe am medizinischen Fortschritt. Festvortrag bei der 8. Jahrestagung der Deutschen Gesellschaft für Zahnerhaltung am 22.April 1994 in Heidelberg. AKFOS Newsl Jg 3(1):3–11

Laufs A, Uhlenbruck W (1992) Handbuch des Arztrechts. CH Beck, München, S 318, 365

Lechler E, Pape HD (1996) Zahnärztlich – chirurgische Behandlung von "Marcumar" – Patienten. Stellungnahme der DGZMK 3/96, Stand 13.7.1996; Diese Fassung ersetzt die frühere Stellungnahme 2/83. Dtsch Zahnarztl Z 51(12):722–723

Linder B (1997) Freie Mitarbeit in Zahnarztpraxen für Zahnarzthelferinnen. Zahnärztl Inform 4/97:58

Lipp MDW, Dick WF, Daubländer M, Hornke I, Fuder H (1988) Examination of the central-venous epinephrine level during local dental infiltration and block anaesthesia using tritium-marked epinephrine as vasoconstrictor. Anaesthesiol 69:A 371

Lüer EM (1948) Beitrag zum Kapitel "Zahnärztlicher Kunstfehler" unter besonderer Berücksichtigung der derzeitigen Auffassung vom "Kunstfehler". Med Dissertation, Halle/Saale

Maeglin B (1981) Die Weiterverwendung angebrauchter Karpulen. Schweiz Mschr Zahnheilk 91:179

Malinverni R, Overholser CD, Bille J, Glauser M (1988) Antibiotic prophylaxis of experimental endocarditis after dental extractions. Circulation 77:182–187

Martin MV, Butterworth ML, Longman LP (1997) Infective endocarditis and the dental practitioner: a review of 53 cases involving litigation. Br Dent J 182:465–468

Marxkors R (1995) Ursachen und Therapie von Prothesenintoleranz. Dtsch Zahnärztl Z 50:704 (Siehe auch: Marxkors R, Müller-Fahlbusch†, Figgener L (1993) Psychosomatisch bedingte Prothesenunverträglichkeiten und Beschwerden im Mund-Kiefer-Gesichtsbereich. Stellungnahme 4/92. Stand September 1992; Diese Fassung ersetzt die frühere Stellungnahme 4/81. Dtsch Zahnärztl Z 48,3: 149)

Marxkors R (1999) Ursachen, Auswirkungen und Behebungen von Mißerfolgen. Dtsch Zahnarztl Z 54:600–610

Marxkors R, Wolowski A (1999) Unklare Kiefergesichtsbeschwerden. Hanser, München Wien

Muschallik TH (1998) Zahnärztlicher Behandlungsfehler – Was kann passieren? In: Linn EW, Eijkman MA (eds) Mißerfolge bei der zahnärztlichen Behandlung. Deutscher Ärzte-Verlag, Köln, p 20

Niesel HC, Kaiser H (1991) Kann durch die Auswahl von Medikamenten und Adjuvantien das Komplikationsrisiko von Lokalanästhesien gesenkt werden? ZWR Jg 100(3):174–177

Nylander M, Freiberg L, Lind B (1987) Mercury concentrations in the human brain and kidneys in relation to exposure from dental amalgam fillings. Swed Dent J 11:179–187

Oehler K (1999) Der zahnärztliche Sachverständige. Behandlungsfehler in Begutachtung und Rechtsprechung. Deutscher Zahnärzte Verlag DÄV-Hanser Köln, München, S 90–92, 219–226

Oskarsson A, Schultz A, Skerfving S, Hallen IP, Ohlin B, Lagerkvist BJ (1996) Total and inorganic mercury in breast milk in relation to fish consumption and amalgam in lactating women. Arch Environ Health 51: 234–241

Otten JE (1998) Zahnsanierung vor und nach Organtransplantation. Stellungnahme der DGZMK. Zahnärztl Mitt 88 (3182) 24:43–45

Otten JE (1999) Zahnsanierung vor und nach Organtransplantation. Stellungnahme der DGZMK. Dtsch Zahnarztl Z 54(9):532–533

Otto F (1998) Kontrollpflicht bei Implantaten. ZMK 14. Jg. 6/98:25

Pippert H, Horstkotte D, Friedrichs W, Rosin W, Bürrig KF (1991) Prevention of streptococcus endocarditis in rats. In: Horstkotte D, Bodnar E (eds) Infective endocarditis. ICR, London, pp 285–290

Ratajczak TH (1994) Zahnärztliche Dokumentation. AKFOS Newsl Jg 1(1):12

Ratka-Krüger P, Gilles C, Raetzke F (1997) Der HIV-Patient in der zahnärztlichen Praxis. In: Fortbildungsteil 2/97, Zahnärztl Mitt 87,Nr.21,1.11.97: 52–57

Richter EJ (1999) Tagungsbericht der Frühjahrstagung 1999 der Deutschen Gesellschaft für Implantologie in Münster v. 18.-20.März 1999. Z Zahnärztl Implantol 15:117

Rinderer L (1981) Zahnunfälle im Milch- und Wechselgebiß. In: Hotz RP (ed) Zahnmedizin bei Kindern und Jugendlichen. G. Thieme, Stuttgart

Rohde ER (1995a) Dokumentationspflicht und Verpflichtung zur Anfertigung einer Röntgenübersichtsaufnahme bei einer komplikationslos verlaufenden Zahnextraktion. AKFOS Newsl Jg 2(1):8

Rohde ER (1995b) Das Gespräch zur Patientenaufklärung vor medizinischen Eingriffen. AKFOS Newsl Jg 2(3):54–56

Rohde ER (1996a) Das Gespräch zur Patientenaufklärung. Dtsch Zahnärztekalender: 163–185

Rohde ER (1996b) Grundzüge des Zahnarzthaftungsrechts in Deutschland mit einem Überblick über die Rechtsprechung des Landgerichts Frankfurt zur Zahnarzthaftung 1990–1995. Vortrag, gehalten auf dem 2. Internationalen Kongress für Zahnarztrecht und Ethik, Kopenhagen, 24.-26.August 1995. AKFOS Newsl Jg 3(1):16–22

Rohde ER (1997) Juristische Aspekte bei der Fehlbehandlung in der Kieferorthopädie. AKFOS Newsl Jg 4(3):53–57

Rohde ER (1999) Regelwidrige und eigenmächtige zahnärztlich-prothetische Behandlungen. Anhang 1. Juristische Dissertation. Göttingen. Eigenverlag Frankfurt am Main: 115–140

Rowland AS, Baird DD, Weinberg CR, Shore DL, Shy CM, Wilcox AJ (1992) Reduced fertility among women employed as dental assistants exposed to high levels of nitrous oxide. N Engl J Med 327: 993–997

Schiel HJ, Besimo CHE (1997) Präoperativ-prothetische Planung und chirurgische Prinzipien in der oralen Implantologie heute. Eine Standortbestimmung. Der Freie Zahnarzt 9:68–74

Schmidt-Westhausen AM, Strietzel FP (1997) Die zahnärztliche Behandlung immunsupprimierter Patienten. In: Fortbildungsteil 2/97, Zahnärztl Mitt 87,Nr.21: 46–51

Scholich P (1997) Ihr Recht in der Praxis. Recht+Praxis. Der Freie Zahnarzt.6: 28

Schorr G (1998) Medizinprodukte-Recht. Wissenschaftliche Verlagsgesellschaft, Stuttgart

Seifert G (1997) Planungs- und Behandlungsfehler in der Kieferorthopädie. AKFOS Newsl Jg 4(3):47–51

Smit H, Schoeppe W, Zickgraf T (1996) Organspende und Transplantation in Deutschland. Informationsschrift der Deutschen Stiftung Organtransplantation

Spiekermann H (1997) Implantologie – heute und morgen. Zahnärztl Mitt 87,Nr.10,16.5.1997 (1226): 34–40

Störtebecker P (1989) Zahnamalgambedingte Quecksilbervergiftung durch direkten Nase-Hirn-Transport. Lancet 335:9

Stratmann KR (1995) Die zahnärztliche Dokumentation. AKFOS Newsl Jg 2(3):70–72

Strietzel FP (1998) Erweiterung der Indikationen in der Implantologie – eine Indikation zur Zusammenarbeit. Dent Implantol 2(2):75

Tiemann S (1982) Das Recht in der Zahnarztpraxis. Quintessenz, Berlin, S 119–125, 136–157

Trube-Becker E (1973) Bißspuren bei Kindsmißhandlung. Beitr Ger Med 31:115

Trube-Becker E (1974) Die Kindsmißhandlung und ihre Folgen. Tägl Praxis 15:449

Trube-Becker E (1977) Bißverletzungen bei mißhandelten Kindern. Z Rechtsmed 79:73

Trube-Becker E (1982) Gewalt gegen das Kind. Kriminalistik, Heidelberg

Uhlenbrock W (1976) Rechtsfragen bei der ärztlichen Behandlung von Minderjährigen. ArztR 11: 301ff

Vetter Ch (1999) Typ-II-Diabetes: "Alterszucker" schon bei Kindern. Neue Erkenntnisse für die Kinderbehandlung. Zahnärztl Mitt 89(14):26–27

Visser H (1997) Laser in der Zahnheilkunde. Der Freie Zahnarzt 11:68–83

Vogel C (1979) Haftpflichtansprüche aus kieferorthopädischer Behandlung. Fortschr Kieferorthop 40(6): 520–523

Vogel C (1980a) Haftpflichtansprüche aus zahnärztlicher Chirurgie und Lokalanästhesie. Dtsch Zahnärztekalender. C. Hanser, München, pp 98–109

Vogel C (1980b) Fehler, die dem Zahnarzt vorgeworfen werden. Dtsch Zahnarztl Z 35:366–368

Vogel C (1982) Prozesse gegen Ärzte. ZWR 91.Jg, Nr.4: 20–25

Wagner I, Schneider W (1998) Die interaktive elektronische Krankengeschichte zur Entscheidungsunterstützung im klinischen Management, Westerburger Kontakte, 1.Hj

Wahl G (1996) Zahnärztlich-chirurgische Eingriffe bei Diabetikern. Stellungnahme 4/96 der DGZMK, Stand 6.9.1996; Diese Fassung ersetzt die frühere Stellungnahme 3/78. Dtsch Zahnärztl Z 51(12):723

Wichmann M (1999) Kronen und Brücken. Gemeinsame Stellungnahme der DGZMK und der DGZPW. Dtsch Zahnärztl Z Jg 54, 8/99:469–470

Will R (1983) Replantation – Das Wiedereinsetzen von Zähnen. Quintessenz, Berlin

Wolf JWA, Courant A (1998) Mißerfolge in der Implantologie. In: Linn EW, Eijkman MA (eds) 8. Mißerfolge bei der zahnärztlichen Behandlung. Dtsch. Ärzte-Verlag, Köln, pp 151–169

16 Child Maltreatment

Jean-Marc Hutt

16.1 Introduction

In about 2,9 million cases of child maltreatment per year in the USA, more than 50 percent of the injuries are on the face or head (soft tissue injury) and neck region. Nevertheless, in Illinois only 9 percent of the cases have been reported by dentists. This low percentage is explicable more by ignorance than by neglect, because dentists are required to report any suspect of child maltreatment to the "*Department of Child and Family Services (DCFS)*" (Becker et al. 1978).

In Norway, in Switzerland and in Spain, the obligation to notify authorities has priority over the medical confidentiality. In Norway, estimated 85 out of 1.000.000 children per year are maltreated and estimated 3-4 children die from such injuries (with a population of 4.4 million).

Dentists freely admit they often do not know what to look for during the examination in suspected child abuse and how to confront the parents with this suspect.

In case of suspected sexual child abuse an immediate physical examination is required. Documentation and interdisciplinary approach (pediatrician, surgeon, gynecologist, forensic physician) is beneficial (Brinkmann and Banaschak 1997).

Although the apparent findings like extensive bruises, marks by objects, cuts and strangulation marks, multiple fractures, burns, frostbites and bite marks are obvious and not to misinterpret, in contrast the legal assessment may be difficult (Trube-Becker 1973, 1974, 1977, 1982; Kenney and Spencer 1995).

A maximum of attention is indicated since the statistics are shocking. Oral injuries include damage of the lip inside, torn labial frenulum or tooth damage. Mainly Children under 3 years are affected. 50% of all cases of child maltreatment are cases of recurrence (Laskin 1973).

16.2 Definition

The term *child maltreatment/abuse* is subject to constant change.

For example, the educational methods of the 1950s appear to be exaggerated.

But how will the following generations judge about our methods of education?

The term *child maltreatment/abuse* is not universally valid.

Children are treated differently from country to country.

What is our opinion about the female genital cutting in African countries?

A distinction between the maltreatment and the educational measure is difficult.

J.-M. Hutt, Dr. med. dent. (Strasbourg),
Dr. for. sciences (Nancy), Association Française d'Identification Odontologique (AFIO)
Private Practitioner, 11, quai des Bateliers,
F-6700 Strasbourg, France
e-mail: jmhutt@hotmail.com

K. Rötzscher (ed.), *Forensic and Legal Dentistry*,
DOI 10.1007/978-3-319-01330-5_16,

16.2.1 Abused Child, Child at Risk, Endangered Child, and Definitions of Terms

The abused child is the victim
Of physical violence,
Of sexual abuse,
Of psychological and emotional violence,
Of neglect, with severe consequences for the physical, mental, and emotional development.

The new French penal code considers it as an aggravating fact if the aggressor is a person of authority.

The child at risk is a child whose living conditions are a risk to his health, safety, education, and morale.

The endangered child is both an abused child and a child at risk. Often these children are known to various social services.

Forms of maltreatment:

- The physical maltreatment
- The psychological maltreatment
- The sexual abuse
- The neglect: failure to provide basic needs like food, hygiene, medical care, appropriate clothing, or supervision

16.3 Epidemiology

In most cases, the perpetrators are parents and other caregivers such as relatives, babysitters, and foster parents.

But a stereotypical perpetrator profile is not possible.

Researches have detected a number of risk factors or attributes commonly associated with maltreatment. Children in families and environments where these factors exist have a higher probability of experiencing maltreatment:

- Teen parenting.
- Parents who have experienced physical violence themselves mistreat their children in 30 % of cases.
- Difficult life circumstances do favor maltreatment: unemployment, death, poverty, health problems, prostitution, alcohol abuse, drug abuse, social isolation, etc.
- Family problems: divorce, remarriage, single parents, and domestic violence.
- Men tend more to physical punishment than females do.
- Mental disorders such as severe depressions, personality disorders, and psychiatric disorders increase the risk of child abuse, neglect, and incest.
- Frequent pregnancies or twin births.
- Miscarriage.
- Unwanted pregnancy.
- Poor education.
- Hyperactive, physically, or mentally disabled children.

16.4 The Role of the Dentist

Surprisingly, the dentist has a strategic importance in the diagnosis of child abuse. Fifty percent of abused children have orofacial lesions or cervical lesions.

The perpetrators change the doctor very often, but they usually are not suspicious of the dentist.

Despite this privileged position of a dentist, the number of detected cases is low.

Possible reasons might be:

- Confidentiality
- The attempt to solve the problem by the dialogue with the family
- Reluctance to report suspected child abuse
- Reluctance to interfere

Child abuse leaves deep and lasting scars. As difficult as reporting child abuse or neglect can be, it is important and also a duty to pursue any suspicious signs.

16.5 The Clinical Orofacial Lesions

1. *The ribbon crack*
   Injuries to the lip frenulum of the upper lip are common. Possible reasons are as follows: the violent insertion of a blunt object into the mouth, e.g., a spoon if the child eats too slow or refuses the food, and beating against the mouth.
2. *Lesions of the soft palate*
   Point to disturbances in swallowing and speaking.

3. *Lesions of the lips*
   Mostly by punches with a blunt object or by impacting against a hard surface, resulting in wounds or bruises (Fig. 16.1).
4. *The tongue*
   The tongue may be squeezed, resulting of a blow to the jaw between the teeth by a punch against the lower jaw.
5. *Lesions of the mouth and nose*
   As a result of repeated microtraumata or a massive punch, the nasal cartilage breaks and causes severe restrictions of facial aesthetics (boxer's nose) (Fig. 16.2).
6. *Dental arches*
   Simple crown fractures to severe crown-root fractures after trauma.

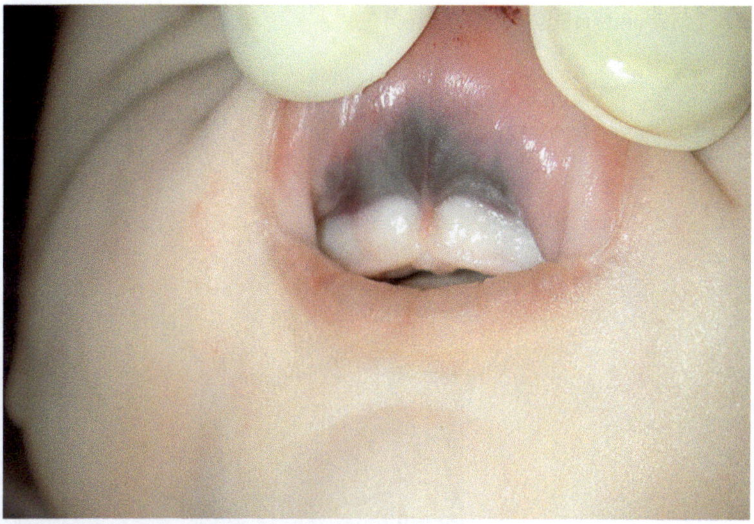

Fig. 16.1 Injury of the lip frenulum

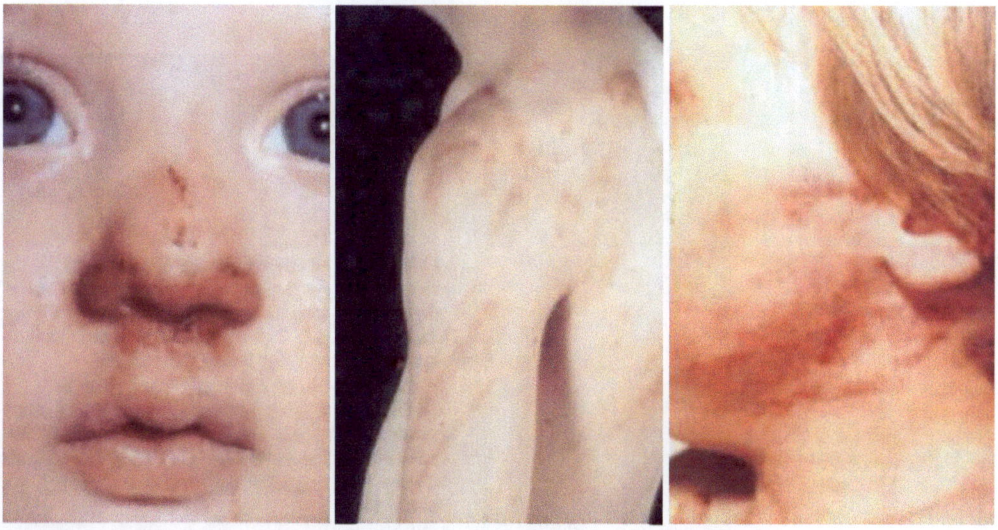

Fig. 16.2 Lesion by nose punch, flagellation, hematoma after slap

7. *The dental neglect*
   Failure to dental care and failure to treatments lead to multiple extractions, difficult food intake, and growth disorders.

16.6 Accompanying Medical Lesions

1. The skin
   1.1 Bruises and hematoma (see Fig. 16.2).
   1.2 Wounds (Figs. 16.3 and 16.4).
   1.3 Burns: about 10 % of abused children show burns by spraying or dipping in hot water.
   1.4 Bites (Fig. 16.5).

Ripped-out hair

2. *The eyes*
   Subconjunctival hematoma
3. *The ears*
   Injuries of the eardrum and bruises (Fig. 16.6)
4. *Fractures* most frequent (after skin lesions), although they are less diagnosed by a dentist.
5. *Behavior disorders*
6. *Growth disorders*

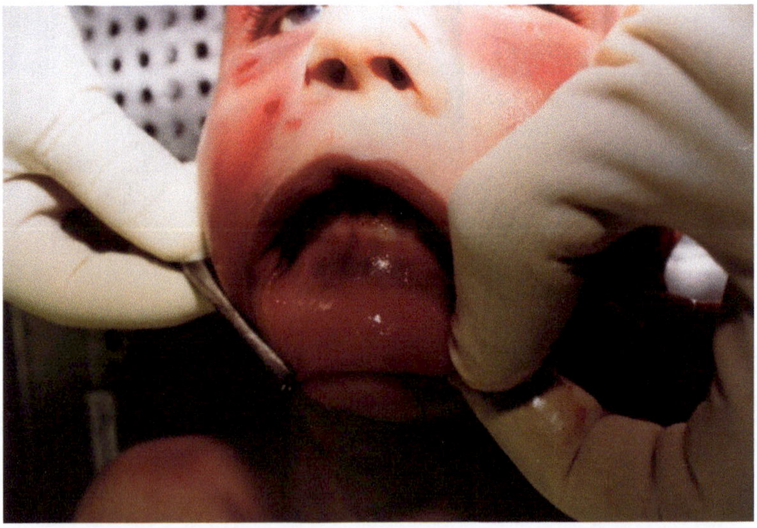

Fig. 16.3 Punch against the chin

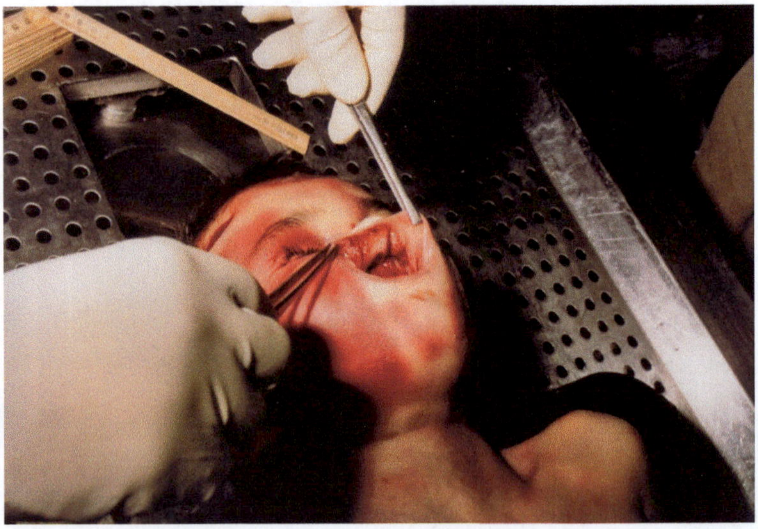

Fig. 16.4 Injuries of the frenulum

Fig. 16.5 Bite mark

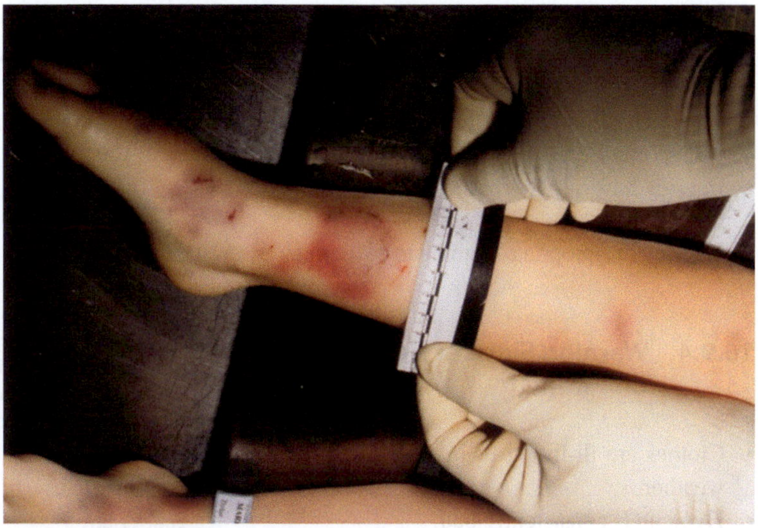

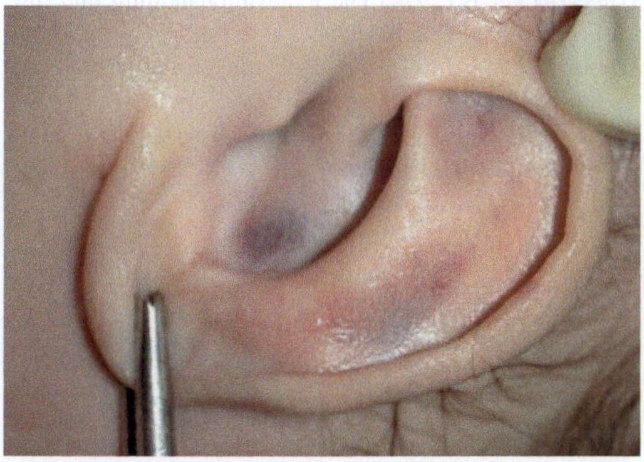

Fig. 16.6 Hematoma by a punch against the ear

16.7 The Differential Diagnosis

All previous images show cases of proven child abuse.

Nevertheless, some systemic diseases have similar symptoms.

In cases of doubt, it is important to carefully objectify the symptoms to avoid serious diagnostic errors.

16.8 The Duties of the Dentist

Failure to report cases of child abuse and failure to render assistance to those children are prosecuted by law. Physician and dentist are obligated to notify the authorities, since child abuse means a releasing exception from the medical confidentiality.

16.9 Reporting Suspicious Cases

16.9.1 In Cases of Suspicion

- Reporting can be done anonymously via a toll free number, e.g., *Aide sociale à l'enfance.*
- Reports can also be done to the chief physician at pediatric wards.

16.9.2 In Severe Cases with Danger to the Child

- Referral to hospital *with the consent of parents.*
- Immediate notification of the prefect.
- In case of possible reprisals by the penetrator, the police must be informed.

It is estimated that an abused child will be abused again in 60 % of the cases.

Abused children are more likely to repeat the cycle as an adult, unconsciously repeating what they experienced as children. On the other hand, many adult survivors of child abuse have a strong motivation to protect their children against what they went through and become excellent parents.

16.9.3 Warning Signs of Physical Abuse in Children

- Frequent injuries or unexplained bruises, welts, or cuts.
- Injuries have a pattern such as marks from a hand or belt.
- Wearing inappropriate clothing to cover injuries.

16.9.4 Warning Signs of Neglect in Children

- Clothes are ill-fitting or inappropriate for the weather.
- Hygiene is consistently bad.
- Untreated illnesses and physical injuries.
- Is frequently left alone.
- Is frequently late or missing from school.

16.9.5 Warning Signs of Sexual Abuse in Children

- Trouble in walking or sitting
- Knowledge or interest in sexual acts
- Wants to avoid a specific person

Sexual child abuse is more common than previously suspected (girls > boys). In an oral sexual trauma, the dentist must consider infectious diseases of the mouth.

References

Becker DB, Needleman HL, Kotelchuk M (1978) Child abuse and Dentistry; Orofacial Trauma and its Recognition by Dentists. JADA 97:24–28

Brinkmann B, Banaschak S (1997) Sexueller Kindesmißbrauch. Editorial. Rechtsmedizin 8;1:1

Kenney JP, Spencer DE (1995) Child abuse and neglect. Chapter 6. Human abuse and neglect

Laskin DM (1973) The battered-child syndrome. J Oral Surg 31:903

Trube-Becker E (1973) Bißspuren bei Kindsmißhandlung. Beitr Ger Med 31:115

Trube-Becker E (1974) Die Kindsmißhandlung und ihre Folgen. Tägl Praxis 15:449

Trube-Becker E (1977) Bißverletzungen bei mißhandelten Kindern. Z Rechtsmed 79:73

Trube-Becker E (1982) Gewalt gegen das Kind. Kriminalistik, Heidelberg

Part III

Forensic Dentistry

Preliminary Comments 17

Klaus Rötzscher

Dental, oral, and maxillofacial medicine is concerned with the regular development, preservation, and rehabilitation of the stomatognathic system, which is the functional system of the teeth, periodontium, jaw, and jaw joint; the jaw and facial muscles, glands, soft tissue, and mucous membranes; and their blood, lymphatic, and nerve supply.

Forensic odontostomatology (different international terms are used: forensic dentistry, forensic dental medicine, forensic odontology, and *odontologie médico-légale*, each with different content and scientific–theoretical functions) as a specific modification of dentistry, oral, and maxillofacial medicine is an independent field of knowledge within the forensic sciences. It provides scientific and research findings of oral and maxillofacial medicine in civil or criminal law cases and has a key role in the context of criminology. Physicians (forensic medicine), dentists (forensic odontologist), and the investigating authorities (criminologists) supply the court (defense, judge, and prosecutor), as well as insurance companies and the students of these disciplines, with their knowledge in the field of forensic odontostomatology.

The main tasks of forensic odontostomatology are (Keiser-Nielsen 1980) scientific processing of criminology, setting up principles that are tested and generally accepted as the standard for dental practice, acquiring legal knowledge for effective cooperation between dentists and lawyers; and identifying unknown dead or living persons with the aid of their teeth by age estimation, gender determination, prophylactic odontological identification aids, assessing the chemical–physical effect on the masticatory system, inferences from the type and material of dental work in certain cases, and the investigation of bite/tooth marks and securing of these evidences (Hahn 1995). Forensic odontostomatology collects the results of dental research for criminological and legal use (Rötzscher 1996).

17.1 Tooth Structure

The development of teeth in the human embryo begins around the age of 6½ weeks. We distinguish three development stages (nodular, cap-shaped, and bell-shaped stage) that are observed both in the milk and the permanent teeth. The cell junctions of the inner enamel epithelium differentiates into palisade-shaped arranged cells (ameloblasts) with a cylindrical shape. These cells are significantly involved in enamel formation. Next, differentiation of dental papilla mesenchymal cells, located on the periphery, starts. They arrange themselves into cylindrical cells (odontoblasts) and are involved in dentinogenesis.

The primary tooth germs initially lie together in a groove of the jaw bone. Later, a branching in the alveoli takes place. The root is formed by the

K. Rötzscher, Dr. med. Dr. med. dent.
German Academy of Forensic Odontostomatology (AKFOS),
Wimphelingstraße 7, 67346 Speyer, Germany
e-mail: roetzscher.klaus.dr@t-online.de

K. Rötzscher (ed.), *Forensic and Legal Dentistry*,
DOI 10.1007/978-3-319-01330-5_17, © Springer International Publishing Switzerland 2014

inner and outer enamel epithelium, which tubularly grows into depth. The number of the tubes determines the number of roots. The shape of the tubes corresponds to the later form of the roots. In addition to the cement and the remaining shares of the periodontium, the periodontal ligament and the alveolar periost are also built by the dental follicle (Taatz 1980).

All animals outside the mammalian family are polyphyodont, that means their teeth are continuously replaced. Mammals (e.g., humans) change their teeth only once. Human dentition is heterodont; three different types of teeth exist in a row of teeth:

- Incisors (I, *dentes incisivi*)
- Canines (C, *dentes canini* = *dentes cuspidati*)
- Bicuspid teeth (P, *dentes praemolares* = *dentes bicuspidati*)

These teeth are replaced, in contrast to the molars (M, *dentes postmolares* = *dentes multicuspidati*), which are formed only once in permanent dentition (Fig. 17.1).

The tooth germs of the first dentition are at the outside of the dental lamina; those of the deciduous dentition (*dentes lactales sive dentes decidui*) are at the inside of the dental lamina with the formula:

$$3I+1C+4P+3M=44 \text{ and } 3i+1c+4p=32;$$

where upper case letters indicate permanent dentition, and lower case letters indicate the primary teeth. Many mammals have more teeth than humans, e.g., canids (dog-like carnivores) and bears have 42, and felids (feline predators) have less 30. Rarely, a phylogenetic hyperodontia (*dentes supernumerarii*) occurs in humans.

The human bite has a bilaterally symmetrical arrangement. Thus, the number of teeth in one jaw is 16, for both jaws it is 32 (in permanent dentition), with the formula:

$$2I+1C+2P+3M=32.$$

Because there are no molars in primary teeth, (as in permanent teeth) the number of teeth for both jaws is 20, with the formula:

$$2i+1c+2m=\text{primary molars}=20.$$

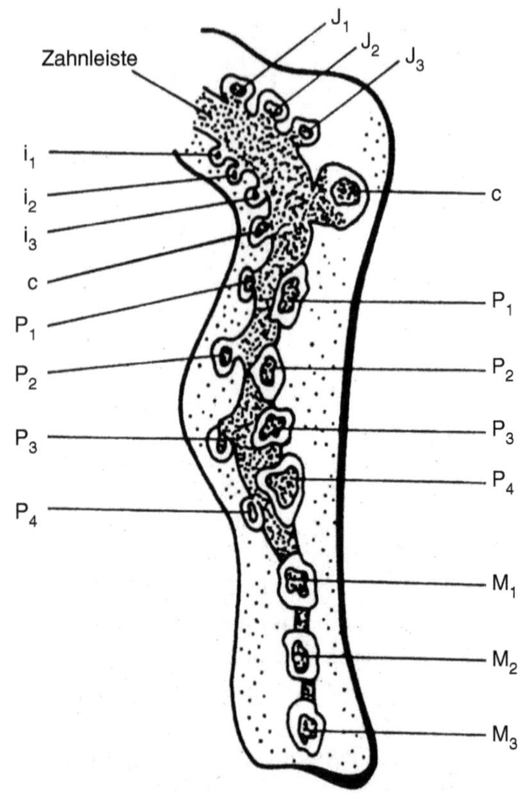

Fig. 17.1 Teeth of the lower jaw of a mammal embryo (pig) (from below) (schematic)

The posterior arising of the three molars of permanent dentition (M1, M2, and M3) is called *growth teeth*. Their tooth germs develop from the blind end of the dental lamina of the deciduous molars, which distally extends itself by proliferative growth (Schroeder 1987).

Human dentition is thecodont; the teeth are fitted with roots that anchor themselves in the jaw. The visible part of the tooth is the crown (*corona dentis*) and the invisible part is stuck in the jaw (*radix dentis*). The passage between crown and root is the tooth neck (*collum dentis*). The crown is covered by tooth enamel (*enamelum dentis*), the hardest substance in the human body (~95 % inorganic substance) (Fig. 17.2).

The root is completely surrounded by the dental cement (*cementum dentis*) and contains the dentin (*dentinum dentis, substantia eburnea*).

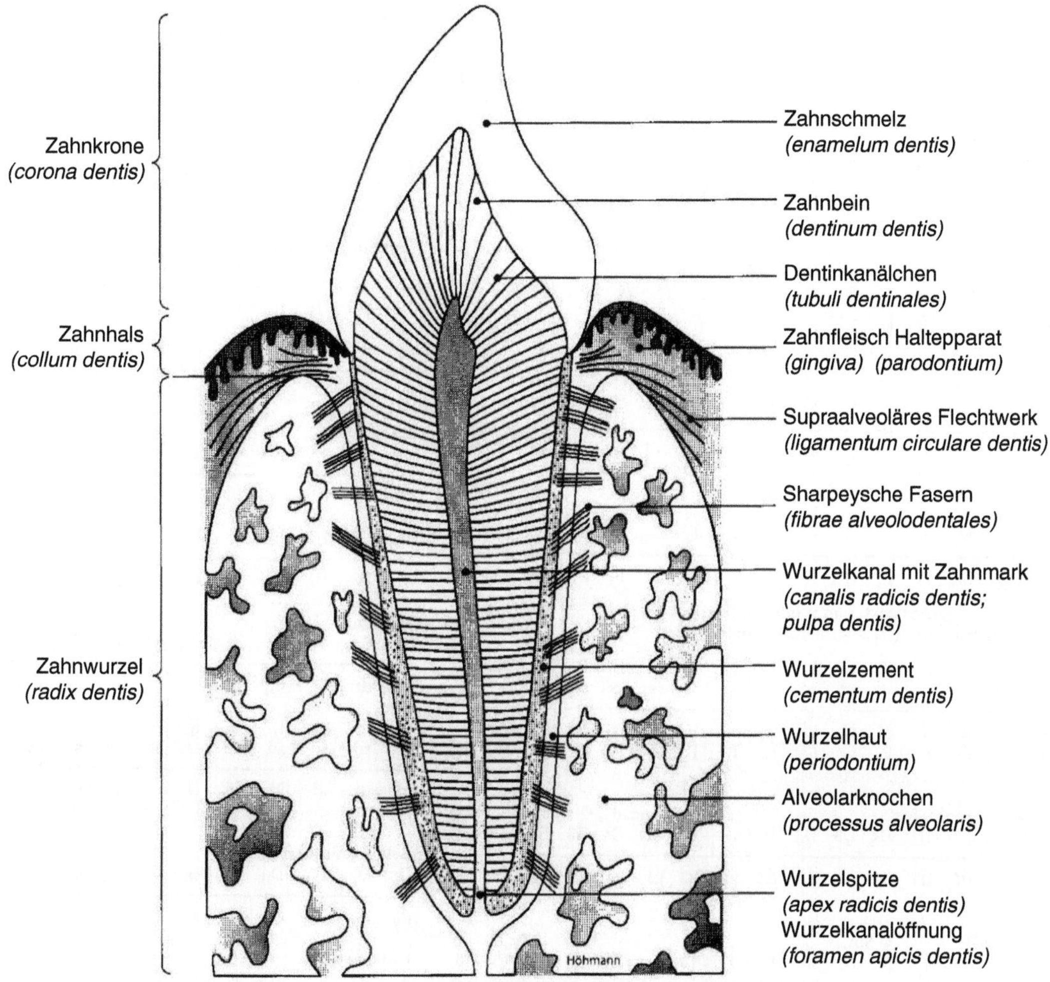

Fig. 17.2 Tooth structure (Drawing Dr. med. dent. B. Höhmann, Munster-Westfalia)

The dentin is quantitatively the largest amount of the dental hard tissue. The interior of the dentin is a cavity filled with the pulpa dentis (*cavum dentis*). The dentin is formed by the odontoblasts, which radially run from the pulp to the dentinal tubules (*dentinal canaliculi*). The pulp proceeds with one or more root canals (*canalis radicis dentis*) past the root apex (*apex radicis dentis*) and ends with an opening (*foramen apicis dentis*) in the depth of a tooth socket (alveolus). All alveoli are located in the teeth-bearing part of the jaw, the alveolar process. The structure of the human thecodont dentition requires the structures parodontium.

17.2 Nomenclature

Lamentably, dental terms are not internationally uniform. Thus, it remains necessary to decipher dental records before they can be evaluated (Alt and Türp 1998).

A dental notation system was created by university professors at the beginning of twentieth century (Zsigmondy 1861, 1874 or Haderup 1887 with his dental shorthand nomenclature). Frykholm and Lysell (1962) have detected that more than 32 different systems for the notation of teeth are in use worldwide. Several common notation systems are used, including Palmer's

Bleibendes Gebiß
Anatomische Zahnformel

rechts								*links*							
M_3	M_2	M_1	P_2	P_1	C	I_2	I_1	I_1	I_2	C	P_1	P_2	M_1	M_2	M_3

F.D.I. (1970)

18	17	16	15	14	13	12	11	21	22	23	24	25	26	27	28
48	47	46	45	44	43	42	41	31	32	33	34	35	36	37	38

Zsigmondy (1861), **Palmer*** (1891)

8⌋	7⌋	6⌋	5⌋	4⌋	3⌋	2⌋	1⌋	⌊1	⌊2	⌊3	⌊4	⌊5	⌊6	⌊7	⌊8
8⌉	7⌉	6⌉	5⌉	4⌉	3⌉	2⌉	1⌉	⌈1	⌈2	⌈3	⌈4	⌈5	⌈6	⌈7	⌈8

Haderup (1887)

8+	7+	6+	5+	4+	3+	2+	1+	+1	+2	+3	+4	+5	+6	+7	+8
8-	7-	6-	5-	4-	3-	2-	1-	-1	-2	-3	-4	-5	-6	-7	-8

Holland

M_3	M_2	M_1	P_2	P_1	C	I_2	I_1	I_1	I_2	C	P_1	P_2	M_1	M_2	M_3
M_3	M_2	M_1	P_2	P_1	C	I_2	I_1	I_1	I_2	C	P_1	P_2	M_1	M_2	M_3

Sive (sd = superior dexter, id = inferior dexter)
(ss = superior insister, is = inferior sinister)

M_3 sd	M_2 sd	M_1 sd	P_2 sd	P_1 sd	C sd	I_2 sd	I_1 sd	I_1 ss	I_2 ss	C ss	P_1 ss	P_2 ss	M_1 ss	M_2 ss	M_3 ss
id M_3	id M_2	id M_1	id P_2	id P_1	id C	id I_2	id I_1	is I_1	is I_2	is C	is′ P_1	is P_2	is M_1	is M_2	is M_3

Belgien, Frankreich D = droit/rechts, G = gauche/links)

D8	D7	D6	D5	D4	D3	D2	D1	G1	G2	G3	G4	G5	G6	G7	G8
d8	d7	d6	d5	d4	d3	d2	d1	g1	g2	g3	g4	g5	g6	g7	g8

Universal* U.S.A.

1	2	3	4	5	6	7	8	9	10	11	12	13	14	15	16
32	31	30	29	28	27	26	25	24	23	22	21	20	19	18	17

Bosworth* U.S.A.

8	7	6	5	4	3	2	1	1	2	3	4	5	6	7	8
H	G	F	E	D	C	B	A	A	B	C	D	E	F	G	H

Milchgebiß
Anatomische Zahnformel (m = Milchmolar)

rechts					*links*				
m_1	m_2	C	I_2	I_1	I_1	I_2	C	m_1	m_2

F.D.I.

55	54	53	52	51	61	62	63	64	65
85	84	83	82	81	71	72	73	74	75

Zsigmondy, Palmer

V	IV	III	II	I	I	II	III	IV	V
V	IV	III	II	I	I	II	III	IV	V

sive

e	d	c	b	a	a	b	c	d	e
e	d	c	b	a	a	b	c	d	e

Haderup

05+	04+	03+	02+	01+	+01	+02	+03	+04	+05
05-	04-	03-	02-	01-	-01	-02	-03	-04	-05

sive

V	IV	III	II	I	I	II	III	IV	V
V	IV	III	II	I	I	II	III	IV	V

Holland

dm_2	dm_1	dc	di_2	di_1	dil	di_2	dc	dm_1	dm_2
dm_2	dm_1	dc	di_2	di_1	dil	di_2	dc	dm_1	dm_2

sive

m_2 sd	m_1 sd	c sd	i_2 sd	i_1 sd	i_1 ss	i_2 ss	c ss	m_1 ss	m_2 ss
id m_2	id m_1	id c	id i_2	id i_1	is i_1	is i_2	is c	is m_1	is m_2

Belgien, Frankfreich

D_V	D_{IV}	D_{III}	D_{II}	D_I	G_I	G_{II}	G_{III}	G_{IV}	G_V
d_V	d_{IV}	d_{III}	d_{II}	d_I	g_I	g_{II}	g_{III}	g_{IV}	g_V

Universal

A	B	C	D	E	F	G	H	I	J
T	S	R	Q	P	O	N	M	L	K

Bosworth

D5	D4	D3	D2	D1	D1	D2	D3	D4	D5
DE	DD	DC	DB	DA	DA	DB	DC	DD	DE

Fig. 17.3 Various dental notation systems (Dorion 1991; Frykholm and Lysell 1962)

Notation (1870, 1891), Cunningham's Universal Notation (see also Parreidt 1882), Bosworth (Fig. 17.3), and the Two-Digit System of the Fédération Dentaire Internationale (FDI) (Goodman 1967; Dorion 1991; Ortiz 1995).

In the current international literature, the four-quadrant method (tooth schema), a two-digit system proposed by Piquet in 1924, is used (Keiser-Nielsen 1971). In 1970, the Working Group for Forensic Odontology (WG/FO) of the Fédération Dentaire Internationale (FDI) varied this system (FDI WORLD 1995).

The FDI Two-Digit System (Fig. 17.4) was adopted in 1955 by the American Dental Association (ADA) and its Commission of Dental Accreditation as an official equivalent of the current universal system (Peck and Peck 1993). The FDI Two-Digit System is also accepted by the International Organization for Standardization (ISO 3950) (1984, 1995), the International Association for Dental Research (IADR), and the World Health Organization (WHO) (1977, 1987), and is used by INTERPOL (1989). For global cooperation, it is recommended

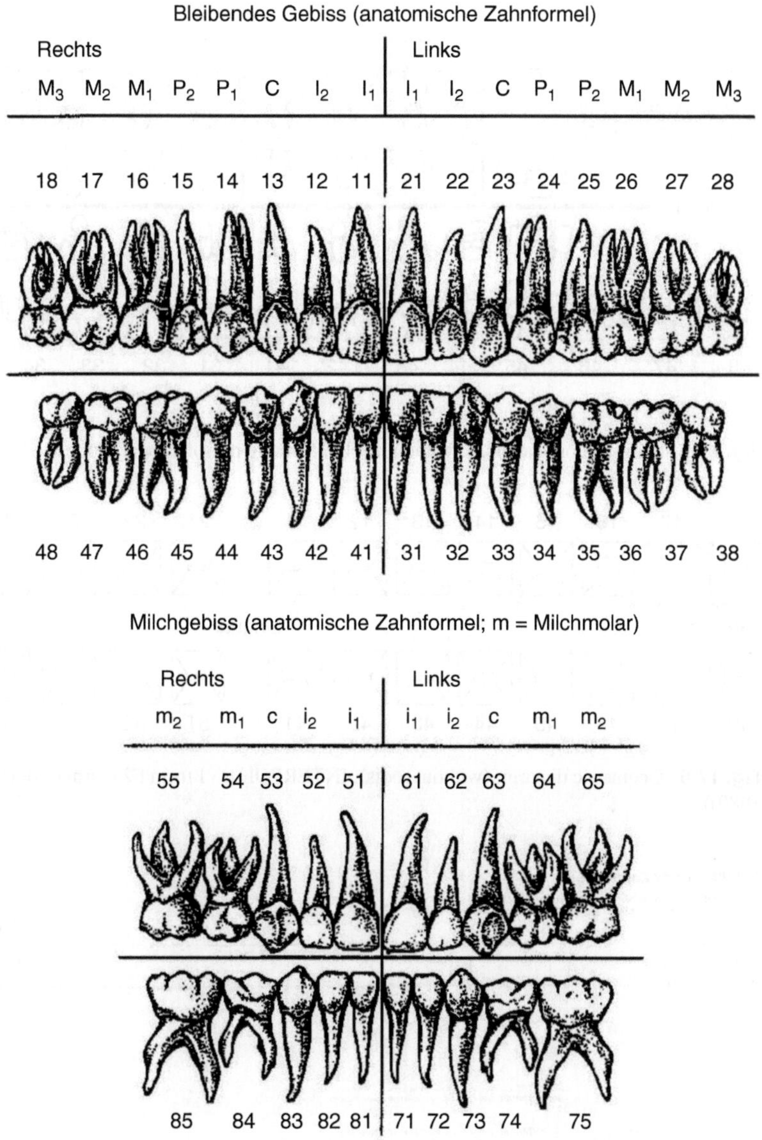

Fig. 17.4 The Two-Digit System; the four-quadrant method (schematic anatomical diagram) (Schumacher 1984)

that the FDI Two-Digit System be used (Rötzscher 1992a, 1992b, 1994).

The first digit of the Two-Digit System identifies the four quadrants of the jaw, clockwise, as 1 = right upper jaw, 2 = left upper jaw, 3 = lower left jaw, 4 = lower right jaw. The second number refers to the teeth (1–8) in each quadrant, counted from the centerline (Schumacher 1984). In the primary dentition, the first digit (5–8) analogy names the quadrant of the jaw, the second number the teeth (1–5) in each quadrant.

Semi-anatomical (Fig. 17.5) or geometric (Fig. 17.6) diagrams without descriptions of root are suitable for rough orientation, but are not recommended for detailed information. Therefore, the German Academy of Forensic Odontostomatology recommends an anatomic diagram (Rötzscher et al. 1999), where the changes in the root zone (diseases, treatments, remaining root fragments, etc.) can also be recorded (Figs. 17.7 and 17.8).

The International Organization for Standardization (ISO) developed a revised version of dentistry (notation system for teeth and regions of the oral cavity)—two-digit tooth and field names of the oral cavity in continuity with

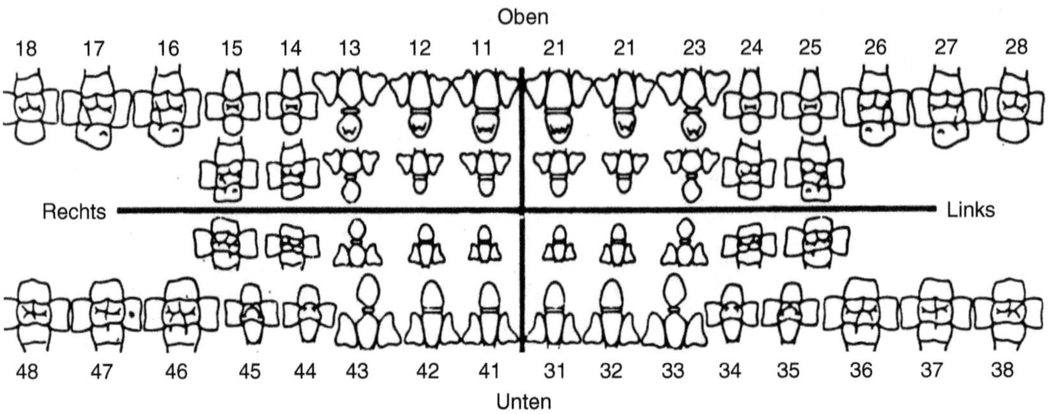

Fig. 17.5 Semi-anatomical chart (without roots). Missing person report (Police) (Pol KP 16 D)

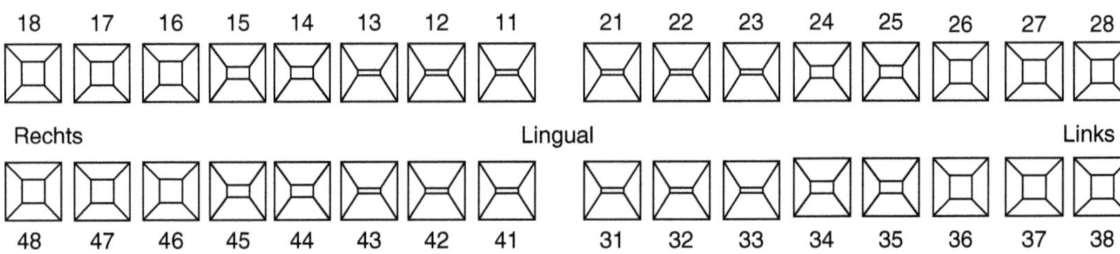

Fig. 17.6 Geometric diagram (without roots). INTERPOL DVI form F2 (form of dental identification (Keiser-Nielsen 1980))

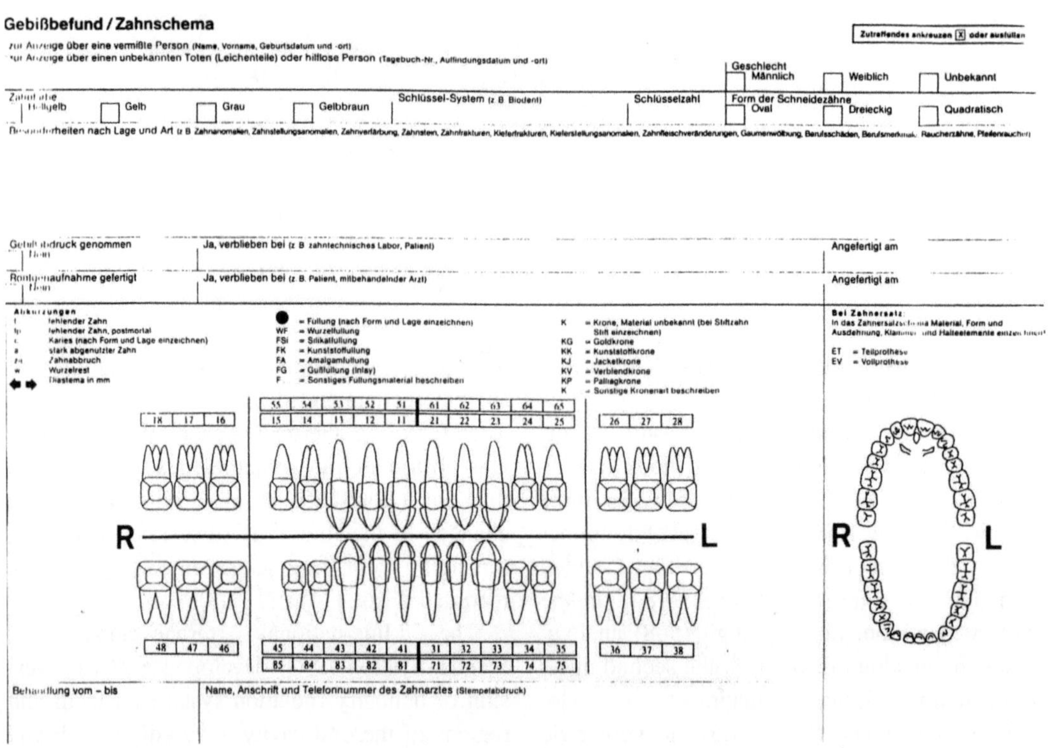

Fig. 17.7 Anatomical chart. Change of Pol KP 16 D (By Dr. B. Höhmann, Munster, Westphalia)

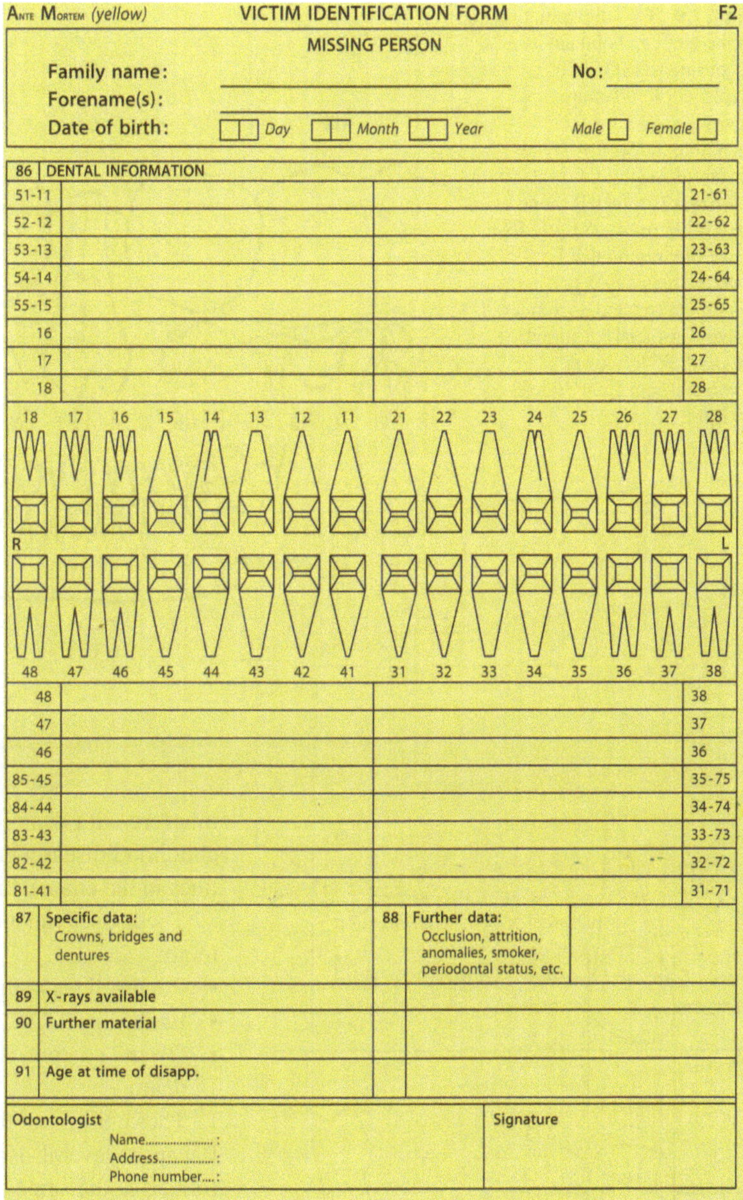

ANTE MORTEM (yellow) VICTIM IDENTIFICATION FORM F2

MISSING PERSON

Family name: No:

Forename(s):

Date of birth: Day Month Year Male Female

86 DENTAL INFORMATION

51-11			21-61
52-12			22-62
53-13			23-63
54-14			24-64
55-15			25-65
16			26
17			27
18			28

48			38
47			37
46			36
85-45			35-75
84-44			34-74
83-43			33-73
82-42			32-72
81-41			31-71

87 Specific data: Crowns, bridges and dentures

88 Further data: Occlusion, attrition, anomalies, smoker, periodontal status, etc.

89 X-rays available

90 Further material

91 Age at time of disapp.

Odontologist
Name...................:
Address...............:
Phone number....:

Signature

Fig. 17.8 Geometric diagram (with root description) INTERPOL DVI form F2. Form of dental identification (Designed by Dr. med. dent. B. Höhman, Munster-Westfalia)

the existing system (ISO 3950). This standard completes the FDI system (FDI World 1995). The names of the teeth and areas of the oral cavity (ISO 3950) are shown in Figs. 17.9 and 17.10)

17.3 Individual Characteristics

The individuality of the teeth is based on many points of comparison (variables) of the 20 or 32 teeth (position anomalies and malformations); each tooth has five anatomical regions. For full dentition, the calculated possible restoration conditions are 3.8×10^4 (Hausmann et al. 1997). The higher the number of quantitative and qualitative points of comparison, the more reliable is the comparison. Computer models have shown that there are greater than 2.5 billion variations (Fiala 1968; Sopher 1986).

Individual characteristic structures are already formed in the enamel and dentin during tooth formation (by layer formation of dental hard

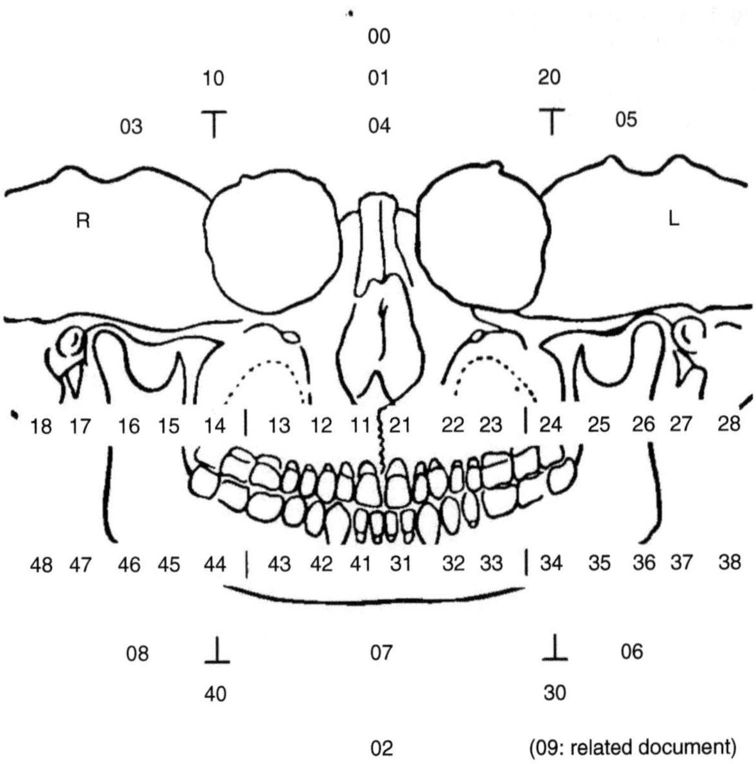

Fig. 17.9 Two-digit notation of the teeth and oral cavity according to ISO 3950. Explanation: *00* entire oral cavity; *01* maxilla; *02* mandible; upper (orofacial) sextant; *03* right; *04* front; *05* left lower (orofacial) range; *06* left; *07* front; *08* right; *09* name of a region that is defined in an annex or document (related document) upper (orofacial) quadrant; *10* right; *20* left lower (orofacial) quadrant *30* left; *40* right

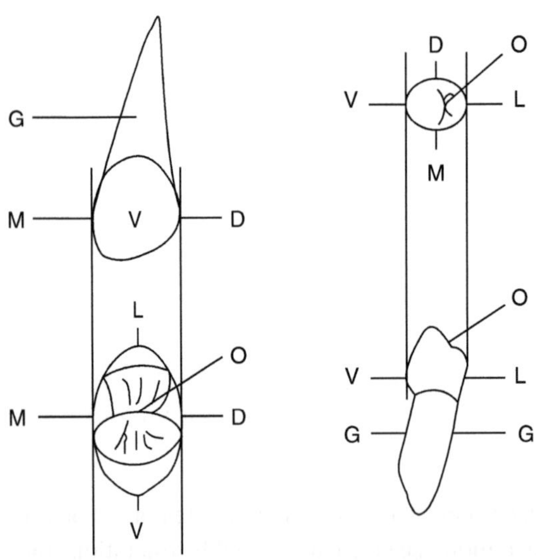

Fig. 17.10 Abbreviations for notations of the dental surface in accordance with ISO 3950. *O* occlusal, *M* mesial, *D* distal, *V* vestibular (labiobuccal), *L* lingual, *G* root surface

tissues). During the prenatal and especially during the postnatal phase of dental development, every individual passes through more or less numerous and intense disease processes that interfere with dental development (birth trauma, childhood diseases) and that leave characteristic lines in the enamel and dentin.

These lines run along the growth layers of the tooth:

- Retzius lines in the enamel prisms
- Ebner-line
- Owen contour lines in the circumpulpal dentin

These lines are broadened by disturbances. Because several types of teeth (groups) are formed at the same time (at the same side in the upper and lower jaw) and because the temporal rhythm of growth disturbances differs from person to person, but is equal for all teeth of an individual, whether two teeth are from the same individual or not can be deduced (Schroeder 1971).

The presence of individual characteristics is duplicated by dental treatment measures, such as conservative dentistry by cavity preparation and the type of filling material (Figs. 17.11 and 17.12), endodontics, jaw and facial surgery by dental extractions and other surgical healing measures, as well as prosthetic dentistry by the

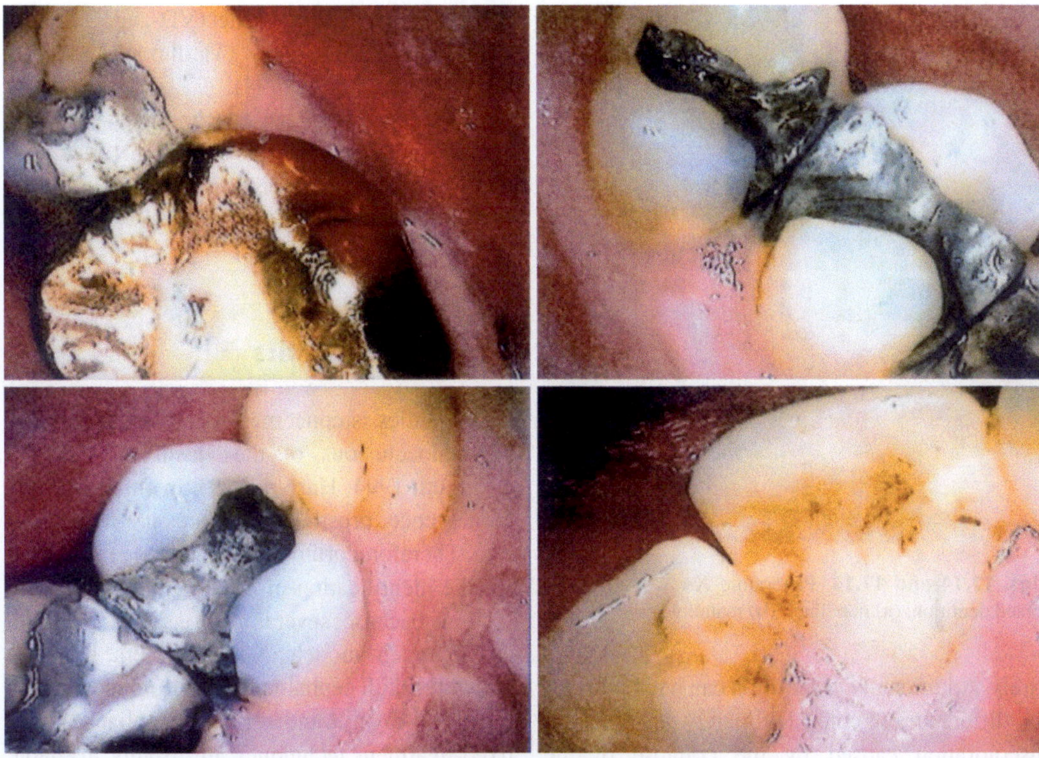

Fig. 17.11 Different filling materials. Sample photos using FLEXISCOPE intraoral camera (Courtesy of Fa. Newtech/ Denzlingen)

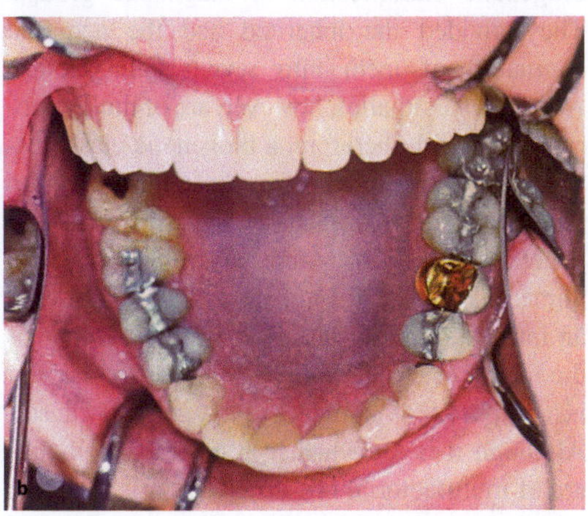

Fig. 17.12 An intraoral color photograph of the upper jaw (with mirror and cheek retractors) (Courtesy of Prof. Gunnar Johanson, Malmö)

type of prosthesis, the implantology (Fig. 17.13), the geriatric dentistry, and orthodontics (Rötzscher and Reimann 1975; Sopher 1986).

On the other hand, modern dental prophylaxis significantly decreases individual characteristics

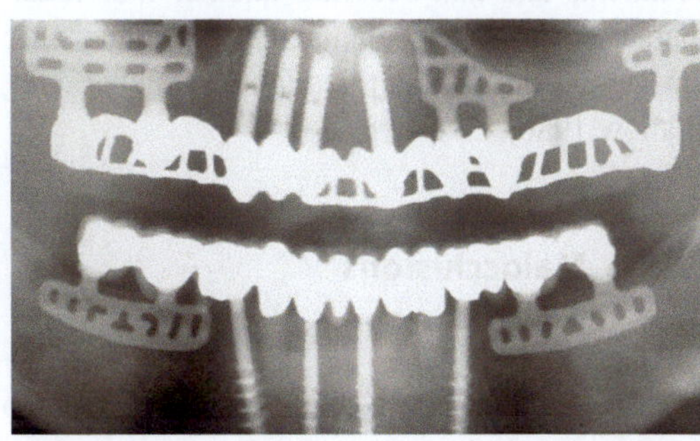

Fig. 17.13 Radiograph of dentition with implants and prosthetics

by pedodontical (pediatric) and periodontical measures (e.g., fluoridation and improved oral hygiene) with reduction of caries and periodontal diseases in the deciduous and mixed dentition (Figs. 17.14 and 17.15) and their consequences in adulthood.

The determination of tooth color has only a low status for identification of living or dead persons. If no prosthetics have been implemented, determination of tooth color takes place only

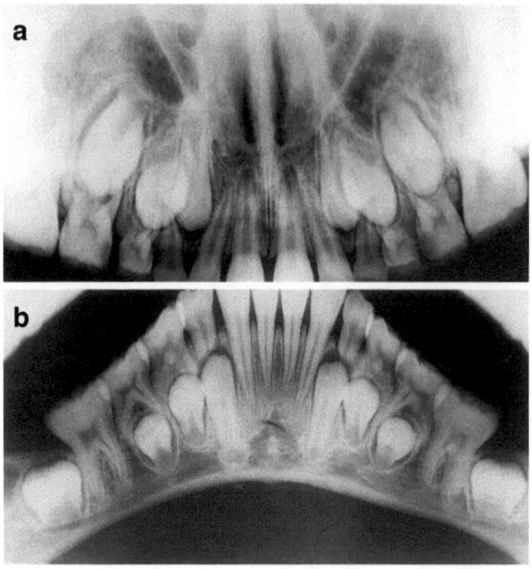

Figs. 17.14 and 17.15 Panoramic X-ray image of a mixed dentition, (**a**) maxillary, (**b**) mandible

rarely. Additionally, a dentition can have substantial differences in color. Ultimately, a slow tooth discoloration caused by the collapse of the necrotic pulp occurs postmortem. In contrast, the tooth color is always specified before prosthetic treatments and that becomes another individual characteristic that is obtained postmortem and can be used for identification (Schuebel and Shallow 1980).

17.3.1 Malocclusions

We distinguish:

1. Congenital, hereditable, or malocclusions occurring during dental development
2. Acquired natural disorder or traumatic injury
3. Presence or absence of one or more of the 20 or 32 teeth
4. Combinations and changing fit of the various restorations and their materials
5. Orthodontic appliances or fixed-treatment techniques for rehabilitation of the stomatognathic system (FKO):
   (a) Activator, modified FKO appliances (FKO-Kybernetor principle)
   (b) Disk-shaped device (Schwarz-plate) with orthodontic screws (i.e., Y plate)
   (c) Feed and return skillet (VD-and RD-plate)
   (d) Fixed appliances (Vardimon and Ant-Baumgartner 1994)
   (e) Standard-edgewise technique
   (f) Removable devices (Schmuth 1994)
   (g) Standard-edgewise technique, straight-wire technique (Andrews), SW appliance (SWA)

17.3.2 Orthodontics

Orthodontics is concerned with the treatment of all malocclusions of the masticatory system (Schmuth 1994; Harzer 1999). In childhood and adolescence, prosthetic measures are the exception. Therefore, orthodontic knowledge is needed for the identification of children and adolescent victims because several photographs, planning and treatment models, X-rays of teeth, the skull structure, skull cephalometric side images (FRS), hand X-rays, and FKO appliances or fixed-treatment techniques are usually available and can be used for comparison.

Kantorowicz and Korkhaus (1926) proposed a biogenetic classification of diagnostic groups. They divided the inherited and the acquired anomalies of teeth into seven main groups. Almost all anomalies, however, are of multifactorial origin and, therefore, a biogenetic classification must be rejected. Note that any attempt to divide malocclusions solely by etiological and genetic aspects will remain incomplete. Despite numerous efforts, it is not yet possible to develop an internationally valid classification because of the nature of the malformations, whose majority is composed of a range of biogenetic causes. Although it is known that almost all anomalies are of multifactorial origin, the variation and the morphological and functional diversity of dental malocclusions and dysgnathia allows no classification in only a few diagnostic groups, or may only be poorly characterized by them. Nevertheless, the indication of Angle class and the use of guiding symptoms with regard to a possible uniform documentation and communication is useful and helpful (Klink-Heckmann 1977; Schmuth 1994; Harzer 1999).

17.3.2.1 Frequency of Dysgnathia

Tooth position and malocclusion are common in the population, and their incidence depends on age. From 3 to 6 years (use-phase of the primary dentition):

(a) the open bite or
(b) the increased overjet (usually as result of sucking or other habits)

are dominant in 30 % of children. Up to the age of 8–10 years, this high frequency decreases by 1–2 % for (a) and by 12 % for (b). However, mandibular prognathism and crossbite, which already occur at 2–4 % in the deciduous teeth are progressive. In the literature, the incidence rate for all kinds of malocclusion ranges between 40 % and 80 % (Harzer 1999).

17.3.2.2 Dentures

During excavations, individual features of dentures are used for the temporal determination of the time of death (Zuhrt et al. 1978; Alt 1997). Individual features can be derived from the production and development data in the field of prosthetic and restorative dentistry (Endris 1982; Heydenreich 1995).

17.4 Anomalies of the Dental Hard Tissue

Usually the teeth are slightly yellow colored and the enamel is translucent; different dentin pigment and anatomically regular tooth thicknesses as well as variations of the shades are found within a tooth and may change in the different regions of the teeth. Now and again, the forensic odontologist is faced with pigmented teeth (tooth discoloration) (Padayachee 1988).

17.5 Pink Teeth Phenomenon

The term pink teeth refers to pink or dark red (port wine) discoloration of the dentin of several teeth, especially in the cervical part (Fig. 17.16), and, rarely, in the apex of the root (Whittaker et al. 1976). Not every tooth must be involved. In some diseases, single pink spots were observed.

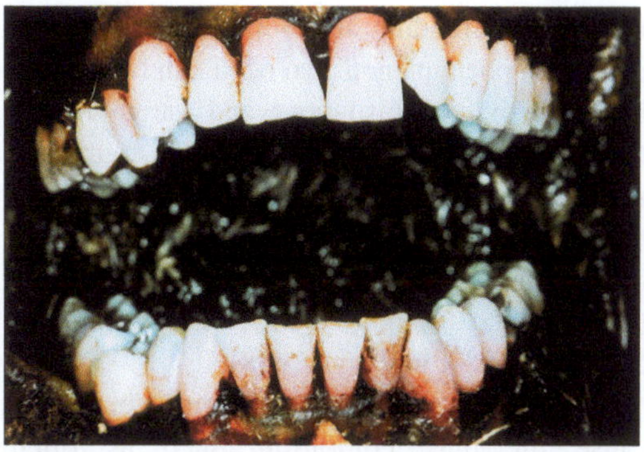

Fig 17.16 Pink teeth phenomenon

First described in 1829 (Bell 1829), the pink teeth phenomenon is repeatedly used in the investigation of homicides (Borrman et al. 1994). Pink teeth are observed earliest at 1–2 weeks after the time of death. The pink teeth phenomenon is caused by the infiltration of hemoglobin and hemoglobin derivatives into dentin, under the precondition of hyperemia or congestion in erythrocyte extravasation based in the pulp capillary, further autolysis, and moist environment.

Permanent or temporary pigmentation of teeth depends on uncharacteristic, not-associated causes but also on associated causes (Padayachee 1988). In typhoid patients, pink discoloration can be observed in single teeth (Miller 1957). During the preparation, individual teeth may have discolorations caused by irritation of the microcirculation of the pulp systems and by vascular stasis and hemorrhage (Grayson et al. 1989; Bergenholz 1991).

Temporary pink/red discoloration can be found after dental trauma. In these cases, the pulp necrosis may cause grey or black discoloration (Giunta and Tsamtsouris 1978). A single tooth can appear pink if the pulp is visible (by internal dentin resorption and stored granulation tissue) (Auslander 1967; Grossman 1984). Pink teeth is not found in cases of natural death (Bröndum and Simonsen 1987).

Most pink teeth findings are found in dead people who lay in the water or in damp conditions; such as with drowning being the cause of death (Bell 1829; Beeley and Harvey 1973; Whittaker et al. 1976; Pilz et al. 1980; Clark and

Law 1984; Bröndum and Simonsen 1987). The pink teeth phenomenon also occurs in burns, carbon monoxide poisoning, and strangulation (Whittaker et al. 1976). However, pink teeth have also been detected in cases without any relation to a specific cause of death. Pink teeth have also been found in death by barbiturate poisoning (Beeley and Harvey 1973; Bröndum and Simonsen 1987; van Wyk 1988).

Basically, certain postmortem conditions cause the pink coloration, such as often described in drowned bodies with the head hanging low in the water. In this respect, the analogy to postmortem hypostasis is obvious. The color intensity depends on the time factor (Gustafson 1966). Pink teeth may easily be overlooked on inspection with the naked eye. For this reason, careful histological examination should be performed in suspect cases, because the dentin may be involved more or less intensively (van Wyk 1988). The appearance of a pink discoloration in certain body regions (including the teeth) depends on specific anatomical terms, but is mostly independent of the actual cause of death.

17.6 Habitual Marks

In many people, you can see marks on the teeth (Alt 1997) caused by their habits, e.g.:

- Grinding (bruxism, bruxomania)
- Excessive tooth abrasion
- Pipe smoking (so-called pipe smoker's hole)
- The habit of holding certain things with the teeth
- Smoking (resulting in a brown/black discoloration of the teeth)
- Tea drinking (resulting in a brown/black discoloration of the teeth)
- Ritual mutilations by extracting or grinding of teeth
- Piercings (modern body piercing) in the orofacial region (lips, tongue, cheek), such as young people of both sexes in the Western world increasingly have (Alt and Pichler 1998)
- Leukoplakia, which may cause irritations in the soft tissues

17.7 Occupational Marks

Today, occupational characteristics of teeth are less common because of improved working conditions, but certain occupations still can influence the dental status:

- People who are constantly in touch with dust have more tooth wear.
- Industrial workers often have tooth erosion caused by contact with acids; metal workers often have discoloration of the teeth.
- Baker's caries is well known, but is declining because of the introduction of modern production methods.
- Musicians, glass blowers, and carpenters often have traces in the cutting edge of the front teeth.

17.8 Social Position

Dental findings and dental restorations allow conclusions regarding social status. People in higher positions and artists (e.g., singers) often pay attention to a good dental status and may undergo complex and expensive treatments (psychosocial aspects). In contrast, socially weak people take less care of their identity and thus less or not at all of their teeth. A Scandinavian study has shown, however, that the SAS airline staff had no better dental status than the average population (Keiser-Nielsen 1980).

References

Alt KW (1997) Odontologische Verwandtschaftsanalyse. G. Fischer, Stuttgart/Jena/Lübeck/Ulm

Alt KW, Pichler SL (1998) Artificial modifications of human teeth. In: Alt KW, Rösing FW, Teschler-Nicola M (eds) Dental anthrology. Fundamentals, limits and prospects. Springer, Wien/New York, p 389

Alt KW, Türp C (1998) Roll call: thirty-two white horses on a red field. The advantages of the FDI two-digit system of designating teeth. In: Alt KW, Rösing FW, Teschler-Nicola M (eds) Dental anthropology. Fundamentals, limits, and perspectives. Springer, Wien/New York, pp 41–55

Auslander WP (1967) Discoloration of a traumatic sequela. NY State Dental J 33:534–538

Beeley JA, Harvey W (1973) Pink teeth as a post-mortem phenomenon. J Forensic Sci Soc 13:297–305

Bell T (1829) Anatomy, physiology and disease of the teeth. Highley, London, p 12,13

Bergenholz G (1991) Iatrogenic injury to the pulpin dental procedures: aspects of pathogenesis, management and preventive measures. Int Dent J 41:99–110

Borrman H, DuChesne A, Brinkmann B (1994) Medicolegal aspects of post-mortem pink teeth. Int J Leg Med 106:225–231

Bröndum N, Simonsen J (1987) Postmortem red coloration of teeth. A retrospective investigation of 26 cases. Am J Forensic Med Pathol 8:127–130

Clark DA, Law ML (1984) Postmortem pink teeth. Med Sci Law 24:130–134

Dorion R (1991) Tooth designation conversion. Manual of forensic odontology. ASFO, AAFS, Colorado Springs, p 329

Endris R (1982) Forensische Katastrophenmedizin. 6.5.3 Technologische IdM. Kriminalistik, Heidelberg, p 86

FDIWorld(1995)Nachrichten.Zahnbezeichnungssysteme. Mai/Juni,11-12; Sept/Okt: 24–25

Fiala B (1968) Identifikace osob podle chrupu - Forensni stomatologie (Identifikation anhand des Gebisses - Forensische Stomatologie). Státní Zdravotnické Nakladelství, Praha, p 43

Frykholm KO, Lysell L (1962) Different systems for the recording of teeth and tooth surfaces. Int Dent J 12(2):194–207

Giunta JL, Tsamtsouris A (1978) Stains and discolorations of teeth: review and case reports. J Pedod 5:175–182

Goodman P (1967) A universal system for identifying permanent and primary teeth. J Dent Child 34:312–315

Grayson A, Kim S, Kim SB (1989) Coronal and apical blood flow of the pulp in response to crown preparation. J Dent Res 65 (Special issue): IADR Abstract no. 422

Grossman LI (1984) Endodontic practice. Lea and Febiger, Philadelphia

Gustafson G (1966) Forensic odontology. Staples Press, London, p 191

Haderup V (1887) Vorschlag zu einer internationalen Bezeichnung der Zähne. Korresp Bl Zahnärzte 16:314

Hahn W (1995) Forensische Zahnheilkunde/Odonto-Stomatologie. In: Hoffmann-Axthelm W et al. (Hrsg) Lexikon der Zahnmedizin: 6. (11.) Aufl. Quintessenz, Berlin, p 243

Harzer W (1999) Lehrbuch der Kieferorthopädie. 4.2 Klassifikationen. 4.3 Häufigkeiten von Dysgnathien. S. 58–60

Hausmann R, Liebler M, Schellmann B (1997) Zur Personenidentifikation mittels Zahnstatus. Rechtsmedizin 7:86–89

Heydenreich HG (1995) Zeitraum der Verwendung verschiedener Materialien. Persönl Mitt

Keiser-Nielsen S (1971) FDI two digit system of designation teeth. Int Dent J 21:104–106

Keiser-Nielsen S (1980) Person identification by means of the teeth. J. Wright & Sons Ltd, Bristol, pp 12–13

Keiser-Nielsen S (1984) Oscar Amoëdo. In: Hill IR (ed) Forensic odontology. Its scope and history. Bicester, Great Britain, pp 14–16

Klink-Heckmann U (1977) Problematik der Klassifikation der Dysgnathien. In: Klink-Heckmann U, Bredy E (Hrsg.) Orthopädische Stomatologie. Thieme Stuttgart, pp 23–24

Miller SC (1957) Oral diagnosis and treatment. Blackstone, New York

Ortiz A (1995) Dental records – a tool in forensic dentistry. In: Bowers CM, Bell GL (eds) Manual of forensic odontology. ASFO, AAFS, Colorado Springs, p 30

Ortmann C, DuChesne A (1998) A partially mummified corpse with pink teeth and pink nails. Int J Legal Med 111:35–37

Padayachee A (1988) Pigmentation of teeth: a review. J Forensic Odontostomatol 6(2):67–76

Palmer C (1870) Proceedings of the 10th annual meeting of the American Dental Association, Nashville, Tennessee. Dent Cosmos 12:209–211

Palmer C (1891) Palmer's dental notation. Dent Cosmos 33:194

Parreidt J (1882) Zählung der Zähne und Benennung der verschiedenen Zahnsorten. In: Zahnärztl Mitt aus der chirurgischen Universitätszahnklinik zu Leipzig. A. Felix, München, pp 10–15

Peck S, Peck L (1993) A time for change of tooth numbering systems. J Dent Educ 8:643–647

Pilz W, Reimann W, Krause DH (1980) Gerichtliche Medizin für Stomatologen. J.A. Barth, Leipzig, p 94

Rötzscher K (1992a) The origins and development of FDI, Interpol and IOFOS: international cooperation in identification. J Forensic Odontostomatol 10(2): 58–63

Rötzscher K (1992b) Postmortem dental chart. IOFOS Newsl Year 14 No 3: 7–12

Rötzscher K (1994) Probleme der zahnärztlichen Befunderhebung und der Zahnregistrierung. AKFOS Newsl Jg 1:6

Rötzscher K (1996) 20 Jahre Arbeitskreis Forensische Odonto-Stomatologie. AKFOS (1976–1996). AKFOS Newsl Jg 3:63–64

Rötzscher K, Reimann W (1975) Die forensische Stomatologie. In: Prokop O, Göhler W (Hrsg) Forensische Medizin, 3.Aufl. Volk und Gesundheit, Berlin, pp 545–564

Rötzscher K, Benthaus S, Höhmann B, Grundmann C (1999) Zur Dokumentation zahnärztlicher Befunde. Kriminalistik 6(99):411–413

Schmuth GPF (1994) a) Dysgnathie und Eugnathie: 1–3, b) Klassifikation der Dysgnathien Befundgruppen:4–18, c) Kieferorthopädische Behandlungstechnik - Herausnehmbare Geräte. In: Schmuth GPF, Vardimon AD (Hrsg) Kieferorthopädie, 3.Aufl. G. Thieme, Stuttgart/New York, pp 237–300

Schroeder HE (1971) Histologische Methoden in der forensischen Zahnheilkunde. Recht Praxis 8:434–436

Schroeder HE (1987) Orale Strukturbiologie. G. Thieme, Stuttgart/New York, p 4

Schumacher GH (1984) Anatomie für Stomatologen. 1.Teil Kopf, Orofaziales System, Auge, Ohr 1.3.3. Kennzeichnung der Zähne und Zahnformeln. JA Barth, Leipzig, pp 10–11

Schwarz AM (1933) Die “Schuld” des Unterkiefers an der Angle-Klasse II und III. Z Zahnärztl Orthop 20:1–22

Schwarz AM (1936) Die kieferbezügliche Untersuchung. Urban & Schwarzenberg, Berlin

Sopher IM (1986) Kap.5: Grundsätzliche Begriffe der zahnärztlichen Identifikation: Der prämortale Befund. Die Individualität des Gebisses. Forensische Zahnmedizin. Quintessenz, Berlin, pp 65–66

Taatz H (1980) Entwicklung der Zähne. Entwicklungsstörungen der Zähne. In: Pilz W, Plathner C, Taatz H (Hrsg) Grundlagen der Kariologie und Endodontie. J.A. Barth, Leipzig, pp 27–32, 96–119

van Wyk CW (1988) Pink teeth of the dead, II. Minor variations. J Oral Pathol Med 17:568–572

Vardimon AD, Ant-Baumgartner H (1994) Festsitzende Techniken. In: Schmuth GPF, Vardimon AD (Hrsg) Kieferorthopädie, 3.Aufl. G. Thieme, Stuttgart/New York, pp 301–338

Whittaker DK, Thomas VC, Thomas RIM (1976) Post-mortem pigmentation of the teeth. Br Dent J 140:100–102

Zsigmondy A (1861) Grundzüge einer praktischen Methode zur raschen und genauen Vermehrung der Zahnärztlichen Beobachtungen und Operationen. Dtsch Vierteljschr Zahnh 1:209–211

Zsigmondy A (1874) A practical method for rapidly noting dental observations. Br J Dent Sci 17:580–582

Zuhrt R, Rottstock F, Winterfeld RI (1978) 14. Möglichkeiten und Methoden der Stomatologie bei der Identifizierung, 14.6. Liegezeitbestimmung. In: Hunger H, Leopold D (Hrsg) Identifikation. J.A. Barth, Leipzig, pp 310

18 Clinical Results

Klaus Rötzscher

18.1 Preliminary Comments to Initial Findings

The chronology of a medical/dental treatment is first to collect the history and then to gather the clinical findings (including X-ray images). From these data, diagnosis, treatment, and finally the course are derived.

When documenting the anamnesis, many practitioners only record whether a tooth is decayed, damaged, or missing. A description of the nature and localization of fillings or bridges that is more detailed is made only for treatments dentists have performed themselves. This incomplete documentation does not meet the requirements of dental standards. Furthermore, many dentists use shortcut formulas, and these hieroglyphs must be deciphered in phone calls, faxes, or emails.

Clinical findings *lege artis* must gather all odontological data in precise and readable form, as taught during university education (Kaatsch and Ritz 1993) (Fig. 18.1, Tables 18.1 and 18.2).

The quality assessment of information regarding the presence of dental documentation is different. Therefore, identifications may be complicated or even impossible (Andersen et al. 1995) (Table 18.3).

K. Rötzscher, Dr. med. Dr. med. dent.
German Academy of Forensic Odontostomatology (AKFOS),
Wimphelingstraße 7, 67346 Speyer, Germany
e-mail: roetzscher.klaus.dr@t-online.de

The acceptance of information technology (IT) in dental practices is increasing. Paperless billing was introduced in 1997; now approximately 80 % of practitioners keep electronic records (Stratmann 1997). According to a statistical survey of the Dentist's Confederation (KZBV) in December 1998, in Germany, 91.31 % of 52,116 dentists, practice owners, or associates in private practice – with a total of 76,766 chamber members (according to the BZÄK statistics from the fourth quarter of 1998) – file their findings for conservative and surgical services in a computer system. This allows a more rapid recall of findings.

In the initial finding, all extractions, fillings (localization and extent), implants, dentures (crowns, bridges, etc.), bars, root residues, localization and extent of carious lesions, apical and conspicuous marginal bone defects, stains, calculus, and periodontal disease must be recorded. Such a complete initial finding with evaluation of all odontological features is the basis of any dental activity (Kaatsch and Ritz 1993).

18.2 01-Finding

For billing of no. 01, the following index Fig. 18.2 (01-finding are made every half year and are paid by health insurance) is used in Germany. It includes a "comprehensive examination of the teeth, mouth and temporomandibular disorders" (Meurer 1988):

1 c=dental caries; 2 z=tooth=destructed; 3 f=tooth=missing (Fig. 18.2).

K. Rötzscher (ed.), *Forensic and Legal Dentistry*,
DOI 10.1007/978-3-319-01330-5_18, © Springer International Publishing Switzerland 2014

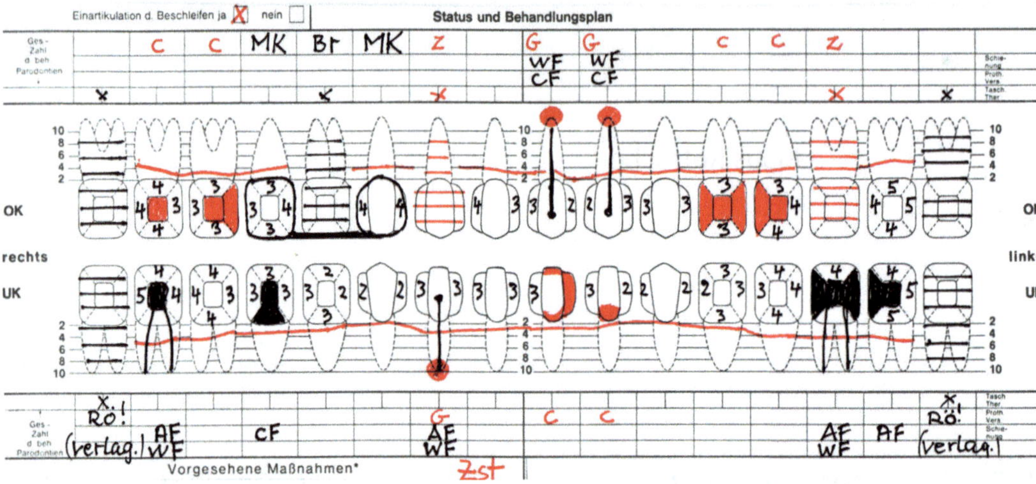

Fig. 18.1 Findings on anatomical chart (see Table 18.1 and 18.2)

Table 18.1 First findings checked at the first visit of the patient (16 June 1994)

Findings	Tooth
Caries	16mo, 17o, 24mod, 25mo, 31cdl, 32c
Missing teeth	14, 18, 28 (Rö!), 38 verlagert, retiniert (Rö.), 48 verlagert, retiniert (Rö.)
Destructed teeth	12, 26 (Rö!)
Filled teeth	21p AF, 22p AF, 36mod AF, 37mo AF, 45ob CF, 47o CF
Crowns	13, 15 (metal ceramic)
Bridges	14 (pontic), 13, 15 (abutment teeth)
Nonvital teeth	21, 22, 26, 31, 36, 42, 47
Root fillings	21, 22, 36, 47 (Rö.)
Trepanation	42
Apical changes	21, 22, 42 (Rö: chronic apicalostitid)
Calculus	16–27, 35–46

Table 18.2 Explanation of abbreviations

Definition	Abbreviation
Caries	C
Missing teeth (not visible teeth)	X (extracted), X-ray! (shifted teeth?)
Destructed teeth	Z
Filled teeth (fillings)	AF (amalgam), CF (plastic)
Crowns, bridges	MK (metal ceramic), Br (bridge)
Negative vitality testing	Vit (–)
Root-treated teeth	WF
Trepanation	trep
Apical changes	G
Calculus	Zst

Table 18.3 Quality assessment of antemortem (AM) information

Category	Definition
Degree 0	No information
Degree 1	Information without patient file (no written documents)
Degree 2	Patient file only
Degree 3	Patient file, with single radiographs (unsystematic)
Degree 4	Patient file, with bitewings
Degree 5	Patient file with a full orofacial review and OPG radiographs (panoramic radiographs or similar)

Six categories, Andersen et al. (1995)

Most dentists in Germany use this index in the recall stage.

Fillings, implants, removable dentures, crowns, bridges, rails, root residues, the localization and extent of carious lesions, apical and conspicuous marginal bone defects, stains, calculus, and periodontal diseases are not gathered in the 01-finding.

Findings according to the DMF index, which are regarded as inadequate, are recorded as D = tooth = decayed (destructed), M = tooth = missing (missing), F = tooth = filled (filled); the so-called decay index, or the EKF-Index (German Version) records findings as E = tooth = extracted, K = tooth = decayed, F = tooth missing (the total

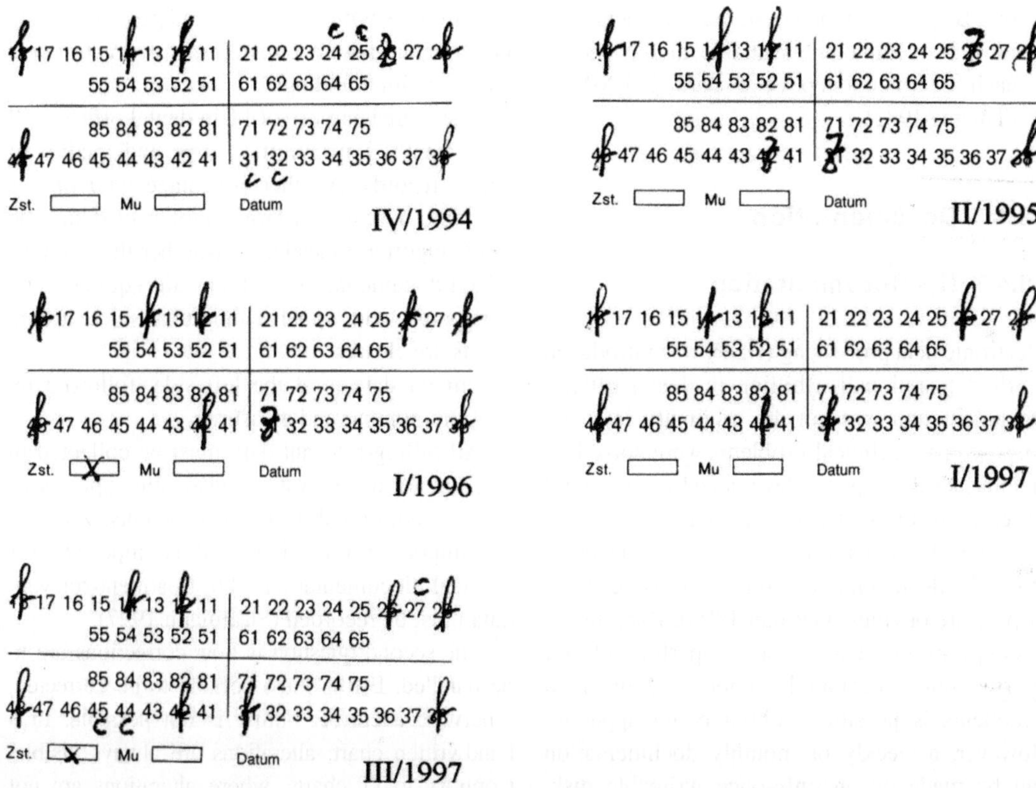

Fig. 18.2 01-findings are made every half year and are paid by health insurance

number of teeth is 28 because the wisdom teeth are not taken into account); or in modification to the DMF-area index (DMF-S [surface]) by dividing the crown into five areas and finally to the DMF-tooth index (DMF-T [tooth]) with a maximum of 32 teeth per bite. The indices are used for caries epidemiology (statistical survey of the number of caries manifestations, up to the time of examination).

18.3 File Management

According to recent jurisdiction, the practitioner has to record all findings and measures. Dental records are not only reminders for the practitioners, but also for proper documentation for their patients. The complete recording of all stages of treatment (in a legal sense) has several functions:

1. To ensure a scheduled further treatment by:
   (a) The same dentist
   (b) An assistant, representative, or successor
   (c) Another dentist/dental specialist by referral
2. Protection against:
   (a) Complications and incidences
   (b) Liability claims because of malpractice
   (c) The accusation of negligence in examination and planning in case of failure or incident
   (d) The accusation of complicating the burden of proof
   (e) The accusation of providing insufficient documentation for assessments by insurance companies or legal authorities
   (f) The risk of rendering a faulty opinion and its legal consequences
3. The practitioner is required to record each treatment step with detailed listing of treated teeth, diagnosis, and date of treatment

(§ 5 BMV-Z). At the latest, the documentation must be completely available at the end of each treatment step (§ 5 para 2 BMV-Z) (Thieme 1982).

18.4 Documentation

18.4.1 IT – Documentation

Electronic data processing (EDP) was introduced in 1968 to rationalize billing in dental offices. Documentation was not the originally intended purpose. The technical problems were solved by an interface description, developed by the Central Research Institute of Ambulatory Health Care in Germany. The risks of IT for an orderly accounting and documentation for a possible legal dispute are obvious (German 1998). Back-up on a tamper-proof disk must be performed. Of course, a subsequent modification of documented treatments is possible without being apparent. However, a weekly or monthly documentation can be made on an only-once writeable disk. Properly performed IT documentation suggests the correctness of its content. The burden of proof is with the practitioner only if the completeness or accuracy of the stored data is doubtful (Walther 1996). Although the fundamental jurisdiction has yet been decided, it is acknowledged that dental documentation may be based on IT as well as on imaging and virtual recordings (Epple 1994).

A survey of 143 dentists in Middle Franconia, Germany (Hausmann et al. 1997) showed that, in 65 %, only a "minimal finding" was recorded; in 19.5 %, findings that also included restorations made by the respondent ("updated finding") were recorded; and, in 15.5 %, findings in which all existing restorations, including preexisting restorations, were documented ("exemplar finding"). The study also inspected the error rate in the treatment of 61 patients, which was 21.36 % in "exemplar findings" and 55.6 % in "minimal findings." The compared dental charts show considerable differences in the scope and quality of the recorded data. As a result, quite often, only a "minimum finding" is available for forensic examinations or assessments in legal disputes. According to this evaluation, IT is increasingly used in dental practice. Interestingly, 82 % of the practitioners with "exemplar findings" have used IT, compared with only 33 % of practitioners with "minimal findings".

The increasing use of IT in dental offices will significantly improve the scope and quality of dental records. Another advantage *inter alia* is the rapid access to a large amount of data. The most important question is whether the computerized documentation includes all required data. Compared with handwritten charts, electronic charts are clearer:

Treatment date is at the left side, followed by tooth number and measures.

All billing-relevant data must be collected in detailed form. IT systems also offer options of entering additional data and comments, which is not important for billing but is important for medical documentation. All treatment-relevant data must be recorded (Stratmann 1997).

The second question is how corrections are to be handled. Errors must be able to be corrected, otherwise a correct billing is not possible. In a handwritten chart, alterations are always visible. Contrary to IT charts, where alterations are not retraceable, information regarding what was altered, by whom, and at what time, can be documented. The original data must be stored in a write-protected file. Modern image processing programs allow alterations of stored data. These corrections must be securely stored. Subsequent retouchings on an original X-ray image cannot be returned to the original condition (Stratmann 1997).

18.4.1.1 Storage Periods (Table 18.4)

Table 18.4 Storage periods for dental records in Germany (March 1995) (Thieme 1982)

1. Medical records (index cards): 3 years after treatment (BMV – Z § 5 (2) EC – Agreement § 4.2)
2. Orthodontics and periodontal disease: 3 years after treatment (BMV – Z § 5 (2) EC – Agreement § 4.2)
3. Dentures (planning models): 2 years after placement (§ 135 para 4, sentence 3 SGB V)
4. X-ray images: much longer storage periods (§ 28 para 3 RöV, valid in the version of 30 April 2003) 4.1. Recordings of X-ray treatments: 30 years after last treatment (§ 28, 3 RöV), e.g., radiation records 4.2. X-ray records: 10 years after last examination 4.3. X-ray images must be available for inspection (§ 28 para 3 RöV valid in the version dated 30 April 2003)

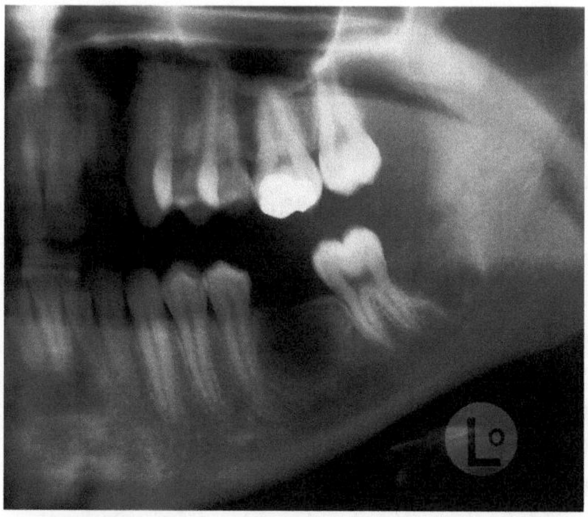

Fig. 18.3 After surgical removal of a cyst in region 36 (see Fig. 18.4) and extraction tooth 36 (OPG-Nr. 3807/92)

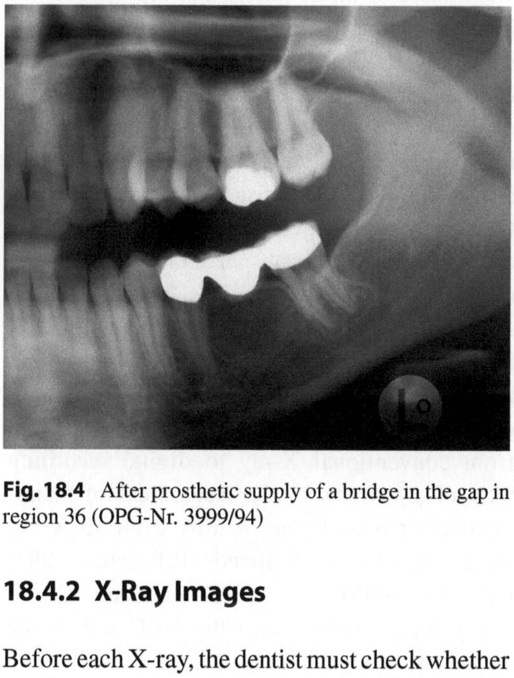

Fig. 18.4 After prosthetic supply of a bridge in the gap in region 36 (OPG-Nr. 3999/94)

18.4.2 X-Ray Images

Before each X-ray, the dentist must check whether and which previous images exist. Date, place, type, and dose of radiation must be documented, as well as the technical data of the X-ray machine (Riepert and Rittner 1989). The X-ray image is the basis for any prosthetic, implant, oral surgery, and orthodontic treatment. For forensic assessment of a proper treatment, X-ray images are essential, because the detection of faulty treatment (e.g., root perforation, incomplete extractions, faulty fillings, or poorly fitted dentures) is possible with their help. Additionally, inflammatory, tumoral (see Figs. 18.3 and 18.4), and traumatic injuries are visible and eventually may exonerate the practitioner from an accusation of faulty treatment. Note that tooth extractions should not be performed without previous X-ray documentation in order to display the region (not only of parts, e.g., impacted wisdom teeth). The X-ray image is approved as evidence (Rohde 1995; Rötzscher 1995a). Digital X-ray images are approved as evidence in court if printed on paper and stored on hard disk (Buitrago-Tellez et al. 1992; Rohde 1995).

Radiation exposure for periodontal diagnosis was investigated by Visser (1997). Typical doses are in the range of 5–332 μSV; reference is the conventional periapical status (Visser 1997). The average annual radiation dose in the Federal Republic of Germany is ~3.93 mSv; of which, 2.37 mSv are from natural radiation exposure and 1.56 mSv are from civilization-related exposure (Federal Office for Radiation Protection); 1 Sv = radiological SI unit of effective dose (equivalent dose or biological effect dose), where SI is the Système International d'Unités), the legal basis for technical units (SI base units = SI units). If correctly used, the benefit (precise diagnosis) of X-ray imaging prevails over the potential risk from radiation exposure (Visser 1999).

In recent years, the quality of X-ray images has significantly increased and X-ray imaging offers a high diagnostic value, whether using an intraoral or a panoramic technique. One rule for selecting the radiographic technique is that the maximum diagnostic information should be reached even if the technique bears a higher risk for radiation exposure. A panoramic layer image with a 400 film-screen system corresponds to four-speed e-gear shots (Sitzmann and Benz 1999).

Currently the following X-ray techniques are available (Visser 1999):

Intraoral dental film images
Bitewings
Panoramic radiographs
Digital X-rays
Computed tomography

18.4.2.1 Archiving

Hardcopies of digital radiographic images can reach the quality of the screen display, even with economy printers. This image data should be archived electronically. This begs the question of compressing, because a loss of data must be avoided. Several scientific studies suggest that the higher compression of lossy methods, e.g., the JPEG algorithm with up to 10 % of the original amount of data, is not clinically relevant.

Bitewing images as well as tooth shots are projection radiographic images with an intraoral image receptor system. A bitewing status generally consists of four X-rays in the posterior region, which means that the front teeth are not shown.

Computed tomography (CT) provides detailed images of the jaw. On axial CT images, a layer thickness of 1 mm is currently at an angle of about 0.3 mm in the layers. The display of the teeth and jaw bone is not interleaved or blurred and is true to scale. Compared with intraoral and panoramic radiographs, CT provides results that are more accurate (Visser 1999).

In cases of broken instruments, needle tips, and root residues, a second X-ray level may be necessary for exact localization. The patient being symptom free is not a criteria! For the second level, the use of a dental CT is reasonable. A dental CT module is additionally required (diagnostic basic knowledge), whereby the depth of cuts for the localization of the foreign body can be determined.

Errors in using radiographic measures may be caused by improper setting of the X-ray tube.

Techniques for digital dental radiography are digital X-ray or subsequent digitization of conventional dental films with video technology and scanner technology (with a line scan camera for scanning the brightness and color or a small imaging scanner for slides and negatives). This method was initially applied for forensic identification purposes in 1992 (Tai et al. 1993). The Kodak Photo CD is commonly used (Visser 1994).

The Federal Criminal Police (BKA) in Wiesbaden uses the X-ray machine BV 25 T, manufactured by Philips Medical Systems. Endris reviewed this in 1989 in an expert opinion for the BKA. Originally developed for the Bundeswehr, this X-ray machine can be disassembled and is portable. It is a non-stationary medical electrical device for diagnostic purposes (Rötzscher 1995b).

In radiographic diagnostic of the skull, the regular X-ray image provides insufficient information. In contrast, radio-stereoscopy offers a three-dimensional image by binocular viewing of objects.

The advantages of extraoral jaw recording methods, such as the panoramic radiograph (OPG) and the teleradiography or cephalometric lateral view X-ray (FRS), are the extensive survey and the orientation ability toward skeletal parts and toward the dentition as a whole (Pashinjan and Ajub 1992). Another advantage is that an extraoral image can replace several intraoral images (whereby the value of single images shall not be decreased).

A major step in the field of data acquisition and transfer is the acquisition of digitized X-ray images (Direct Digital Radiography [DDR]) using the Radio-Visio-Graphy (RVG), DEXIS MobilRöntgen, or GENDEX DIGORA (without cable and sensor) or VISUALIX (HD-CCD) in a computer system. This becomes a valuable aid in the event of a disaster because it saves time in identification of unknown living or dead. Simplicity of transport makes them superior to conventional devices because X-ray films no longer need to be developed. GENDEX DIGORA offers "DenOptix combo," a scanner that simultaneously develops intraoral and panoramic images and allows an easy transition from conventional X-ray to digital recording technology (Benz 1997). Regardless of manufacturer or model year, results from all X-ray machines can be digitized (Rötzscher 1991; Hinrichs 1997). The RVG program allows X-ray images taken with the RVG unit to be stored and analyzed (Figs. 18.5, 18.6, 18.7, and 18.8) (Rötzscher 1995b).

X-ray images can be easily combined with almost any currently available dental EDP (patient files). Many years of experience in digital image reproduction technology have developed the RVG system as a PC version (plug-in card, sensor, and software) (Mouyen et al. 1989). The installation of this equipment in the dental practice computer converts the computer into a complete X-ray diagnostic system (van Thiel 1994). The hard disk is able to print the RVG

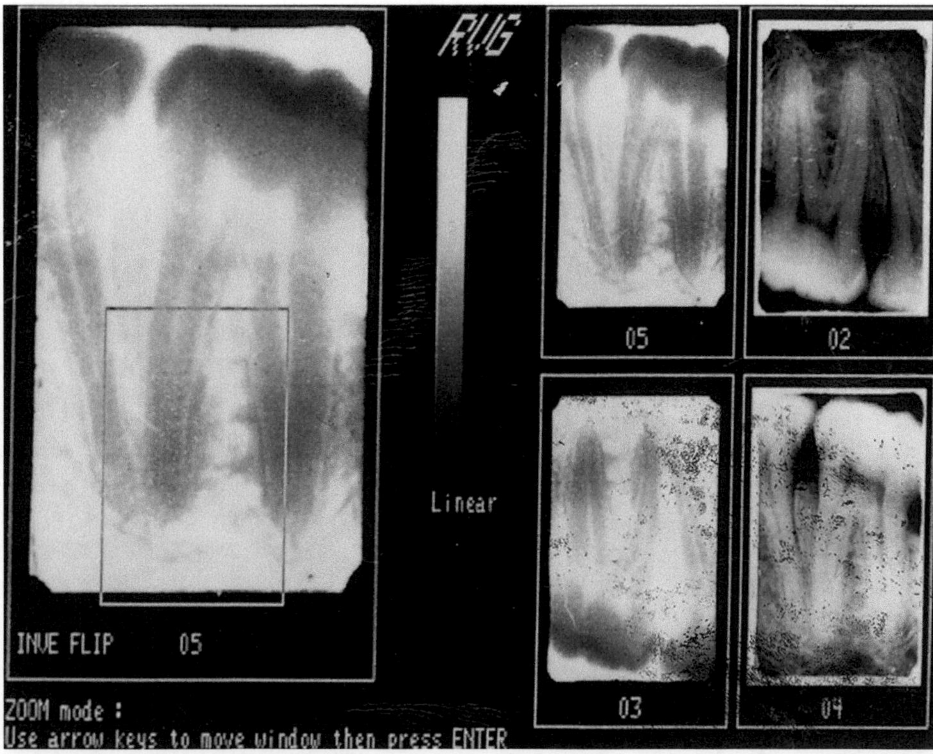

Fig. 18.5 Print of an x-ray image from the screening

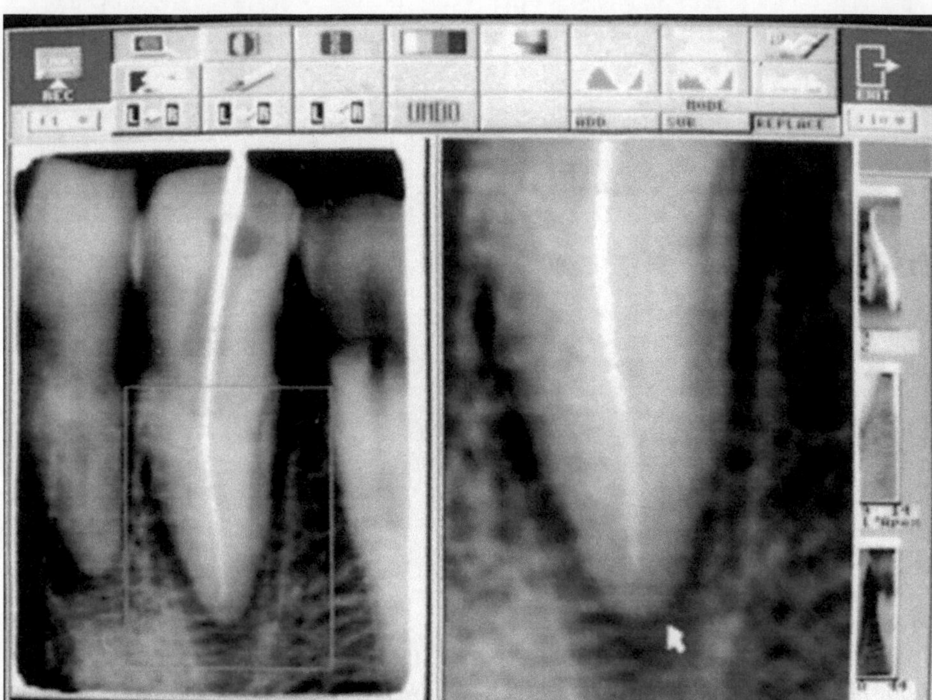

Fig. 18.6 Enlargement of any image portion

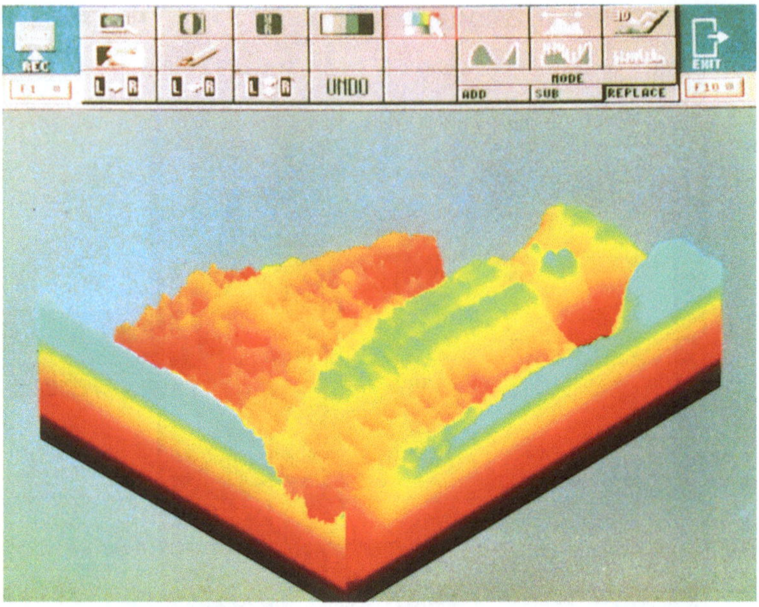

Fig. 18.7 Pseudo-3D representation on the screen

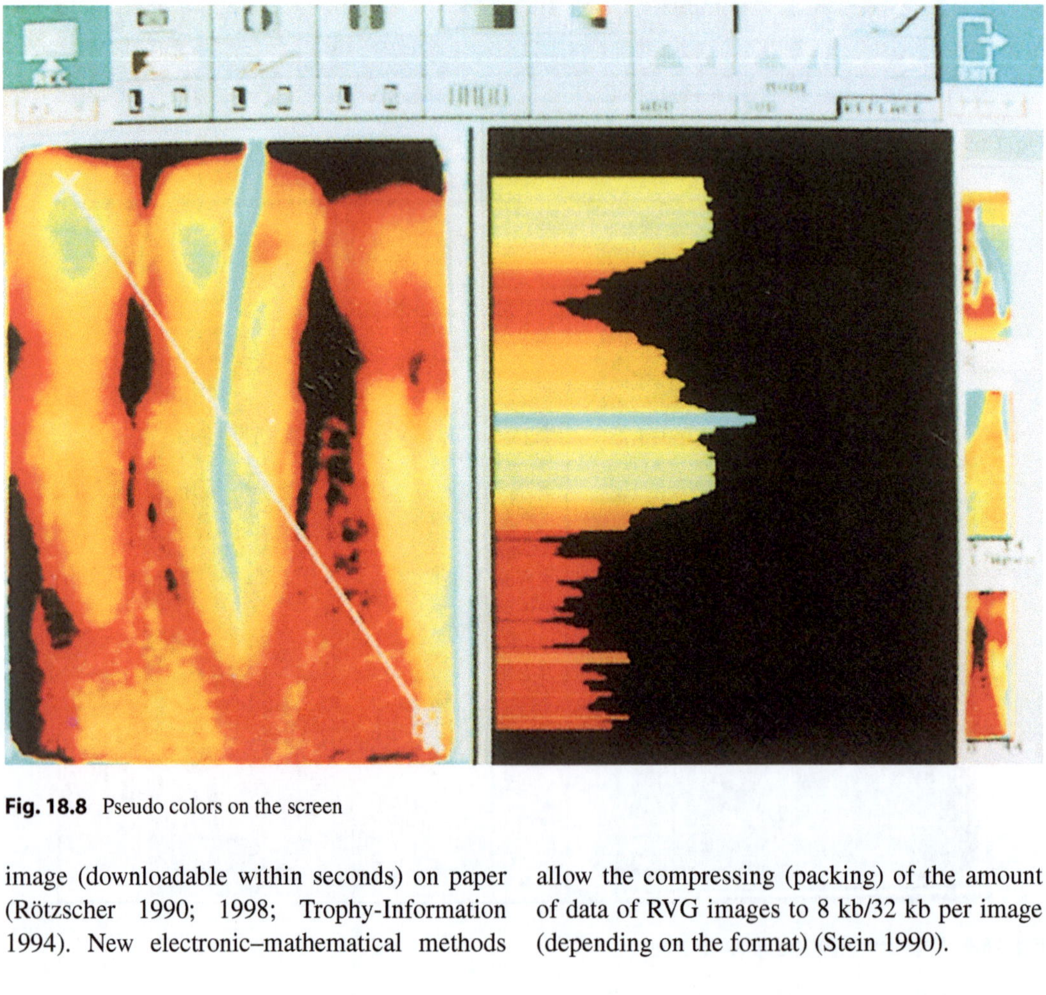

Fig. 18.8 Pseudo colors on the screen

image (downloadable within seconds) on paper (Rötzscher 1990; 1998; Trophy-Information 1994). New electronic–mathematical methods allow the compressing (packing) of the amount of data of RVG images to 8 kb/32 kb per image (depending on the format) (Stein 1990).

By the introduction of Stomavision (STV), a component of a complex IT solution for practices, intraoral color photographs can be enlarged, printed, and archived up to 20 times (van Thiel 1994). Subdirectories allow X-ray images of different people to be distinguished (as files within XRAY). The results of the processing can be stored as new images. Once stored, images can be displayed or printed on the high-resolution black-and-white monitor of the RDC or on the VGA monitor of the computer.

Trophy offers a peripheral X-ray machine with a portable RVG-Cell phone; the size of an A4 sheet of paper, equipped with a VGA LCD screen and all necessary X-ray image-editing keys. The machine can be used for 20 min on a rechargeable battery and can be used independently at each processing station (Trophy-Information 1994).

Electronic filing provides the most secure storage of dental radiographs: no loss of quality, copying of floppy disks, streamer, etc. Instead of the conventional dental films, the RVG system uses a sensor, an intraoral camera (which detects the X-ray radiation), and scintillators (light) of rare earth screen with charge-coupled device (CCD) sensors made of silicon as the active element.

The advantages over traditional X-rays are:

- Superiority of its transport
- No need to develop film material
- The capability of digital images to be stored in the computer
- Global availability
- Economic efficiency (reduction of radiation exposure up to 80–90 %)

The minimum IT requirements are a frame grabber card, a VGA card, a monitor, MS-DOS 4.01 or later, 640-kb RAM, a free 8-bit slot, a Microsoft-compatible mouse, and a hard disk with at least 80 Mb (Malengrez 1991). In 1994, Trophy presented the first digital pocket-ray system. The image is displayed on the monitor and is wirelessly transmitted via the base station to the printer (Trophy-Information 1994).

Additionally, the digital X-ray system, DEXIS MobilRöntgen, allows for wireless X-rays via laptop with a PCMCIA slot, which is basic equipment in any laptop. Thus, any modern notebook can become a mobile digital X-ray station. The DEXIS Sensor can be connected to the computer or the laptop and the images can be immediately viewed on the screen with no development time, in large format, with excellent image quality (Fretzschner 1997). The DEXIS RöntgenSensor can be used both in horizontal and long format as well as for bitewings. All X-ray images can be stored in the X-ray archive, accessed, and sent worldwide at the touch of a button.

18.4.3 Photography

In photographs of documents and photographs for identification purposes, the following principles must be considered:

1. Reproducibility, preferably standardized
2. Simple lighting, also reproducible
3. Reduction of image contents, dividing of complex image contents into several images
4. Plain and non-reflecting backgrounds
5. Displaying of images as a whole, detailed views only in combination with overview images
6. Uniform display of images series: same camera angle, same background, etc.
7. An identification (ID) number should always be on the photo
8. Use of scales in models; the ABFO No. 2 metric angle plus Kodak color scale (Fig. 18.9) and grid (Fig. 18.10) is recommended

To exploit the usually very short depth of focus region, the focus should be on the area of the canines (Fig. 18.11). An ideal camera is not available. The camera system of choice is a miniature single-lens reflex (SLR) camera with through-the-lens (TTL) control (where the light output of the flash is directly controlled by the camera) and autofocus.

The film material of choice for medical documentation is color diapositive film with medium speed (ISO 100/21 DIN and 200/24). Agfa DigiPrint provides an inexpensive and high-quality copying process. Consistent color reproduction is of significant importance. Thus, a film

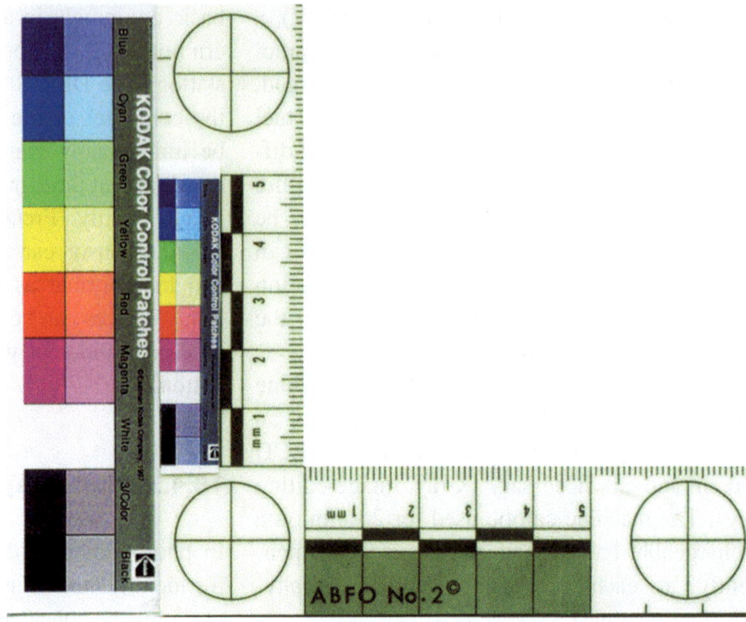

Fig. 18.9 ABFO No. 2 metric angle plus Kodak color scale

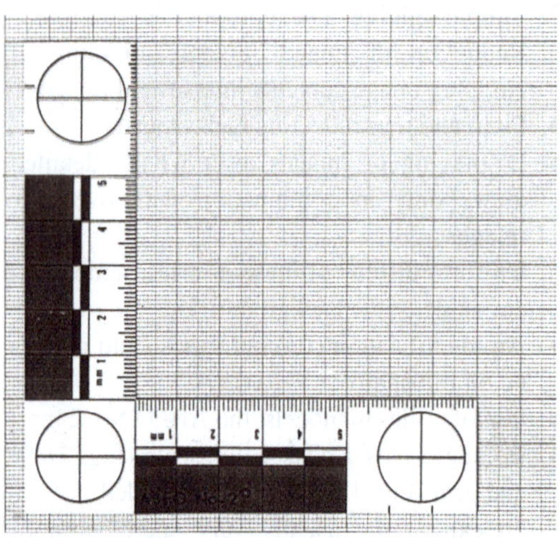

Fig. 18.10 Metric angle with grid

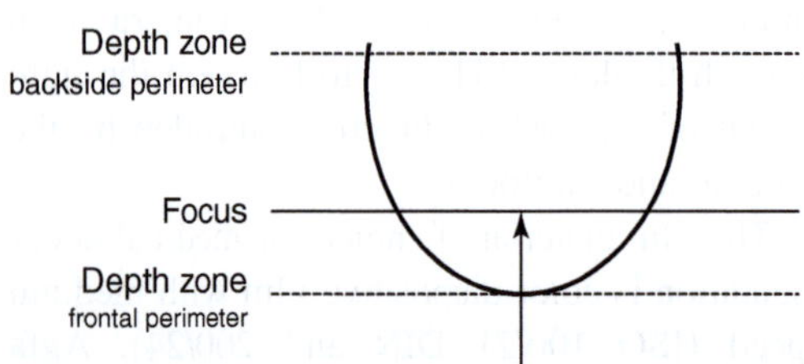

Fig. 18.11 Depth zone

with only a small color tolerance range is recommended (e.g., Kodak professional T 400 CN T-max black and white).

The standard focusing screens, which contain a microprism and a sectional image range finder as an adjustment, should be replaced by a disc with an engraved grid line for better axial alignment. Medical lenses are macro lenses with a built-in ring flash. The light source of choice for intraoral photography is the electronic flash. The side-flash is more powerful than ring flashes and it provides vivid images that are rich in contrast. Since 1 January 1997, new CE manufacturing standards exist for electronic flash units.

The combination of side and ring flash by Yuzo (Fig. 18.12) appears suitable for dental photography and allows a great variety of individual system combinations. The system can be connected to any standard SLR camera (Benthaus 1998). Photographs into the oral cavity may be difficult because of partial shade.

Currently, the lightest camera for use in dentistry is the Yashica Dental Eye II with permanently fitted 100-mm medical lens and selectable image scale. Tools for intraoral photography are plastic or metal cheek retractors and a photo mirror (surface-coated glass or metal mirror) for oral, occlusal, and buccal views. It is recommended that several pictures be taken. Photos taken under specified and comprehensible conditions have the highest value. The goal is not to take congruent but similar images. The intraoral status usually consists of five pictures (horizontal format):

- Frontal view of both rows of teeth in occlusion (with cheek retractors)
- Left and right lateral views (with mirror)
- Upper and lower occlusal views (also with mirror) (Luntz 1991; Bengel 1994)

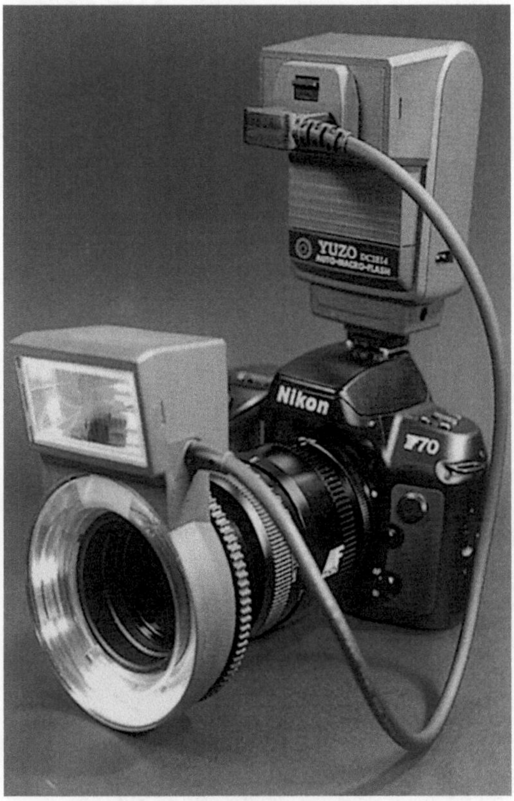

Fig. 18.12 Yuzo ring-side blitz in the survey. Despite the cable connection between the generator and lighting system, the camera is compact (Image courtesy of Dr. S. Benthaus, Munster-Westfalia)

Digital camera systems with digital image processing and global communication technology are perfect for transmission. After coupling the camera to the computer, a black and white control image can be obtained after approximately 3 s, and a color image is available after 6 s. All images can be archived in a storage medium; a 250-MB (1.2 GB) Mesial (M), Occlusal (O), and Distal (D) are sufficient for 4,000 (20,000) color images in full video quality (Fig. 18.13). The more complicated and extensive the information to be transmitted, the more difficult is the transmission. Data of the macro area in highest quality should be available to a computer far away (various tooth shapes, colors, finishes, etc.).

The Dürr conferencing system uses LAN and ISDN for data transfer. VistaCam is also established. It is built on the ProShare technology for Intel processors. This latest standard ensures a new quality for long-distance connections, including the video presentation (Miedke 1998). The DEXIS Image-Program (with an intraoral camera) offers the options of adding notes and comments via microphone and sending these images worldwide via telephone. Thus, telemedicine (teleradiology) increasingly gains in importance in the rapidly evolving field of technology of data storage and transmission.

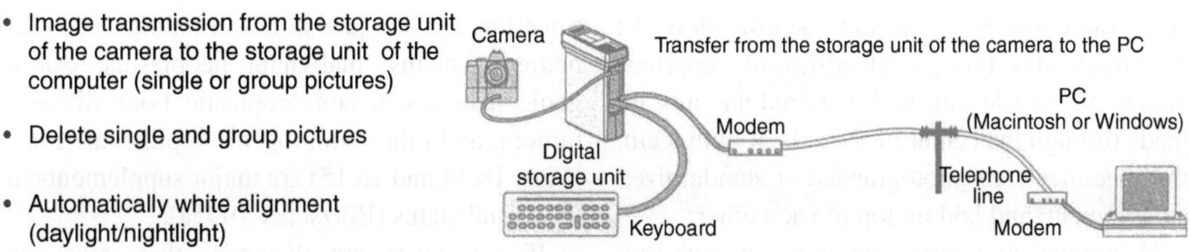

Fig. 18.13 Image transmission from the storage unit of the camera

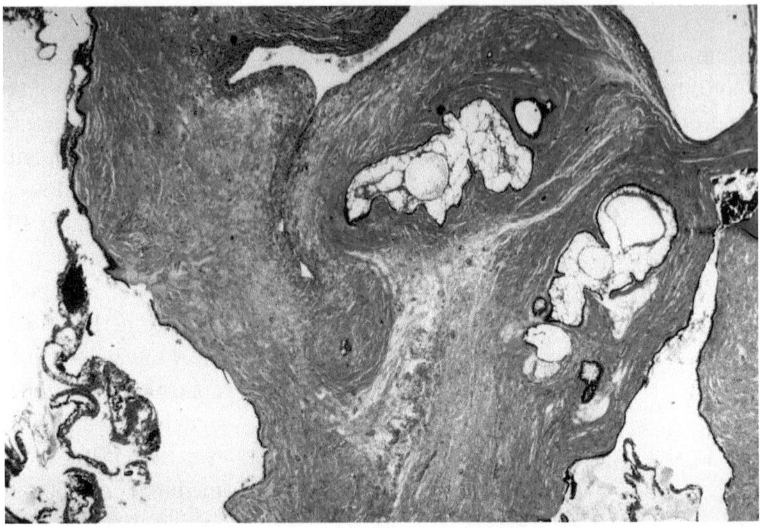

Fig. 18.14 Magnification 25:1

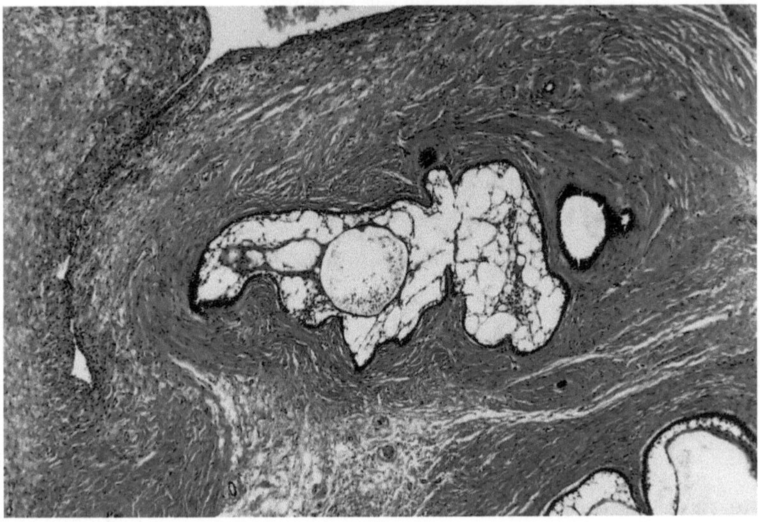

Fig. 18.15 Magnification 50:1

18.4.4 Histology

The lines (Retzius lines in the enamel prisms, Ebner lines, Owen contour lines in circumpulpal dentin) in the tooth structure are arranged in the same direction; this can aid identification. To investigate this type of identification, approximately 50- to 100-μm-thick longitudinal cuts are made through the center of the axis of both teeth, the specimens are photographed at standardized enlargement, and laid on top of each other.

A comparison microscope, in which both sections can be simultaneously observed, is much easier to use. This technique shows whether the lines in the enamel or dentin have the same location, width, and frequency. Gustafson (1946, 1966) were able to match growth and failure patterns of hard tissue to one or several individuals with this method (Schroeder 1987).

Histological examination is required for identification by the jaw bones. Findings such as benign growths, malignant neoplasms, osteogenic neoplasms, non-neoplastic bone disease, tumors, and other odontogenic (epithelial) cysts (Figs. 18.14 and 18.15) are major supplements to the dental status (Rötzscher 1995a).

If jaw cysts are detected, they must be recorded according to the code of the International Classification of Diseases of Dentistry and Stomatology (ICD-DA), the

International Classification of Diseases for Oncology (ICD-O), the Systematic Medical Nomenclature (SNOMED), and the Classification of Tumours of the World Health Organisation (WHO) (Mittermayer 1984; Kramer et al. 1992).

Jaw cyst (E-No. 30/789-94) diagnosis: Cystic follicular ameloblastoma (typing: ICD-DA 213. XI; ICD-O 9310.0. Histological Odontogenic Tumours); as shown in Figs. 18.14 (magnification 25:1) and 18.15 (magnification 50:1). Previously used synonyms are adamantinoma, adamantoblastoma or multilocular cyst; a benign tumor derived from parts of the tooth germ with locally destructive growth and the characteristic histological development of the enamel organ (Mittermayer 1984). Histologically, these are mainly found as micro cysts and macro cysts whose glades are confined by a prominent cubic to cylindrical cell layer. The adjacent cell layers are separated and located in the glade. These cells are spindle-shaped in the middle section and only the surface displays a suggested epidermoid differentiation. The smaller cell slides are confined by a prominent high cylindrical cell layer, whose nuclei have radially oriented nuclear vacuoles (for the histological assessment of the cyst region 36, the author thanks Prof. Dr. K. Donath, Department of Oral Pathology, University of Hamburg).

To evaluate the hard tissue (e.g., teeth with fillings or crowns, teeth with thickened cortex, or jaw bone with metal or ceramic implants), Donath recommends the EXACT cutting-grinding system, which enables extremely thin slices (<10 µm) to be obtained for histological diagnosis. For routine samples, the fast and user-friendly toluidine blue stain is used. Metachromasia yields good staining results for hard and soft tissue. Tissues embedded in Technovit 7.200 VLC can be colored with hematoxylin eosin stain, van Giesen stain, or periodic acid–Schiff (PAS) reaction; cryo or paraffin techniques are not applicable here (Donath 1985, 1988, 1990).

References

Andersen L, Juhl M, Solheim T, Borrman H (1995) Odontological identification of fire victims – potentialities and limitations. Int J Leg Med 107:229–234

Bengel W (1994) Fotografieren im Mund leicht gemacht. Zahnarztl Mitt 84(15):16–22

Benthaus S (1998) Ringblitz-Seitenblitz-Kombination – eine sinnvolle Ergänzung für die zahnärztliche Fotografie? Quintessenz 49:69–72

Benz C (1997) Die digitale Röntgenaufnahme-heute und morgen. ZMK Jg 13(Okt):26–28

Buitrago-Tellez C, Wenz W, Friedrich G (1992) Digital x-ray image processing as an aid in forensic medicine. Radiologe 32:87–89

Donath K (1985) The diagnostic value of the new method for the study of undecalcified bones and teeth with attached soft tissue. Sawing and grinding technique. Pathol Res Pract 179:631–633

Donath K (1988) Die Trenn-Dünnschliff-Technik zur Herstellung histologischer Präparate von nicht schneidbaren Geweben und Materialien. Der Präparator 34(1):197–206

Donath K (1990) Preparation of histologic sections – equipment and methodical performance. EXAKT-Kulzer-Publication, Norderstedt

Endris R (1989) Begutachtung der Leistungsfähigkeit des Röntgengerätes BV 25 T der Firma Philips Medical Systems. Brief an das BKA Wiesbaden, 9 Aug 1989

Epple (1994) Der Einsatz von EDV und die ärztliche Haftung passim: Deutsch, Medizinrecht 3 Rschr 355

Fretzschner M (1997) Trends in der Zahnheilkunde, Digitales Röntgen heute. Zahnarzt-Wirtschaft-Praxis. Anwenderbericht. COLLEGmagazin 2/3:57–60, 104–108

Gustafson G (1946) Mikroskopisk undersökning av tänder som hjälpmedel inom rättsodontologien (The microscopic examination of teeth as a means of identification in Forensic Odontology). Odont Tidskr 54:470–479

Gustafson G (1966) Forensic odontology. Sex and race. Staples Press, London, pp 78–90

Hausmann R, Liebler M, Schellmann B (1997) Zur Personenidentifikation mittels Zahnstatus. Qualität und Quantität zahnärztlicher Befunddokumentation. Rechtsmedizin 7:86–89

Hinrichs K (1997) Die Speicherfolientechnik in der Dental-Radiologie. ZMK Jg 13(Okt):29–30

Kaatsch HJ, Ritz S (1993) Dokumentation des Zahnstatus als Identifizerungshilfe. Rechtsmedizin 3:120–127

Kramer IRH, Pindborg JJ, Shear M (1992) Histological typing of odontogenic tumours. Springer, Berlin/Heidelberg, pp 11–51

Luntz LL (1991) Dental photography. In: Averill DC (ed) Dental identification, manual of forensic odontology. ASFO, Colorado Springs, p 36

Malengrez P (1991) Informationsblatt der Fa. TROPHY-Radiologie, Kehl

Meurer A (1988) Gebührenordnung für Zahnärzte – GOZ. Kommentierung des Zahnärztlichen Gebührenrechts für die Privatliquidation. Kohlhammer, Köln/Stuttgart/Berlin/Mainz, p 88

Miedke ED (1998) Das conferencing-system von Dürr dental. Dent Mag 1(98):52–54

Mittermayer C (1984) Oralpathologie X, 2.Aufl. Schattauer, Stuttgart/New York, p 220

Mouyen F, Forest D, Lodter PH (1989) RVG-Röntgen. Dent Mag 2:100–103

Pashinjan GA, Ajub F (1992) Einsatz von Odontogrammen und Panoramaröntgen zur Identifikation. UDK, Moskau, 340.62: 616,314-073.755.4

Riepert T, Rittner C (1989) Zur Röntgenidentifizierung unbekannter Leichen bei fortgeschrittenen postmortalen Veränderungen. Z Rechtsmed 102(11):207–216

Rötzscher K (1990) Radiovisiography. The electronic camera in use. The forensic Odontology as well as the dental practice need information. Poster, 12th Meeting IOFOS, Adelaide, Australien, 28 Okt 1990

Rötzscher K (1991) Die Radio-Visio-Graphie im Einsatz mit Computer-Systemen. Identifikation durch Datenspeicherung und Datenübertragung. Internationales Symposium über Massenkatastrophen, Poster S48, 70. Jahrestagung Dtsch Ges Rechtsmedizin, Lausanne, 10–14 Sept 1991

Rötzscher K (1995a) Identification by an operated mandibular cyst – not only teeth that tell: The WHO Classification of Tumours – a special help in identification. In: Jacob B, Bonte W (eds) Advances in forensic sciences. Forensic Odontology and Anthropology, vol. 7, in coop. with Alt KW, Pieper P. Köster, Berlin, S 74–75

Rötzscher K (1995b) Die Röntgenübersichtsaufnahme, Hilfsmittel und Dokumentation. AKFOS Newsl Jg 2(1)

Rötzscher K (1998) Prothesenmarkierung – Eine kurze Darstellung. AKFOS Newsl Jg 5(1):14–15

Rohde ER (1995) Dokumentationspflicht und Verpflichtung zur Anfertigung einer Röntgenübersichtsaufnahme bei einer komplikationslos verlaufenden Zahnextraktion. AKFOS Newsl Jg 2(1):8

Schroeder HE (1987) Orale Strukturbiologie. G. Thieme, Stuttgart/New York, p 4

Sitzmann F, Benz Ch (1999) Einzelbildstatus oder Orthopantomogramm. Stellungnahme der DGZMK. Nachdruck Dtsch. Zahnärztl Z 53/1998, H.12, Zahnärztl Mitt 89(1):33

Stein FW (1990) RadioVisioGraphie: eine Innovation in der zahnärztlichen Röntgentechnik. Zahnarztl Mitt 6(90):586–588

Stratmann KR (1997) EDV-Dokumentation in der zahnärztlichen Praxis. AKFOS Newsl Jg 4(3):58–59

Tai CE, Blenkinsop BR, Wood RE (1993) Dental radiographic identification utilising computerised digital slice interposition: a case report. J Forensic Odontostomatol 11:1

van Thiel R (1994) Radiovisiographie (RVG) und intraorale Kamera (STV) in Praxis-EDV integriert. Zahnärztl Inform Rheinland-Pfalz III:64–66

Thieme S (1982) Das Recht in der Zahnarztpraxis. Quintessenz, Berlin, S 157ff

Trophy-Information (1994) RVG-jet. Zahnärztl Mitt 84:16

Visser H (1994) Ein einfaches Verfahren zur Digitalisierung von Zahnfilmen. ZWR 103(5):282–287

Visser H (1997) Untersuchungen zur Optimierung der parodontologischen Röntgendiagnostik. Habilitationsschrift, Göttingen

Visser H (1999) Zeitgemäße parodontologische Röntgendiagnostik. Dtsch Zahnärztl Z Jg 54(2):64–72

Walther W (1996) Hilfen zur Karteiführung mit dem Praxiscomputer. In: HZB 11:6ff

Age Estimation

19

Klaus Rötzscher

19.1 Introduction

Forensically estimating age is an important part of forensic odontostomatology, not only in terms of identity verification but also in living persons who do not know their own age or make false age statements for various reasons. Age estimation is also central to anthropology and archeology. An age estimation based on tooth status is possible.

By the nineteenth century, teeth were used to determine the age of a person (Saunders 1897). Determining age by using the teeth was needed for admission of children to factory work. Saunders used the dental eruption times in children aged 9–13 years and 5–16 years (Ewald 1992).

The dental age of humans can be classified in two phases:

1. The first phase, childhood, runs up to the age of 18 years, while the teeth are developing in the jaw. This takes place in a regular progression, which is only slightly affected by external factors.
2. The second phase, adulthood, starts after the completion of tooth development. After this phase, degenerative and age-dependent changes, which may be variable, must be given attention. However, in this period, other age-related indicators are even more variable.

For forensic estimation of age in living persons, three main methodological procedures are available:

1. Tooth morphologic procedures
2. Biochemical procedures
3. Radiological procedures

These methods significantly differ in their capabilities, limitations, and risks. They include medical/dental procedures or tests such as dentin isolation or X-ray examinations, for which no medical indication is usually given (Ritz and Kaatsch 1996).

Because of frequently updated guidelines on the basis of tooth-morphological investigations in white people, a relatively precise age estimation is possible; however, it is questionable whether these standards are also applicable in other ethnic groups (Marré and Hetzer 1999).

Dental age estimation in children and young people of foreign origin cannot provide any details (with the currently available methods). Early extraction of deciduous teeth, nutrition, and other outside influences can affect the timing of tooth eruption. The older a child is, the less accurate is the estimation. The existing literature explicitly shows that the average time of tooth eruption varies among ethnic groups.

Several authors point out that conclusions regarding chronological age based on the number of teeth is a variable criterion that does

K. Rötzscher, Dr. med. Dr. med. dent.
German Academy of Forensic Odontostomatology (AKFOS),
Wimphelingstraße 7, 67346 Speyer, Germany
e-mail: roetzscher.klaus.dr@t-online.de

K. Rötzscher (ed.), *Forensic and Legal Dentistry*,
DOI 10.1007/978-3-319-01330-5_19, © Springer International Publishing Switzerland 2014

not allow a reliable estimation (Liliequist and Lundberg 1971; Preece 1983; Towlson and Peck 1990). A blanket application of values for whites to other ethnic groups is not possible. In age estimation, for social reasons, bone maturity is decisive (Helm 1990). Ritz and Kaatsch (1996) have listed the methods for age estimation of living persons in the recent literature (Table 19.1).

19.1.1 ad 1: Stages of Dentition

For morphologic (anatomical) purposes, the following main stages of dentition are significant (Thoma 1953):

- The time of formation of dental germ, development, and calcification
- The time of eruption of milk teeth and permanent teeth

During the second dentition stage, between the age of 6 and 12 years, determination of age should not be based on only the eruption of permanent teeth. The progress of resorption of deciduous tooth roots up to the total loss and the progressive formation and calcification of the roots of the permanent teeth are helpful features and are displayed on the radiograph.

19.1.2 ad 2: Determination of Racemization of Aspartic Acid in Dentin

The aging phenomenon of intravital racemization of aspartic acid in human proteins was first described in the 1970s. Since then, the level of racemization of aspartic acid is used to determine the age of fossil materials (Pfeiffer et al. 1995). The racemization of aspartic acid in dentin is, compared with other methods, a very accurate measure for age estimation.

Like all amino acids, aspartic acid may occur in two forms: in a L-and in a D-form. In the biosynthesis of human proteins, exclusively L-amino acids are used. From the time of protein synthesis, a spontaneous, non-enzymatic conversion of L-aspartic acid residues into their D-form may occur. This in vivo racemization may lead to an age-dependent accumulation of D-aspartic acids in long-living, "aging" proteins, if they cannot be replaced after synthesis (they are permanent) (Ritz-Timme 1999). With advancing age, this accumulation is observed in bradytrophic tissues and gives objective information about the age of a person (Pfeiffer et al. 1995). In this respect, dentin tissue is the optimal tissue with its extremely bradytrophic metabolism and a relatively homogeneous and stable anatomic

Table 19.1 Age estimation of living persons

Methods	Age range	Reliability	Authors (selection)
I. Tooth development			
Development of several types of teeth	<ca. 14 years	<2 years	Gustafson and Koch (1974), Hägg and Matsson (1985), Mörnstad et al. (1994) and Saunders et al. (1993)
II. Dental morphology			
Macroscopically (in situ)	All ages	Rough estimate only	Endris (1979)
Morphology of permanent teeth	Adulthood	±10–24 years ±10 years cannot be reproduced	Endris (1979), Lode and Reimann (1985), Solheim (1993a, b) and Lucy and Pollard (1995)
III. Biochemistry			
1. Racemization of aspartic acid in dentin			
(a) Extracted teeth	All ages	±3–8 years	Ogino et al. (1985), Ohtani (1994), Ohtani and Yamamoto (1987, 1990a, b, 1991, 1992a, b) and Ritz et al. (1993a, b)
(b) In dentin biopsies	All ages	±6 years	Ritz et al. (1995)

Methods in recent literature (Ritz and Kaatsch 1996)

and biochemical structure. In forensic practice, the analysis of dentin is the standard method for biochemical age estimation (Ritz et al. 1990; Pfeiffer et al. 1995; Ritz-Timme 1999), because dentin analysis yields a wide range of basic data at a reasonable cost and has the advantage that it can also be used in examination of living persons (the examination of other kinds of tissues is reserved for special cases). In Germany, age estimation in living persons by this method was not applied until 1995 (Ritz et al. 1995). The main application is the adult age (Ritz-Timme 1999).

19.1.3 Methodology

- Tooth preparation must be standardized (preferably by a dentist).
- The prepared root dentin is washed in several steps.
- The washed dentin is hackled (after freeze drying).
- The resulting dentin powder is aliquoted.
- The acid extraction is carried out with 0.6 N hydrochloric acid (the acid-soluble fraction is freeze dried).
- This sample preparation results in a total dentin sample per tooth and an acid extract.
- The total dentin sample and the acid extract are hydrolyzed and derivatized, and amino acids (as *N*-trifluoracetylisopropylester) are separated by gas chromatography on a chiral capillary column.
- The D-/L-aspartic acid ratio is determined (Ritz-Timme 1999).

Dentin extraction is permitted only with active consent of the person, namely:

- In extracted teeth
- After tooth extraction with existing clinical indications

Otherwise, dentin biopsy will be performed. Dentin biopsy is legitimized in legal and social indications (Ritz and Kaatsch 1996). The testing laboratories must meet minimum requirements. A postmortem age estimation by the level of racemization of aspartic acid is possible with good results, because of a close relationship between the level of racemization and the age of root dentin, especially if a majority of coronal dentin is missing (Ritz et al. 1993a, b).

19.1.4 ad 3: The Radiological Investigation

According to § 24 RöV, a radiological investigation is permissible only if medically indicated and, according to § 81a STPO, permitted only by judicial decision. Following the principle of proportionality, a radiological investigation in suspected criminal offense (§ 81a STOP) may be performed by force, in contrast to asylum procedure, where empowerment is not given.

In this context, the dental panoramic radiograph (OPG) is based on the following technical parameters (Vendura et al. 1998):

- OPG (orthopantomograph/radiograph): tube voltage: 63–81 kV
- Maximum radiofrequency current: 9 A at 80 kV
- Film size: 15 × 30 cm
- Radiation exposure: dose equivalent 750–800 micro-Sievert. The radiation-sensitive organs (eye, thyroid gland) are outside of the useful radiation

Events, methods, and legal aspects of age estimation according to Ritz and Kaatsch (1996) are given in Table 19.2.

In cases of suspicion of an obvious abuse, whether the suspect is older or younger than 16 years (if no other data is available) is important, and thus an investigation for age estimation is legally admitted. The legal occasions for age estimation of living individuals are usually for criminal, administrative, civil, and social issues (Ritz and Kaatsch 1996):

Criminal law

- Criminal responsibility – age > 14 years – § 19 StGB
- Applicability of adult criminal law – age > 18 or 21 years – §§ 1, 105 AJC)

Administrative Law

- Asylum – § 16a para 1 GG, § 12 para 1 and 3 AsylVfG
- Ability to submit applications and declarations, Aliens Act – § 68 age estimation without or with invalid identity documents

Table 19.2 Age estimation in living persons

Occasions	Methods	Legal aspects
Criminal responsibility of young offenders: >14 years old (§ 19 StGB)	Radiological assessment of the dentition	X-rays (§ 24 RöVO) only by judicial decision (§ 81a StPO)
Young asylum seekers aged >16 years old (§16 of the Asylum Procedure Act, § 68 of the Aliens Act)	Radiological assessment of the development of the 3rd molar	X-rays (§ 24 RöVO) only by judicial decision (§ 81a StPO)
Applicability of the adult criminal law for young offenders: >18 or 21 years old? (§ § 1, 105 JGG)	Radiological assessment of the development of the 3rd molar (Thorson and Hägg 1991)	X-rays (§ 24 RöVO) only by judicial decision (§ 81a StPO)
	Determination of racemization of aspartic acid in dentin	Dentin recovery only with effective consent
	On extracted teeth	Tooth extraction only with existing clinical indication, otherwise dentin biopsy
	In dentin biopsies	Legitimized dentin biopsies with “legal and social” indications
Clarification of pension claim	Determination of the racemization level of aspartic acid in dentin	Dentin recovery only with effective consent
	On extracted teeth	Tooth extraction only with existing clinical indication, otherwise dentin biopsy
	In dentin biopsies	Legitimized dentin biopsies with “legal and social” indications

Methods and legal aspects (Ritz and Kaatsch 1996)

Civil Law

Changes of age in the family book – § 47 PStG

Social Law

Clarification of pension claims of foreign citizens whose date of birth is not or allegedly not known – §§ 35, 33a SGB VI

19.2 First Dentition (Deciduous Dentes)

Tooth development can be divided into four stages (Gustafson and Koch 1974):

1. Root development
2. Tooth eruption
3. Crown formation
4. Beginning of dentin enamel production (Fig. 19.1)

Every stage of the eruption is declared (the tip of the triangle corresponds to the average), and the largest variation is also declared (the legs of the triangle point to the respective time limit of the eruption). Gender differences are not taken into account.

Many forensic odontologists use the scheme (Figs. 19.2 and 19.3) developed by Schour and Massler (1958) and varied by Ferembach et al. (1979). The fact that the data originated from children who have died from diseases is not considered here. For this reason, the table of the chronology of dental development and tooth growth by Schour and Massler (1940) is of limited suitability (Rötzscher and Reimann 1975). Gender differences are also not included. The schemes are based on the work of Logan and Kronfield (1933) and are often quoted. The American Dental Association (ADA) periodically updates and publishes this table.

Ciaparelli (1985) compared the data with subject groups (schoolchildren) and found that the information corresponded with boys at the age of 4–16 years; in girls this development takes place 3–6 months earlier. The variables were similar at the age of 4–6 years; in boys at the age of 12 years, they doubled, and they tripled at the age of 16 years. Rösing (1994) used this scheme as does Ferembach et al. (1979) (see Figs. 19.2 and 19.3).

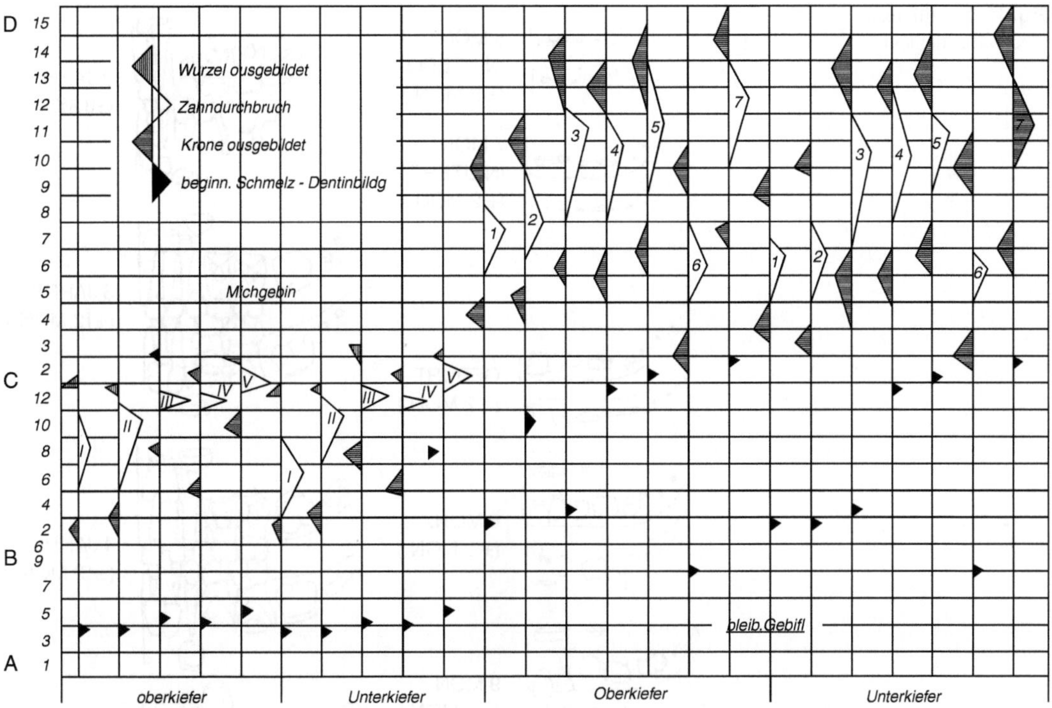

Fig. 19.1 Stages of the teeth of the dentition (Gustafson 1947, 1950, 1955); Chronology of tooth development. Explanation: A1-9: embryonal months, B2-12: months of the first year, C2-day: 2–15; age (I–V: milk teeth) (1–7: permanent teeth – without wisdom tooth) (Courtesy of Prof. Dr. Gösta Gustafson, Lund)

19.3 Second Dentition (Permanent Teeth)

In contrast to the deciduous tooth eruption, the eruption of the permanent dentition extends over a time period that is much longer with many more irregular intervals. In addition, the eruptions have considerable fluctuations, especially the last erupting teeth (Künzel 1976).

Figure 19.4 shows the variability of age groups where certain stages of development are reached (Moorrees et al. 1963). Average ages with a single (+1) and double (+2) standard deviation (s) are shown, in which the complete crown formation (Kk), certain fractions of the root length (1/4, 1/3, 1/2, 2/3, 3/4), total root length (Wx), and the apex half or full circuit (A1/2 k) of the permanent upper and lower central (I1) and lateral (I2) incisors are achieved (black symbols and lines = boys, red = girls) (Moorrees et al. 1963).

Most effective is a classification of the tooth development in as many stages as possible. Moorrees et al. (1963) divided the stages into 14 steps, but the tables are difficult to read.

Dental development is very regular and only slightly dependent on diet, hormones, and disease (Crossner and Mansfeld 1983). Hormones such as growth hormone can affect tooth development, but less than bone development (Garn et al. 1965). Children in warmer regions develop earlier (~6–14 months), according to a study of Arabian children by Fahmy (1974). In an Indian investigation, Kumar and Sridhar used (1990) the Probitt analysis for the eruption and, thus, could calculate the probability for each deviation: up to the age of 9 years, the discrepancy is approximately 1 year, and a little longer up to the age of 13 years. After 13 years, attention must be paid to the wisdom teeth, which have a greater range of variation, of approximately 2–3 years (Haavikko 1974). Note that the dental age may differ from

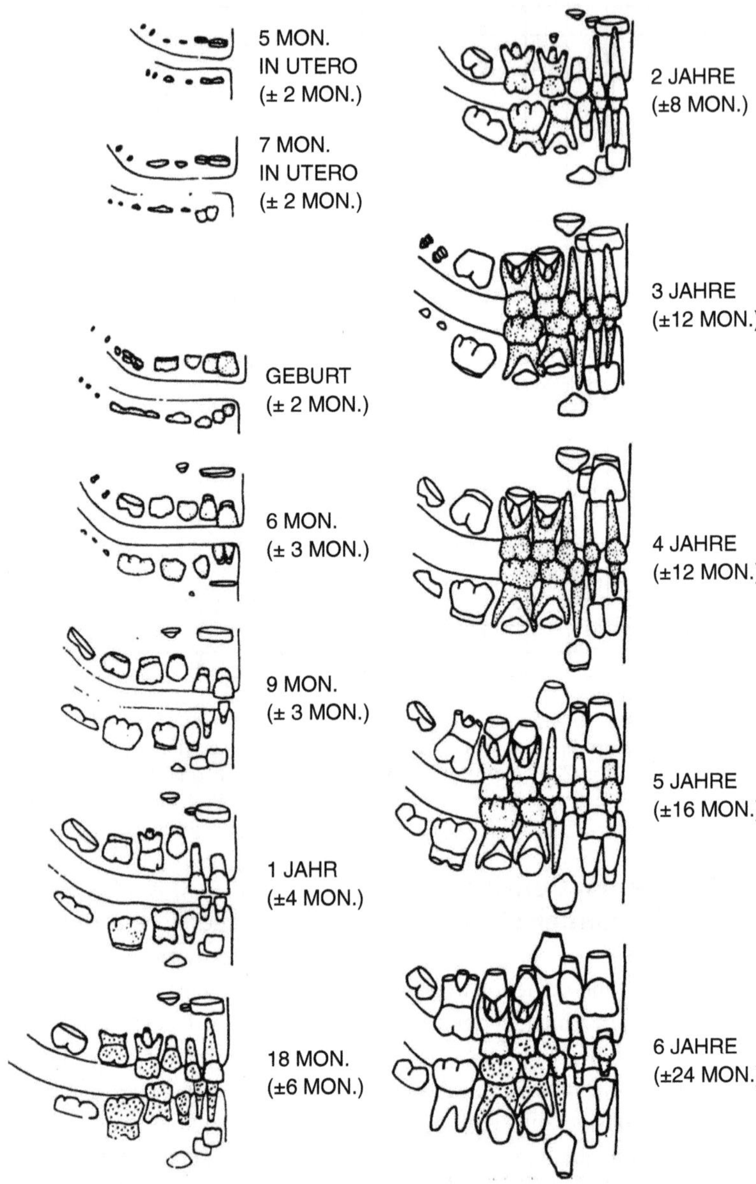

Fig. 19.2 Milk teeth (deciduous dentes)

the "chronological" age (Hurme 1957; Schranz 1958, 1959).

The first molar tooth is the first tooth of the permanent teeth that erupts at the end of the milk teeth; it is also called the 6-years molar, because of its eruption at the age of 6 years. The first phase of the dentition is complete with the eruption of the first molars and the permanent incisors (early mixed dentition) between the age of 6 and 9 years. The eruption of the premolars, the canines, and of the second molars takes place in the second phase, between the age of 9 and 13 years.

Adler (1957a, b, 1959a, b, 1963) collected the eruption events in the permanent teeth in a Hungarian subject group and according to international literature. Estimating dental age in children and young people of foreign origin exclusively by their teeth is difficult, as the tables by Adler (1957a) show. Both the date of the eruption and the frequency of the occurrence of changes in the number of teeth are variable (Hägg

Fig. 19.3 Permanent teeth

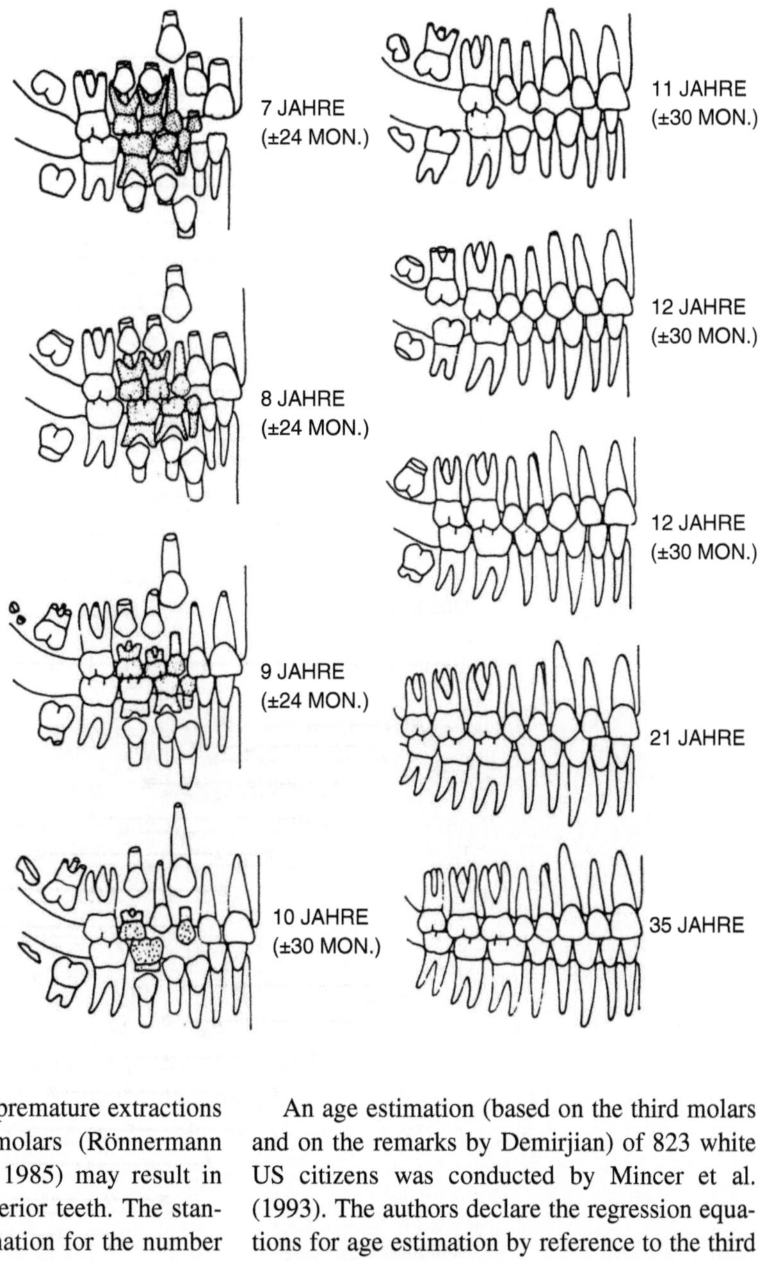

and Matsson 1985). Thus, premature extractions of primary molars and molars (Rönnermann 1977; Hägg and Matsson 1985) may result in premature eruption of posterior teeth. The standard deviation in age estimation for the number of teeth according to Helm (1990) is 1 year, in 5 % of all cases an age difference of up to 2 years is expected.

According to several authors, conclusions regarding age are not reliable because the number of teeth is a variable criterion (Liliequist and Lundberg 1971; Preece 1983; Towlson and Peck 1990). A literature research by Marré and Hetzer (1999) shows the ages (average in years) of tooth eruption.

An age estimation (based on the third molars and on the remarks by Demirjian) of 823 white US citizens was conducted by Mincer et al. (1993). The authors declare the regression equations for age estimation by reference to the third molars, but they also point to the marked variability in the development of third molars. Demirjian et al. (1973, 1976) describe the eight stages of mineralization. Each stage is described by a scale value. The values are added and assigned to a certain age (Demirjian 1994). The authors quote differences of up to 3 years from the actual (from 3rd to 97th percentile).

Haavikko (1974) modified this method by assigning 12 mineralization stages to four teeth,

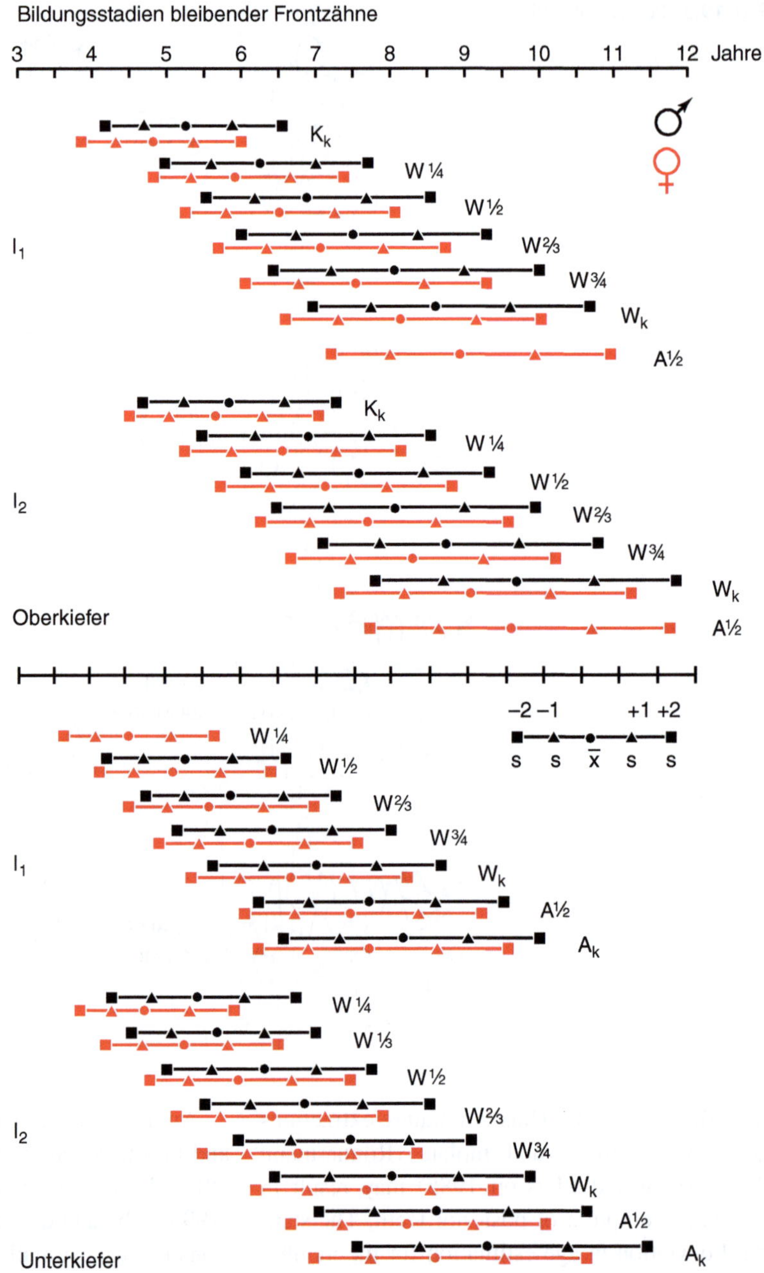

Fig. 19.4 Formation stages of permanent teeth

always six for the root and the crown. The values are added and divided by the number of the assessed teeth and so the age is determined (accuracy of ±2.3 years between the 10th and 90th percentile).

Liliequist and Lundberg (1971) have differentiated seven development stages of a tooth. Each stage also receives a scale value here. The values are added and assigned to an age with the help of an age table.

The most widespread method in practice probably is the method by Demirjian. Davis and Hägg (1994) have applied the method by Demirjian et al. (1973) in 975 Chinese children of preschool age, taking into account the standards of 1982 and 1986. The most distinctive deviations between actual and estimated age occurred in the older age groups, and were more frequent in boys than in girls.

Staaf et al. (1991) compared the accuracy of these three methods in 514 Swedish children from 5.5 to 14.5 years. They noted that in the application of the study by Demirjian et al. (based on Canadian values) for a Scandinavian subject group, the age was overestimated by an average of 6–10 months. The 95 % confidence interval was, depending on the method, up to ±2.1 years.

A new approach for age estimation was developed by Mörnstad et al. (1994). Based on orthopantomograms of 541 Swedish children from 5.5 to 14.5 years, the following parameters were digitized, metrically recorded, and mathematically and statistically elaborated: canopy height (coronal height) width, the distal apical foramen, and the mesial and distal root length of molars, premolars, and single-rooted teeth. A multiple correlation model was developed that provides values that are more precise than other methods, with an accuracy of ± 1.5 to 2.0 years in the 95 % confidence interval.

Tooth development is initiated in the fifth embryonic week (after ovulation). However, even the wisdom tooth, whose germ is formed several years after birth and whose crown is completed before the middle of the second decade of life, is formed by the same biological rules as the prenatal development of deciduous teeth (Schroeder 1987). The third molar, the so-called wisdom tooth, is the most flexible tooth in the permanent dentition, but there are situations in which the third molar is the only available age criterion.

Otuyemi et al. (1997) evaluated the eruption times of third molars in 1,071 13–21-year-old children and young people from rural areas of Nigeria. Of the 4-year-old children, 1.1 % already had all four wisdom teeth. The eruption took place at the average age of 14 years in boys and 13 years in girls. The eruption of the third molar is earlier in contrast to European and American values. This fact is, according to the authors, attributable to nutrition that is more fibrous. Ajmani et al. (1986) detected similar values for the time of eruption in a study of 1,238 15–21-year-old children and young people from northern Nigeria, but the average age was found to be 18 years. Hassanali (1985) determined in (a) 1,343 African and (b) 1,092 Asian students in Nairobi, Kenya, that the eruption time of the third molar was 17.6–18.9 years for (a) and 19.9–21.0 years for (b). This difference is significant.

Thorson and Hägg (1991) applied the method by Demirjian (1986) to 372 adolescents with ages from 14.5 to 24.5 years. In girls, the age of the 14- to 17-year-old girls was underestimated by 6 months, and in 20- to 25-year-old women, by up to 3.5 years. The standard deviation in all age groups was approximately 24 months. In male subjects, ages younger than 20 years old were underestimated by 10–17 months. In the 20-year-old men, the root development was already completed in 33 out of 34 subjects, found that 10 % of the root growth of third molars is already completed at the age of 17 years.

From the age of 16 years, the number of subjects with completed root development increases. Because of agenesis of the third molar, in 20 % of the cases, conclusions about the development state are not possible. Thorson and Hägg (1991) note, that based on the development of the third molars, a definitive statement regarding the age of 18 years is not possible. They refuse an age estimation for legal purposes that is based on the development of the third molars.

The available data in the international literature shows that the average time of tooth eruption varies in different ethnic groups. A blanket application of the values for whites to other ethnic groups is not possible. The determination based solely on the third molars should only be performed if no other criteria are available.

Interdisciplinary cooperation for age assessment in a consortium of experts is required and desirable to provide a quality assurance system. Age estimation should not be made solely on the basis of tooth development, but rather in collaboration with anthropologists, orthodontists, pediatricians, forensic scientists, and radiologists, especially if criminal liability (Schmeling et al. 1999a, b) (age > 14 years – § 19 StGB) must be assessed.

The skeletal development of the hand and wrist (representative for the entire skeleton) in the X-ray image can be used as *pars pro toto* and provides information about the skeletal age (Greulich and Pyle 1988). The limit of this method is reached at the age of 18 years. Together with the panoramic radiograph, it can limit the range of variations of the possible age of the child/youth from different ethnic groups.

Cavalli-Sforza et al. (1994) divide the genealogical relationship of the world population into four main groups: Africans, Australians, Europeans (whites), and Mongolians. Greulich and Pyle (1988) apply the so-called Atlas method. It is the most common method for determining skeletal maturity (Cole et al. 1988; Milner et al. 1986).

However, ethnicity is not the only influence on the development of a child. Rather, it is believed that genetic factors are also responsible for the potential of skeletal maturity. A low socio-economic standard of living and poor environmental conditions lead to retardation (development delay) of skeletal maturity (Schmeling et al. 1999a, b).

For adults, the time-independent level of racemization of aspartic acid can be especially assessed, whereby the reconditioning of a tooth (otherwise a dentin biopsy) is necessary (Rösing and Kvaal 1998).

Investigations by Schmeling et al. (1999a, b) have demonstrated that skeletal maturation takes place in the same (identical) levels in all major ethnic groups. The risk of an age estimation below the actual age should serve to protect that person.

If a tooth is completely developed, all age-related changes at the tooth structure must be studied (Solheim 1988b). Often, they are described as degenerative or regressive, and attrition, color, and periodontal shrinkage are assessed by the naked eye. Although there is a correlation between age and size of the pulp chamber, it is not significant enough for age estimation (Prapanpoch et al. 1992). The tooth structure is subject to physiological and pathological influences and occurs as a consequence of tooth loss.

The main causes for hard tissue loss are:

Chemical–bacterial processes of decay

Extradental and intradental absorption rather than cellular processes

Factors leading to *abrasio dentis* (Schneider and Hampel 1966); dental abrasion is an important and indispensable finding

Interstitial friction surfaces (adjacent teeth in the middle decades of life), changes in the interior of the tooth (increasing narrowing of the lumen in crown-pulp-cavum and the root canals) and the alveolar process (atrophy with exposure of cervical and coronary artery root parts) provide valuable information.

From the statistical view, forensic age diagnosis is a bivariate problem with the two variables being signs of maturity and chronological age. Of great importance is the scattering of the bivariate distribution area (Riepert and Rittner 1989).

The studies of Gustafson (1947, 1950, 1955, 1956) provided the first statistical methodology. The “Gustafson method” was the basis of age estimation by teeth and hand. He assessed six factors of changes of dental hard tissue (Figs. 19.5, 19.6 and 19.7):

1. A = attrition (*abrasio dentis*)
2. S = residue of secondary dentin in the pulp chamber
3. P = periodontal shrinkage
4. Z = cement residue
5. R = cement and dentin resorption
6. T = root transparency

The changes are microscopically examined on thin sections of slides embedded in canada balsam. The strength of each change is divided into four stages (0–3). Points are dependent on the degree of change, and adding all points of a tooth results in the sum of the changes (An + Pn + Zn + Sn + Rn + Tn = total). The relation between scores and age is expressed by a line (chart). The calculated formula is: $age = 4.56x + 11.43$. The correlation with age is 0.91 (Maples and Rice 1979).

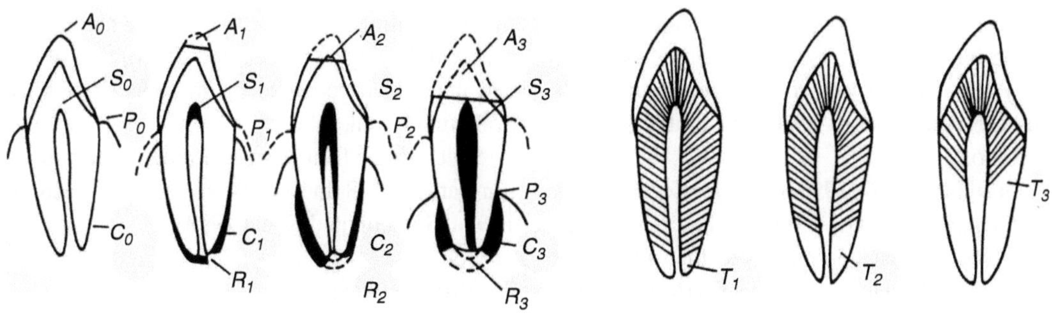

Fig. 19.5 Tooth grinding – six factors (changes in dental hard substance)

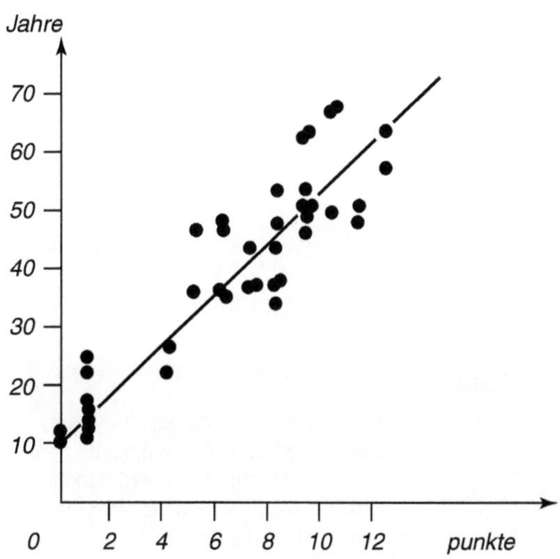

Fig. 19.6 The regression line between observed values is marked

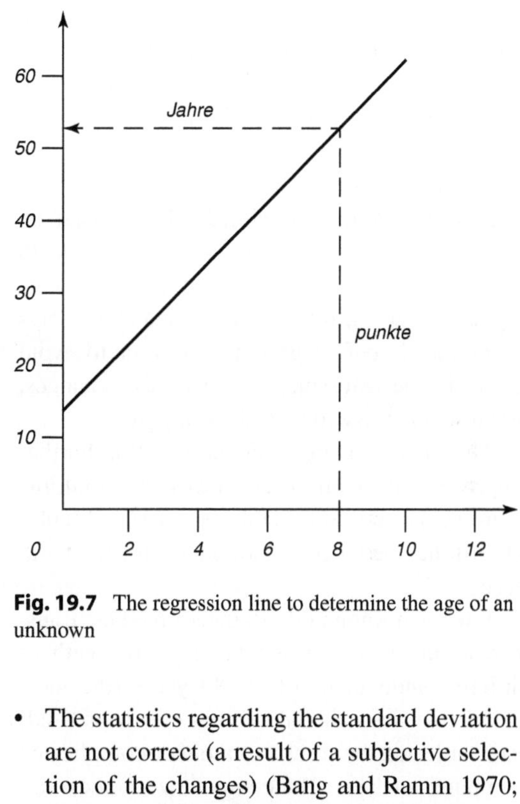

Fig. 19.7 The regression line to determine the age of an unknown

The accuracy of the determination is increased if two or more teeth are available. Then the average of the teeth is used as a total. The Gustafson method has the advantage that it evaluates several features, in comparison with a single feature, which is more error prone. Although several improvements have been published, e.g., in the USA, many forensic odontologists still use the original method. Thus, the Gustafson method was applied for many years as the method of choice by many forensic odontologists.

Nevertheless, this method is criticized (Schmeling et al. 1999a, b):

- The evaluation of the points is the result of a subjective selection of the changes; it is based on too many factors that are pathologically influenced and not only related to age.
- The statistics regarding the standard deviation are not correct (a result of a subjective selection of the changes) (Bang and Ramm 1970; Maples and Rice 1979; Rötzscher 1998).
- The standard deviation is larger than calculated in an independent collection of examples (Burns and Maples 1976; Maples and Rice 1979; Solheim 1988b).

– Gender was not considered.

The examined material of 40 teeth of different individuals (Gustafson 1947, 1950, 1955) is a relatively small selection and it may be possible that some teeth are from the same individual, as in other investigations (Burns and Maples 1976; Johanson 1971; Lode and Reimann 1985).

Because the variability of age-related changes in the teeth from the same individual is apparently less than in teeth of different individuals, this can contribute to a more favorable standard deviation.

Gustafson (1947, 1950, 1955) developed a single formula that should be valid for all groups of teeth. However, it must be considered that age-related changes can lead to different results (Maples 1978; Schulze 1982) as much as tooth position (Schulze 1982), or a formula separately calculated for each tooth type (Bang and Ramm 1970; Schulze 1982). The regression formula by Gustafson was incorrect. Later it was amended to: $age = 13.45x + 4.26$ and the correlation between estimated and actual age $r = 0.912$ (Maples and Rice 1979). Nevertheless, it is not appropriate to skip Gustafson's method and not to mention its results.

Biedow (1963) modified the Gustafson method by assessment of one-sided cut teeth under the stereomicroscope with the same scoring as Gustafson. It is recommended that X-rays be obtained before grinding in order to avoid errors in the assessment of regressive changes, because not every root canal is straight.

The front teeth are particularly useful. Further improvements with seven stages and multiple regressions were added (Johanson 1971). Maples (1978) included a correction factor for the tooth type.

Bang and Ramm (1970) determined the transparent root dentin in a total of 1,200 teeth of different individuals of 10–80 years (the most comprehensive material that has ever been used) and subjected the results to a rather complicated computer analysis. The computerized index values can be correlated with the age.

The method of Solheim (1993b) provides another improvement. He studied only one tooth from each individual and used a stepwise multiple regression so factors that are not significant for the regression are excluded. After studying age-related changes of 1,000 teeth of Caucasian/white origin (100 of each group of teeth, molars excluded), whose age was known, he selected the measurements with the highest correlation of each group.

First, the teeth were measured uncut and then ground along the pulp center and evaluated, and finally additional measurements were made with a stereomicroscope. A detailed description of the test material is recorded in previous studies by Solheim (1988a, b).

Seven single factors, measurements, or evaluations are used (Solheim 1988a, b, 1990, 1992a, b, 1993a; Solheim and Kvaal 1993):

1. Color
2. Attrition (wear)
3. Root translucence
4. Cement thickness
5. Secondary dentin
6. Periodontal shrinkage
7. Irregularities of the root surface

Solheim represents new methods for age estimation in a chart (Chart 19.1).

Chart 19.1
New methods for age estimation (Solheim 1993a)

Results	
Color	The Pearson correlation varies from 0.59 to 0.84 in different dental groups. The tooth color will darken with advancing age, male teeth tend to be darker than female teeth (Solheim 1988a)
Attrition	The biggest correlation with age was found in premolar bicuspids, with a correlation coefficient of $r = 0.68$ for the second mandibular; the canines were not significantly correlated ($r = 0.23$ mandibular and 0.25 maxillary). The attrition in men was more pronounced than in women (Solheim 1988b)
Root transparency	The degree of translucency showed only slight variations between each dental group. The length of the translucent zone of not-sectioned teeth showed, in most dental groups, the closest relationship to age. If more than one method of measurement for regression analysis was used, a high correlation to age was seen ($r = 0.68$–0.86). Slightly more translucent areas were detected in the teeth of men, with darker teeth and increasing density of cementum (Solheim 1989)

Results	
Cement density	The dental cement density is less related to age than color and apical translucency (Solheim 1990)
Secondary dentin	Although the correlation is not very strong, time is the decisive factor for the continuous formation of secondary dentin, the correlation for age varied from 0.58 to 0.75 for the various dental groups (Johanson 1971). The size of the pulp cavity, more influenced by external factors, is not closely related to age (Solheim 1992a)
Periodontal shrinkage	The weakest correlation ($r=0.22$–0.64) was found in the canines; the strongest in the premolars (Solheim 1992b)
Irregularity of the root surface	The measurements of the irregularity of the root surface (SRS) showed, compared with older evaluation systems, a stronger correlation with age ($r=0.44$, $r=0.68$). The SRS did not vary between genders. However, teeth with narrow pulp chambers had a higher SRS. These age-related changes appear of great value in a multiple regression method of age determination (Solheim and Kvaal 1993)

Analyses with and without color and gender resulted in two different formulas for each tooth type. In archaeological material, the color changes postmortem and gender determination is difficult. The strongest correlation was found with age $r=0.91$ for the maxillary central incisor (including gender and color).

Selected factors (codes) of each tooth type for the multiple regression analysis method (Solheim 1993b) are given in Tables 19.3 and 19.4. For the second premolar of the mandibula, the age correlation with $r=0.76$ was the weakest (sex and color were irrelevant for this tooth). In most cases, only one tooth is sufficient. Correlation in the central maxillary incisors is strongest, but removing and grinding cannot always be taken for granted. The second maxillary premolar shows a strong correlation to age (indicator tooth). Because the latter does not need to be sanded, it can be stored and reintroduced into the socket.

Table 19.3 Formula for age calculation of maxillary incisors (11/21, 12/22) and the second premolars (15/25)

Tooth	Formula	*r*	SEE
11/21	Age = 24.3 + 8.7 CEST + 5.2 D – 2.3 CAP – 4.3 SEX	0.91	7.0
	Age = 25.3 + 7.1 TD – 3.1 CAP + 5.3 SRS – 7.5 EX3 + 0.2 Cl	0.89	7.9
12/22	Age = 38.7 – 126 ST + 4.7 CEST + 4.2 TD + 0.05 Cl	0.90	8.0
	Age = 46.7 – 142 ST + 6.5 TD + 0.05 Cl	0.88	8.7
15/25	Age = 14.2 + 2.5 TID + 4.1 AJ + 8.9 LPMEAN	0.84	9.6

Solheim (1993a)
Standard error *r* Pearson correlation, *SEE* estimation (in years)

Table 19.4 Selected factors and methods (codes) of each tooth type (Solheim 1993b) for the multiple regression analysis

LPMEAN	Logarithmic transformation of the means PMEAN *periodontal shrinkage* at the four tooth surfaces (in millimeters) (Solheim 1993a)
AJ, ARA CL,	Level of *attrition* according to the evaluation of Johanson (1971), in square millimeters and crown length (in millimeters) (Maples 1978)
CEST	*Color value* in its system(Solheim 1988a, b)
CAP, ST, SJ	Crown pulp area in square millimeters (Solheim 1988a, b), large pulp/root width in four levels (Solheim 1992a, b), *secondary dentin*, evaluation by Johanson (1971)
TD, TID	*Translucency evaluation* in millimeters of translucency on non-grounded, dried teeth (Bang and Ramm 1970)
C1, LC1	Total *density of the cement* on the lingual and vestibular surfaces of the apical root third, logarithmic transformation of C1 (Solheim 1990)
SRS	Rating of the *surface unevenness of the root*
EX3	*Extracted tooth* (caries diagnosis or apical periodontitis)

The Solheim method has been proven in practice, but it has not yet been compared with other methods. It seems to be more complicated than other methods. However, if the required equipment and the corresponding descriptions in the literature are available, only a few measurements for each tooth are sufficient. A stereomicroscope must be set for the tests and measurements. For the evaluation of other teeth and the detailed descriptions, the reader is referred to the original work (Solheim 1993b).

If extractions are not desired, X-ray images are used for age estimation, especially in archaeological material and material from identification cases, but mainly for living persons. Matsikidis and Schulz (1982) used the Gustafson method but without root transparency and root resorption.

Another radiographic method is based on the ratio of pulp and root width and length measurements, evaluated on 452 front, eye, and cheek teeth (Kvaal and Solheim 1994). For each tooth type, formulas using multiple regression are calculated. The correlation to the age varies from tooth to tooth ($r=0.86$ for the upper second molar).

In archaeological material and material of special cases of identification, methods were needed in which the teeth do not need to be sanded. Length measurements of the transparent root tip (*apex radicis dentis*) may be performed without grinding. According to the method of Bang and Ramm (Bang and Ramm 1970), the maximum correlation with age was 0.84 for the upper right central incisor. Shade and color of the root dentin may also be involved (Ten Cate et al. 1977).

The cement lines in mammals usually are deposited once a year and can be counted to determine the age. In humans, this method is difficult because there are many lines close together. However, some authors have achieved good results in humans, even in bodies of fire victims (Grosskopf 1990).

The difference between the individual age and the biological age varies depending on the type of the examined tooth (incisor, premolar, molar), the standard deviation is 5.69 years (Prapanpoch et al. 1992). Recent studies on tooth roots of the third molars showed a close relationship between the racemization degree of aspartic acid and age-standard error of estimate (SEE; in years) in 70 patients (2.3 years with total root dentin; in the other material, 2.5 years).

An increasingly interesting method to determine the age (even in fossil materials) is the racemization degree of aspartic acid in dentin, not only for the total amino acid (TAA) but also for the insoluble collagen (IC) and the soluble peptide (SP) fractions. The fastest racemization took place in the IC, but was significantly slower in the SP group (Ohtani and Yamamoto 1990a, 1991, Prapanpoch et al. 1992; Rao et al. 1989). The specification of the initial examination of age estimation using racemization degree of aspartic acid in dentin is by Ogino et al. (1985). With this method, results that are highly accurate with a correlation to the real age and $r=0.99$ are possible.

This was confirmed also for bradytrophic tissue by Pfeiffer and Mörnstadt with HPLC technique (Mörnstad et al. 1994; Pfeiffer et al. 1993). However, this method is expensive, labor intensive, and needs special equipment.

Biological development criteria are especially helpful in the first half of life, while epidemiological criteria are more useful in the second half of life. Zuhrt et al. (1996a) used the main criteria given in Chart 19.2 for odontological age estimation.

Chart 19.2

Main odontological criteria for age estimation (Zuhrt et al. 1996b)

1. **Biological development**	2. **Epidemiological criteria**
1.1. The dentition	2.1. The DMF index
1.2. Presence of third molars	2.2. The dentition
1.3. Extent of root dentin transparence	2.3. The number of healthy teeth
1.4. Abrasion	2.4. The condition of marginal periodontium

The internationally accepted DMF index indicates the average number of decayed (D), missing (M) and restorative powered teeth (F = filled). The inter-individual variability of tooth decay is about the dimension of the average. In evaluating the data, especially of the Berlin morbidity study of 1972 (Schrimer 1977), we use the following rule of thumb: 20 years, 10 DMF teeth; growth in 5 years by 2 teeth; men −1; and women +1.

Because of dental caries and from the age of 40 years, there is a reduction of the dentition by periodontitis (the M component of the DMF index). This fact can be used as a criterion when biological (caries, periodontal disease) and psychosocial (health behavior) aspects are to be considered. As reference material, the studies by Harder and Spaniel (1976), Felgendreher and Twelkmeyer (1977), and Endris (1979) are used.

Because of the gradual spread of caries, the number of healthy teeth is dependent on age. The average number of healthy teeth decreases nonlinearly from 18 teeth at the age of 20 years to 2 teeth at the age of 70 years.

In evaluable soft tissue, because of postmortem changes, different pathological conditions are described: atrophy and profound periodontitis. According to Pawlik, periodontitis occurs in less than 20 % of 20-year-olds, in approximately 50 % of 30-year-olds, and in 90 % of 70-year-olds. The age-related generalized atrophy significantly increases during the second half of life (Zuhrt and Geserick 1996).

After collecting the postmortem findings on a special form, the findings are verbally and graphically (dental chart) documented and individually evaluated. The comparison of usable criteria with the actual age highlights the problem of postmortem age estimation: only rarely is the entire criteria usable and only rarely does a single criterion correspond to the actual age.

Except for two children, the root dentin transparence was determined in all cases. There was low competence of this feature, especially in the early and middle adulthood. In contrast, abrasion was rarely used, but of high significance. Conversely, the assessment of third molars was possible and useful only in early and middle adulthood. In the epidemiological criteria, a useful competence was found only in old age, although hardly in the number of DMF teeth, but rather in the dentition and in the assessment of the marginal periodontium.

Contrary to expectation, dentures are not significant for identification of individuals. In more than half of the cases, a self-imposed strict standard for correct age estimation within a range of up to 10 years could be reached.

Erroneous determinations occur particularly in the early and middle adulthood and particularly in persons from the Far East. Zuhrt and Geserick (1996a) attribute the small influence of the extent of root dentin transparence to the following facts:

- The overassessment of the coefficients from 0.64 to 0.83 and between 0.40 and 0.95 (Bang and Ramm (1970) and Wegener and Albrecht (1980)).
- Neglecting standard deviations depending on tooth position, from 9.3 to 13.6 years and 10.8 and 16.1 years, with ranges from 10 to 32 years for the actual age.
- Improper extrapolation of the concrete specimens for one calculated linear regression.
- Assuming a linear development of root dentin transparence.

Because of our self-critical analysis of forensic odontological age estimation, we feel confirmed in our overall process supported by the findings and suggest even greater caution. In assessing the root dentin transparency, it is critical to consider the standard deviation of the reference values (Zuhrt and Geserick 1996; Zuhrt et al. 1996).

In his evaluation of 350 teeth of live/dead people of either sex (without preselection), Lampe (1977) concluded that malocclusions, one-sided stress (caused by gaps or pain), and even uneven articulation can lead to different abrasion. Parametric functions (grinding) can cause an early severe abrasion. The different levels of dental care with regard to periodontal changes should not be underestimated. In addition, the effects of more or less qualified dental prostheses on the general condition of the dentition should be assessed. As an episode of a local inflammation, an overloading of the tooth or

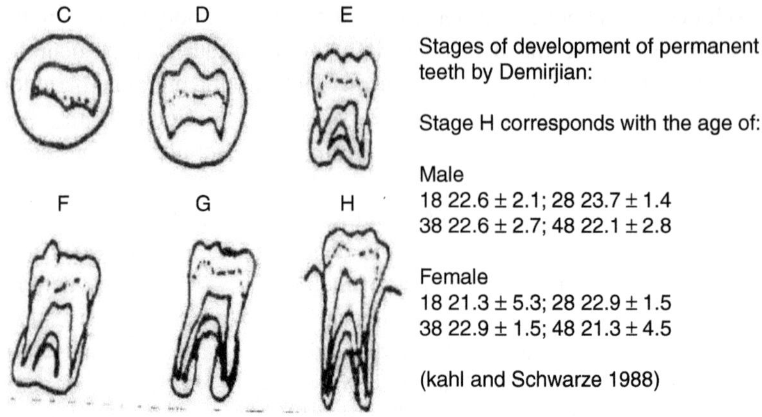

Fig. 19.8 Stages of development of permanent teeth by Demirjian

as a symptom of a general osteopathy, hypercementosis may occur, resulting in an incorrect age estimation because of "cementum". For preparation of the tooth sections, Donath recommends the EXACT cutting-grinding system (Donath 1988; Lampe 1977; Lampe and Rötzscher 1994).

19.3.1 Examination of the Degree of Mineralization of Third Molars in a European Population

The first part of a complex study in which data about the mineralization of the third molars of different ethnic groups will be compiled (Olze et al. 2011) is presented here.

19.3.1.1 Materials and Methods

Out of a total of approximately 6,000 panoramic radiographs (Charité hospital, Berlin), 1,437 orthopantograms of Central Europeans between 12 and 25 years of age were selected; 860 female and 577 male individuals were examined. The average age of the total sample was 20.27 years. The finding of the mineralization of the arranged third molars was separated into sexes and teeth. For characterization of the mineralization, staging according to Demirjian et al. (1973) was used (Fig. 19.8).

19.3.1.2 Results

The evaluation of the radiographs was performed without exception by one and the same examiner. Tables 19.5 and 19.6 show their own examination results in comparison with the data published by Kahl and Schwarze (1988). For the wisdom teeth of all four quadrants, in each case, the average and the standard deviation of the stages were shown.

After evaluation of our data by help of the Mann-Whitney U and Wilcoxon tests, no significant differences regarding the temporal passing of the mineralization stages of the third molars in the maxilla and mandible were found. Significant differences between the sexes were also not noticed.

19.3.1.3 Discussion

For characterization of the development status of an individual, the mineralization is more suitable than the dental eruption (Gleiser and Hunt 1955). Dental eruption is a process that may be influenced by exogenic factors such as early loss of primary tooth, infections, or space conditions. Furthermore, there are various definitions for dental eruption, which reach from eruption of the first cusp through the gingiva to the arrangement of the respective tooth into the dental plane. On the other hand, tooth mineralization displays a process that is largely independent from external influences (Demirjian 1986).

Table 19.5 Third molars, stages according to Demirjian, male

	Kahl and Schwarze (1988)				Olze et al. (2011)			
Dental phase	18	28	38	48	18	28	38	48
A	10.1	10.3	10.0	10.1	–	–	–	–
	1.0	1.7	2.0	1.5	–	–	–	–
B	10.3	10.6	10.7	10.7	14.4	15.5	13.3	–
	1.3	1.5	1.3	1.8	2.7	3.3	2.1	–
C	11.4	11.2	11.5	11.6	13.6	14.5	14.6	14.5
	1.6	1.6	1.4	1.5	0.7	1.9	1.7	1.5
D	12.7	12.6	12.4	12.5	16.5	16.3	16.3	16.7
	1.7	1.6	1.4	1.4	3.1	3.2	3.1	3.1
E	14.2	14.5	14.8	15.0	16.7	16.6	16.7	16.7
	2.0	1.5	1.4	1.9	2.6	2.3	2.3	2.1
F	16.5	16.5	16.0	16.4	17.8	17.7	18.3	18.2
	1.1	1.5	1.7	1.7	2.0	2.0	2.2	2.1
G	18.6	18.8	18.9	17.8	20.6	20.6	21.3	21.3
	1.2	1.1	1.1	2.3	2.4	2.4	2.0	2.1
H	22.6	23.7	22.6	22.1	22.5	22.6	22.7	22.7
	2.1	1.4	2.7	2.8	1.9	1.9	1.9	1.9

First line: average; second line: standard deviation in years

Table 19.6 Third molars, stages according to Demirjian, female

	Kahl and Schwarze (1988)				Olze et al. (2011)			
Dental phase	18	28	38	48	18	28	38	48
A	10.3	10.2	10.2	9.9	–	–	–	–
	1.7	1.4	1.4	1.3	–	–	–	–
B	10.2	9.9	9.9	10.3	14.5	12.6	14.0	13.8
	1.6	1.4	1.4	1.4	3.8	0.9	2.9	1.6
C	11.0	11.0	11.0	11.5	14.2	15.1	14.5	14.1
	1.8	1.7	1.7	1.8	1.7	2.3	1.6	1.5
D	12.8	12.6	12.6	13.1	15.7	15.7	15.5	15.7
	2.1	1.8	1.8	1.8	2.8	2.5	2.6	2.6
E	15.6	15.9	15.9	15.9	16.8	17.0	16.8	17.2
	1.9	1.2	1.2	1.2	2.3	2.7	2.3	2.4
F	17.5	16.7	16.7	17.4	18.6	18.7	19.1	19.0
	4.0	3.5	3.5	3.1	2.5	2.5	2.5	2.5
G	20.1	19.8	19.8	19.9	20.7	20.7	21.7	21.7
	2.5	3.7	3.7	2.7	2.6	2.6	2.1	2.1
H	21.3	22.9	22.9	21.3	22.7	22.7	23.0	23.1
	5.3	1.5	1.5	4.5	1.9	1.9	1.8	1.8

First line: average; second line: standard deviation in years

References

Adler P (1957a) Korrigierte Tabellen zur Bestimmung des dentalen Alters nach dem Verfahren von Matiegka. Dtsch Zahn- Mund- und Kieferheilk 27:190–195

Adler P (1957b) Die Eignung der normalen Wahrscheinlichkeitskurve zur Darstellung der Elimination und Eruption der einzelnen Zähne während des Zahnwechsels. Ost Z Stomatol 54:449–462

Adler P (1959a) Studien über den zeitlichen Verlauf der Zahnung. Med Hyg 17:107–117

Adler P (1959b) Der Geschlechtsunterschied im Zahnwechsel. Dtsch Zahn- Mund- und Kieferheilk 31:20–33

Adler P (1963) Effect of some environmental factors on sequence of tooth eruption. J Dent Res 42:605–616

Ajmani ML, Jain SP, Joshi SD (1986) Age and wisdom teeth in Nigeria. Anthropol Anz 44(2):143–148

Bang G, Ramm E (1970) Determination of age in humans from root dentin transparency. Acta Odontol Scand 28:3–35

Biedow J (1963) A modified method of age estimation in teeth. Excerpta med London, International congress Ser No 80, pp 37–38

Burns KR, Maples WR (1976) Estimation of age from individual adult teeth. J Forensic Sci 21:343–356

Cavalli-Sforza LL, Menozzi P, Piazza A (1994) The history and geography of human genes. Princeton University Press, Princeton

Ciaparelli L (1985) An assessment of dental age in Essex schoolchildren using panoral radiographs with forensic applications. Dissertation, Diploma in Forensic Odontology, London Hospital Medical College

Cole AJL, Webb L, Cole TJ (1988) Bone age estimation: a comparison of methods. Br J Radiol 61:683–686

Crossner CG, Mansfeld L (1983) Determination of dental age in adopted non-European children. Swed Dent J 7:1–10

Davis PJ, Hägg U (1994) The accuracy and precision of the "Demirjian system" when used for age estimation in Chinese children. Swed Dent J 18(3):113–116

Demirjian A (1986) Definition. In: Falkner F, Tanner JM (eds) Human growth. Academic, New York/London, pp 269–298

Demirjian A (1994) Dental development on CD-ROM. SilverPlatter Education, Newton

Demirjian A, Goldstein H (1976) New systems for dental maturity based on seven and four teeth. Ann Hum Biol 3:411–421

Demirjian A, Goldstein H, Tanner JM (1973) A new system of dental age assessment. Hum Biol 45:211–227

Donath K (1988) Die Trenn-Dünnschliff-Technik zur Herstellung histologischer Präparate von nicht schneidbaren Geweben und Materialien. Der Präparator 34(1):197–206

Endris R (ed) (1979) 2.0 Zahn – Zahnbogen – Kausystem, 2.3.2. Bleibende Zähne, Dentes permanentes. In: Praktische Forensische Odonto-Stomatologie. Kriminalistik, Heidelberg, S 15–20

Ewald G (1992) Beitrag zur Bestimmung des Lebensalters durch Auswertung von Röntgenaufnahmen der bleibenden Zähne des Menschen. Inaugural dissertation. Ruprecht-Karls-Universität, Heidelberg

Fahmy MS (1974) The estimation of age of Arabs from their dentitions. An orthopantomographic study of the permanent dentition of different Arab nationalities. J Kuwait Med Assoc 8:145–162

Felgendreher H, Twelkmeyer J (1977) Altersabhängige Untersuchung der Morbidität der bleibenden Zähne des menschlichen Gebisses. Stom. Dipl. Arbeit. Humboldt-Universität zu Berlin

Ferembach D, Schwidetzky I, Stloukal M (1979) Empfehlungen für die Alters- und Geschlechtsdiagnose am Skelett. Homo 30:1–32

Garn SM, Lewis AB, Blizzard RM (1965) Endocrine factors in dental development. J Dent Res 44:243–258

Gleiser I, Hunt EE (1955) The permanent mandibular first molar; its calcination, eruption and decay. Am J Phys Anthropol 13:253–284

Greulich WW, Pyle SI (1988) Radiographic atlas of skeletal development of the hand and wrist. Stanford University Press, Stanford

Grosskopf B (1990) Individualaltersbestimmung mit Hilfe von Zuwachsringen im Zement bodengelagerter menschlicher Zähne. Z Rechtsmed 103:351–359

Gustafson G (1947) Åldersbestämningar på tänder. Odontol Tidskr 55:556–568

Gustafson G (1950) Age determination on teeth. J Am Dent Assoc 41:45–54

Gustafson G (1955) Altersbestimmung an Zähnen. Dtsch Zahnarztl Z 10:1763–1768

Gustafson G (1956) Die Bestimmung des Alters von unbekannten Toten durch den Zahnarzt. Arch Kriminol 117:121–122

Gustafson G, Koch G (1974) Age determination up to 16 years of age based on dental development. Odontol Rev 25:297–306

Haavikko K (1974) Tooth formation age determination on a few selected teeth. Proc Finn Dent Soc 70:15–19

Hägg U, Matsson L (1985) Dental maturity as an indicator of chronological age: the accuracy and precision of three methods. Eur J Orthod 7:25–34

Harder BI, Spaniel M (1976) Analyse der Morbidität der ersten bleibenden Molaren. Med. dissertation, Humboldt-Universität zu Berlin

Hassanali J (1985) The third permanent molar eruption in Kenyan Africans and Asians. Ann Hum Biol 12(6):517–523

Helm S (1990) Relationship between dental and skeletal maturation in Danish schoolchildren. J Dent Res 98:313–317

Hurme VO (1957) Time and sequence of tooth eruption. The human dentition in forensic medicine. J Forensic Sci 2:442–447

Johanson G (1971) Age determination from teeth. Odontol Rev 22(Suppl 21):1–126

Kahl B, Schwarze CW (1988) Aktuakisierung der Dentitionstabelle von I. Schour und M. Massler von 1941. Fortschr Kieferorthop 49:432–443

Kumar CL, Sridhar MS (1990) Estimation of the age of an individual based on times of eruption of permanent teeth. Forensic Sci Int 48:1–7

Künzel W (1976) Querschnittsvergleich mittlerer Eruptionstermine permanenter Zähne bei Kindern in fluorarmen und kariesprotektiv optimierten Trinkwassergebieten. Stomatol DDR 26:310–321

Kvaal S, Solheim T (1994) A non-destructive dental method for age estimation. J Forensic Odontostomatol 12:6–11

Lampe H (1977) Möglichkeiten der Alters- und Identitätsbestimmung an Zähnen. Inaug. Dissertation, Ruprecht-Karl-Universität zu Heidelberg

Lampe P, Rötzscher K (1994) Forensic odontology: age determination from adult human teeth. Med Sci Law 13:623–628

Liliequist B, Lundberg M (1971) Skeletal and tooth development. A methodological investigation. Acta Radiol 11:97–112

Lode F, Reimann W (1985) Altersbestimmung am Zahnhalbschliff. Zahn-Mund-Kieferheilk 73:132–136

Logan W, Kronfield D (1933) Development of the human jaws and surrounding structures from birth to the age of fifteen years. J Am Dent Assoc 20:379–427

Lucy D, Pollard AM (1995) Further comments on the estimation of error associated with the Gustafson dental age estimation method. J Forensic Sci 40:222–227

Maples WR (1978) An improved technique using dental histology for estimation of adult age. J Forensic Sci 23:764–770

Maples WR, Rice PM (1979) Some difficulties in the Gustafson dental age estimations. J Forensic Sci 24:168–172

Marré B, Hetzer G (1999) Altersschätzung bei Kindern und Jugendlichen. Grundsatzfragen. Newsl AKFOS Jg 6(3):41–46

Matsikidis G, Schulz P (1982) Altersbestimmung nach dem Gebiß mit Hilfe des Zahnfilms. Zahnarztl Mitt 72:2524–2528

Milner GR, Levick RK, Kay R (1986) Assessment of bone age: a comparison of the Greulichand Pyle, and the Tanner and Whitehouse methods. Clin Radiol 37:119–121

Mincer HH, Harris EF, Berryman HE (1993) The A.B.F.O. study of third molar development and its use as an estimator of chronological age. J Forensic Sci 38(2):379–390

Moorrees CFA, Fanning EA, Hunt EE Jr (1963) Age variation of formation stages for ten permanent teeth. J Dent Res 42:1490–1502

Mörnstad H, Staaf V, Welander U (1994) Age estimation with the aid of tooth development: a new method based on objective measurements. Scand J Dent Res 102:137–143

Ogino T, Ogino H, Nagy B (1985) Application of aspartic acid racemization to forensic odontology: post mortem designation of age of death. Forensic Sci Int 29:259–267

Ohtani S (1994) Age estimation by aspartic acid racemization in dentin of deciduous teeth. Forensic Sci Int 68:77–82

Ohtani S, Yamamoto K (1987) Age estimation using the racemization of aspartic acid in human dentin. Nippon Hoigaku Zasshi 41:181–190

Ohtani S, Yamamoto K (1990a) Racemization velocity of aspartic acid in dentine. Nippon-Hoigaku-Zasshi 44(4):346–351

Ohtani S, Yamamoto K (1990b) Estimating age through the amino acid racemization of acid-soluble dentinal peptides. Nippon Hoigaku Zasshi 44:342–345

Ohtani S, Yamamoto K (1991) Age estimation using the racemization of amino acid in human dentin. J Forensic Sci 36:792–800

Ohtani S, Yamamoto K (1992) Estimation of age from a tooth by means of acemization of an amino acid, especially aspartic acid – comparison of enamel and dentin. J Forensic Sci 37:1061–1067

Olze A, Schmeling A, Geserick G, Rieger K, Kalb G (2011) Untersuchungen zum Mineralisationsstand der dritten Molaren an einer europäischen Population. AKFOS Newsl J 8(2):47–48

Otuyemi OD, Ugboko VI, Ndukwe KC, Adekoya-Sofowora CA (1997) Eruption times of third molars in young rural Nigerians. Int Dent J 47:266–270

Pfeiffer H, Teivens A, Mörnstadt H (1993) A new method of chiral separation of aspartic acid in teeth with HPLC technique. 13. IOFOS Meeting, Düsseldorf, 24/15/00/3H

Pfeiffer H, Mörnstad H, Teivens A (1995) Lebensaltersbestimmungen durch Ermittlung des Racemisierungsgrades von Asparaginsäure mit Hilfe der HPCL-Technik. AKFOS Newsl Jg 2(2):35

Prapanpoch S, Dove SB, Cottone JA (1992) Morphometric analysis of the dental pulp chamber as a method of age determination in humans. Am J Forensic Med Pathol 13(1):50–55

Preece MA (1983) Are the number of teeth any help in assessing development. Arch Dis Child 58(11):849–850

Rao NG, Rao NN, Pai ML, Kotian MS (1989) Mandibula canine index – a clue for establishing sex identity. Forensic Sci Int 42:249–254

Riepert TH, Rittner CH (1989) Zur Röntgenidentifizierung unbekannter Leichen bei fortgeschrittenen postmortalen Veränderungen. Rechtsmed 102(11):207–216

Ritz S, Kaatsch HJ (1996) Methoden der Altersbestimmung an lebenden Personen: Möglichkeiten, Grenzen, Zulässigkeit und ethische Vertretbarkeit. Rechtsmed 6:171–176

Ritz S, Schütz HW, Schwarzer B (1990) The extent of aspartic acid racemization in dentin: a possible method for a more accurate determination of age at death? Z Rechtsmed 103:457–462

Ritz S, Schütz HW, Peper C (1993a) Postmortem estimation of age at death based on aspartic acid racemization in dentin: its applicability for root dentin. Int J Leg Med 105:289–293

Ritz S, Turzynski A, Schütz HW, Martz W (1993b) Postmortem estimation of age at death based on aspartic acid racemisation in dentin and bone. Sect. 18; 27/10/05/2A, 13. Meeting IOFOS, Düsseldorf

Ritz S, Stock R, Schütz HW, Kaatsch HJ (1995) Age estimation in biopsy specimens of dentin. Int J Legal Med 108:135–139

Ritz-Timme S (1999) Lebensaltersbestimmung aufgrund der Razemisierung von Asparaginsäure: Grundlagen, Methodik, Möglichkeiten und Grenzen, Vortrag, X. Lübecker Gespräch Deutscher Rechtsmediziner:“Osteologische Identifikation“. 3./4. Dezember, Lübeck

Rönnermann H (1977) Effect of early loss of primary molars on tooth eruption and space conditions. A longitudinal study. Acta Odontol Scand 35:229–239

Rösing FW (1994) Forensische Osteologie. 6. Aufl. Erbbiologie/Osteologie, Uni. Ulm, S 13–14

Rösing FW, Kvaal S (1998) Dental age in adults. A review of estimation methods. In: Alt KW, Rösing FW, Teschler-Nicola M (eds) Dental anthropology. Fundamentals, limits, and prospects. Springer, Wien, pp 443–458

Rötzscher K (1998) Gentest identifiziert Bormann-Skelett – Anmerkungen. AKFOS Newsl Jg 5(2):36

Rötzscher K, Reimann W (1975) Die forensische Stomatologie. In: Prokop O, Göhler W (Hrsg) Forensische Medizin 3. Aufl. Volk und Gesundheit, Berlin, S 545–564

Saunders E (1897) The teeth as a fact of age considered with reference to the Factory Children. Addressed to the members of both Houses of Parliament, London

Saunders S, DeVito C, Herring A, Southern R, Hoppa R (1993) Accuracy tests of tooth formation age estimations for human skeletal remains. Am J Phys Anthropol 92:173–188

Schirmer G (1977) Gebissgesundheit, Gesundheitswissen und-verhalten in einer repräsentativen Bevölkerungsstichprobe aus der Hauptstadt der DDR Berlin 1972. Med. Diss. Humboldt-Universität zu Berlin

Schmeling A, Vendura K, Olze A, Reisinger W, Geserick G (1999a) Altersschätzung und ethnische Zugehörigkeit. Vortrag X. Lübecker Gespräch, 3. und 4. Dezenber 1999 in Lübeck

Schmeling A, Reisinger W, Loreck D, Vendura K, Markus W, Geserick G (1999b) Effects of ethnicity on skeletal maturation – Consequences for forensic age estimations. Int J Leg Med (in Druck) 113(5):253–258

Schneider H, Hampel W (1966) Die Einschleiftherapie nach Jankelson. Dtsch Stomat 16:614–623

Schour I, Massler M (1940) Studies in tooth development: the growth pattern of the human teeth. J Am Dent Assoc 27(1778–1793):1918–1931

Schour I, Massler M (1958) Chronology of the development of the dentitions, 2nd edn. American Dental Association, Chicago

Schranz D (1958) A fogak életkorjelzö adatai igazságügyi orvostani szempontból (Die Altersbestimmungsmerkmale bei Zähnen aus dem Gesichtspunkt der gerichtlichen Medizin). Fogorv Szemle Budapest 10–12:390–394

Schranz D (1959) Kritik der Auswertung der Altersbestimmungsmerkmale von Zähnen und Knochen. Dtsch Z Gerichtl Med 48:562–575

Schroeder HE (1987) Orale Strukturbiologie. G Thieme, Stuttgart/New York, p 4

Schulze C (1982) Lehrbuch der Kieferorthopädie. 3 Aufl Quintessenz, Berlin

Solheim T (1988a) Dental color as an indicator of age. Gerodontontics 4:114–118

Solheim T (1988b) Dental attrition as an indicator of age. Gerodontontics 4:299–304

Solheim T (1989) Dental root translucency as an indicator of age. Scand J Dent Res 97:189–197

Solheim T (1990) Dental cementum apposition as an indicator of age. Scand J Dent Res 98:510–519

Solheim T (1992a) Amount of secondary dentin as an indicator of age. Scand J Dent Res 100:193–199

Solheim T (1992b) Recession of periodontal ligament as an indicator of age. J Forensic Odontostomatol 10:32–42

Solheim T (1993a) A new method for dental age estimation in adults. Forensic Sci Int 59:137–147

Solheim T (1993b) Dental age – related regressive changes and a new method for calculating the age of an individual. Thesis, University of Oslo

Solheim T, Kvaal S (1993) Dental root surface structure as an indicator of age. J Forensic Odontostomatol 11:9–21

Staaf V, Mörnstad H, Welander U (1991) Age estimation based on tooth development: a test of reliability and validity. Scand J Dent Res 99:281–286

Ten Cate AR, Thompson GW, Dickinson JB, Hunter HA (1977) The estimation of age of skeletal remains from the colour of roots of teeth. J Can Dent Assoc 43:83–86

Thoma A (1953) Alters-und Geschlechtsbestimmung aus dem Gebiß. Kriminalistik 7:222–225; 252–255

Thorson J, Hägg U (1991) The accuracy and precision of the third mandibular molar as an indicator of chronological age. Swed Dent J 15:15–22

Towlson KL, Peck D (1990) Assessment of chronological age of third world children: can a simple tooth count help? Int Dent J 40:179–182

Vendura K, Schmeling A, Reisinger W, Loreck D, Olze A, Geserick G (1998) Altersschätzung bei Lebenden – Steigende Gutachtenzahlen in Berlin. Posterdemonstration, 7. Frühjahrstagung Region Nord Dtsch Ges Rechtsmed Bonn, 5. U. 6. Juni 1998

Wegener R, Albrecht H (1980) Zur Schätzung des Alters an Hand der Zahnwurzeltransparenz. Z Rechtsmed 86:29–34

Zuhrt R, Geserick G (1996) Forensisch-odontologische Altersschätzung – eine kritische Bilanz unter besonderer Berücksichtigung der Wurzeldentintransparenz. Rechtsmedizin 7:6–14

Zuhrt R, Geserick G, Marré B (1996) Kritische Überprüfung der Altersschätzung bei unbekannten Toten. AKFOS Newsl Jg 3(3):66–69

Identification

20

Klaus Rötzscher and Dieter Leopold

20.1 Introduction

Identification is based on the polymorphism of different individuals. These differences can be highly diverse; they may be acquired or inherited and rooted in biological structures. Requirements for their applicability (intravital and postmortem) are interindividual and intraindividual constancy, classificability, and accessibility.

For the identification of an unknown person, fingerprint data, radiology, dental status, and deoxyribonucleic acid (DNA) analysis are valuable, but only if appropriate research material and corresponding (good quality) reference material is available within a reasonable time. Under certain circumstances, this can be difficult (e.g., in mass disasters involving multinational victims). The more time that has passed between the event and the identification, the more medical and political pressure rises.

The 100th anniversary of the fire of 13ème Bazar de la Charité in Paris, Rue Jean-Gaujon was on 4 May 1897. Approximately 1,600 people were in this bazar at 4:10 pm when a defective projector lamp exploded and turned the bazaar into a sea of flames. One hundred twenty-six people lost their lives and more than 200 people were injured (Amoëdo 1897). Among them was the Duchesse d'Alençon, Sophie Charlotte von Wittelsbach, sister of Elisabeth von Wittelsbach, Empress "Sissi" of Austria. Thanks to the notes of Dr. Davenport, her dentist, she could be identified with certainty (Hutt 1998). Oscar Amoëdo (1863–1945), professor at the *École Odontotechnique* in Paris, described his work in a book that was translated in 1900 by Gottlieb Port, professor of dentistry at the University of Munich and published by Arthur Felix in Leipzig as "*L' art dentaire en médecine légale*" (Amoëdo 1897; Bezymenski 1968; Fig. 20.1). This was the beginning of forensic odontology and disaster victim identification (DVI) management. It was left to Oscar Amoëdo to sift through existing literature, individual works, and to unite this material in a systematic work. He is, thus, the founder of modern forensic odontostomatology.

Forensic odontologists of 27 national societies founded the International Organisation for Forensic Odontostomatology (IOFOS) in Paris (1973) and another 23 societies are associated. In Germany, an interdisciplinary working group of forensic odontostomatology, the German Academy of Forensic Odontostomatology (founded 1976) is a member of the IOFOS.

In various areas of forensic disciplines, the teeth are significant indicators used for age estimation and sex determination because of their individual character. The main application of forensic odontostomatology is the identification of victims in the wake of disasters and crimes

K. Rötzscher, Dr. med. Dr. med. dent. (✉)
German Academy of Forensic Odontostomatology (AKFOS),
Wimphelingstraße 7, 67346 Speyer, Germany
e-mail: roetzscher.klaus.dr@t-online.de

D. Leopold, Univ.-Prof. (em) Dr. med.
Institute of Legal Medicine,
Turmweg 22, Leipzig 04277, Germany

K. Rötzscher (ed.), *Forensic and Legal Dentistry*,
DOI 10.1007/978-3-319-01330-5_20,

(Alt 1997a; Alt et al. 1995; Alt and Türp 1998; Alt and Vach 1995). It is part of a multidisciplinary complex of identification methods.

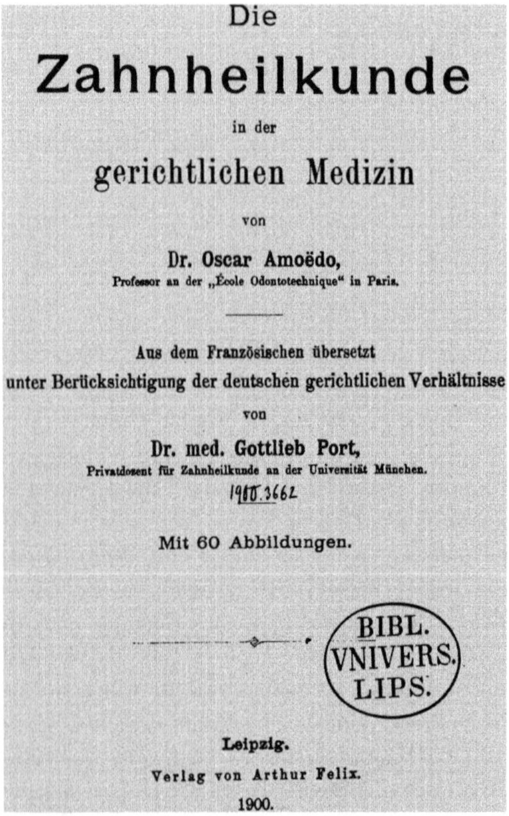
Die

Zahnheilkunde

in der

gerichtlichen Medizin

von

Dr. Oscar Amoëdo,

Professor an der „École Odontotechnique" in Paris.

Aus dem Französischen übersetzt

unter Berücksichtigung der deutschen gerichtlichen Verhältnisse

von

Dr. med. Gottlieb Port,

Privatdozent für Zahnheilkunde an der Universität München.

1900.3662

Mit 60 Abbildungen.

BIBL. VNIVERS. LIPS.

Leipzig.

Verlag von Arthur Felix.

1900.

Fig. 20.1 Oscar Amoëdo's book in German translation by Gottlieb Port (1900)

Among the most spectacular odontological identifications in recent German history is the identification of Adolf Hitler, who was Chancellor from 30 January 1933 to 30 April 1945, when he committed suicide in the bunker of the Reich Chancellery with his wife, Eva Braun, and Martin Bormann, his secretary. Adolf Hitler and Eva Braun were identified beyond doubt by their dental status, while the identity of Martin Bormann could only be confirmed by mitochondrial DNA analysis (Rötzscher 1998a).

Their identification is based on documents from Soviet and American archives, photographs (Fig. 20.2), diagrams, descriptions (interrogations), and skull X-rays (US National Arch and Rec Services: APO 757, 01-FIR/31). Five X-rays of Adolf Hitler were used to identify his odontological status (Figs. 20.3 and 20.4). The X-ray image was taken on 19 September 1944 (Fig. 20.5) after the failed assassination attempt of 20 July 1944.

20.1.1 The Identification of Adolf Hitler

Berlin-Buch, 8 May 1945, Army Surgical Hospital morgue, Nr. 496.

Thirteen bodies were examined (Sognnaes and Strøm 1973). Bodies no. 12 and 13 were

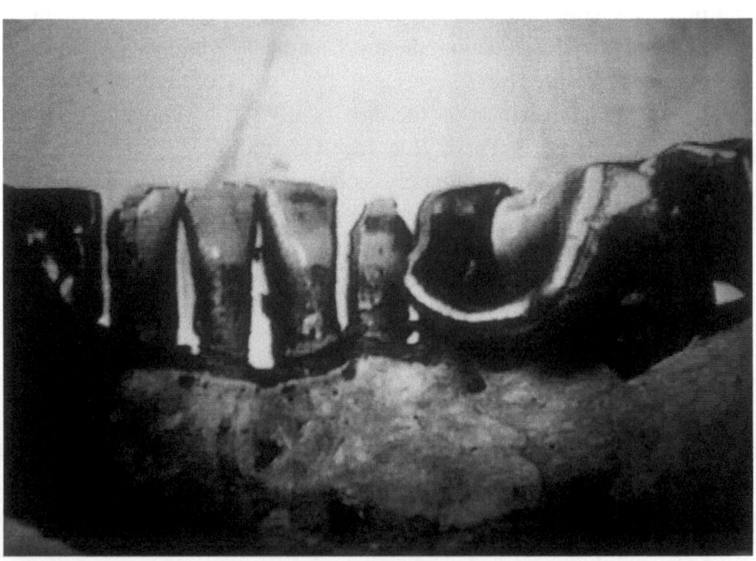

Fig. 20.2 Adolf Hitler: Lingual view of mandibular incisors and the right quadrant, with the characteristic lingual bridging of the intact first premolar (Sognnaes and Strøm 1973) (Courtesy of Dr. Michel Perrier, Lausanne, Switzerland)

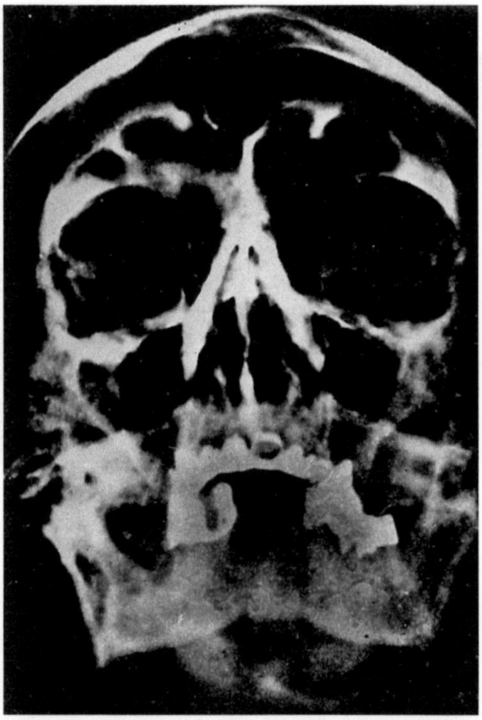

Fig. 20.3 Skull X-rays of Hitler from 21 October 1944

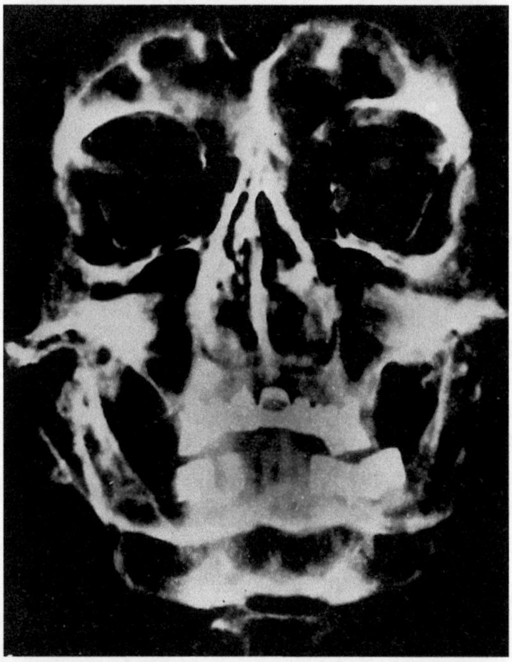

Fig. 20.4 Chin–nose projection of Hitler (Courtesy of Dr. R. F. Sognnaes, Dr. F. Strøm, Prof. Dr. T. Solheim, Oslo, Norway, and Dr. Michel Perrier, Lausanne, Switzerland)

the most demolished by fire. A commission of five medical experts, army anatomists, forensic experts, and pathology anatomists of the First White Russian Front, the Red Army, and the 3rd Shock Army examined, by order of the Military Council of the First White Russian Front, the male body (presumably Hitler's body).

Act No. 12 is the forensic examination of a burnt male body (probably Hitler's body) (documents from Moscow archives) (Bezymenski 1968). The corpse is badly burnt. A portion of the skull is missing. Parts of the occipital bone, the left temporal bone, the lower parts of the cheek and nasal bone and the upper and lower jaw are preserved. The nose and the upper jaw bone show many small fractures. The tongue is burnt, the tip of the tongue firmly stuck between the teeth of the upper and lower jaw.

Sognnaes compared the final report (Soviet Army Surgeon) of the dental status with the details of the dentist Blaschke and his own list compiled in 1975. Sognnaes and Strøm (1973) graphically presented the dental status of Hitler (Fig. 20.6).

The record of the hearing of Käthe Heusermann (assistant of Dr. Hugo Johannes Blaschke) confirms the assumption that the described teeth and bridges are assigned to Hitler. In a meeting with the chief forensic expert, Lieutenant Colonel Shkaranskij, on 11 May 1945 in the premises of CAFS Nr. 496 (see above), Heusermann and Echtermann, the dental technician, described in detail the condition of Hitler's teeth.

20.1.2 The Identification of Eva Braun

Act No. 13 is of the forensic examination of a burnt female body (probably Eva Braun) (Bezymenski 1968):

> Protocol No. 13: Results of the forensic examination of a female body: Yellow glass fragments of a thin-walled ampoule were found in the mouth. The death was a result of poisoning with Cyanide. The most important anatomic findings were the gold bridge of the mandible and the outer four teeth.

Gorbushin (assistant of the chief of the 3rd Army) stated:

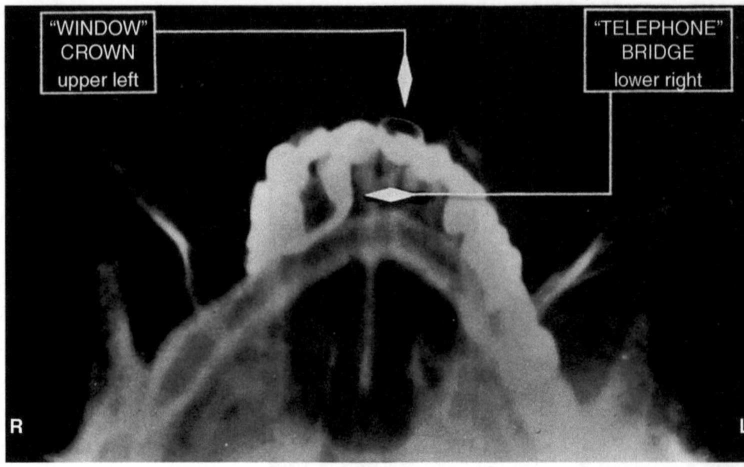

Fig. 20.5 Jaw X-ray of Hitler with extensive crown and bridge work of unusual construction (Courtesy of W. B. Saunders Company, Philadelphia, PA, USA)

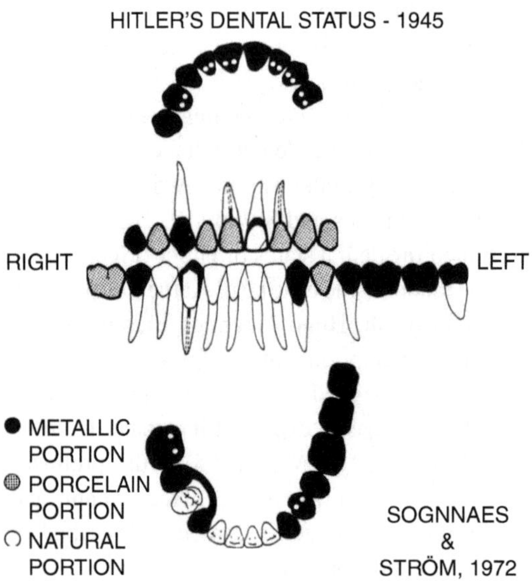

Fig. 20.6 Dental status of Hitler (*drawing*) at time of death (Courtesy of Sognnaes and Strøm 1973)

The evidence to establish the identity of the bodies should be sought due to medical recommendations. In the clinic of Prof. Blaschke, we were welcome by Dr. Bruck. As Bruck learned that we wanted to talk to Prof. Blaschke because of an identification matter, we were told that Professor Blaschke is not in. Mrs. Heusermann handed me the medical history of Adolf Hitler. The X-ray images of Hitler's teeth were supposed to be in the office of Prof. Blaschke in the Chancellery. We found them in the basement of the dental treatment room by help of Mrs. Heusermann. We also detected several gold cups for Adolf Hitler. Käthe Heusermann informed me that crowns and bridges for Hitler and Eva Braun were made by the dental technician Fritz Echtmann. We met him at his home. His information about the bridges, crowns and fillings exactly corresponded with the medical history and X-ray images. Then Mrs. Heusermann and Mr. Echtmann were submitted for identification of the jaw bone of the male body. They both identified it as Adolf Hitler's.

Then we asked Mrs. Heusermann and the dental technician Fritz Echtman to describe the teeth of Eva Braun. We showed them the gold bridge we found in the female body. Fritz Echtermann added that the unique design is the bridge made for Eva Braun. The experts came to the final conclusion that these teeth belong to Eva Braun.

20.1.3 The Identification of Martin Bormann

On 7 and 8 December 1972, during excavation work near the Weidendamm bridge at Lehrter Subway station (Berlin), two relatively well-preserved skeletons (Martin Bormann and Dr. Ludwig Stumpfegger?) were found (Figs. 20.7 and 20.8). Later, some teeth and a gold dental bridge were found (Fig. 20.9). There were uncertainties concerning the identification of one of the bodies, because no X-ray images of Martin Bormann existed, only a dental chart by Prof. Blaschke, drawn from memory in 1945. Prof. Blaschke had been Bormann's dentist (1937–1945) (Fig. 20.10).

Prof. Dr. Wolfgang Eisenmenger, Director of the Institute, and Mrs. Dipl.-Biol. Katja Anslinger of the Institute of Legal Medicine, Ludwig-Maximilians-University, Munich, confirmed the

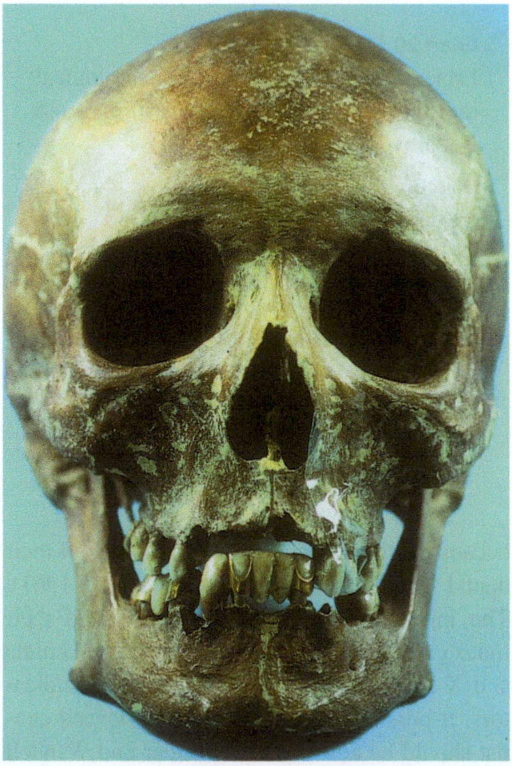

Fig. 20.7 Martin Bormann, a front shot of the skull

positive identification of Martin Bormann with a mitochondrial DNA analysis from femurs and tibias only in 1998; two approximately 5-g bone pieces were extracted from each for the analysis. All four bone samples identically matched with mtDNA sequences of two blood samples of a family member of Martin Borman. This proves, together with all other findings, that the skeletal parts are Martin Bormann's (time of death: early morning hours of 2 May 1945).

Dr. Johannes Hugo Blaschke, a graduate of the University of Pennsylvania (1911), was owner of a dental practice in Berlin Kurfürstendamm and became Hitler's dentist (1934–1945). After his capture in 1945, in the headquarters of the US Armed Forces in Europe, Military Intelligence Service Center, APO customized-757, he recorded the medical history of Hitler (Final Interrogation Report [OI FIR/31, 1946]). Another document contains information about the dentition of Eva Braun and Martin Bormann (Sognnaes and Strøm 1973). One of his first patients was Hermann Goering. Soon after, the "elite" of the Third Reich was his clientele.

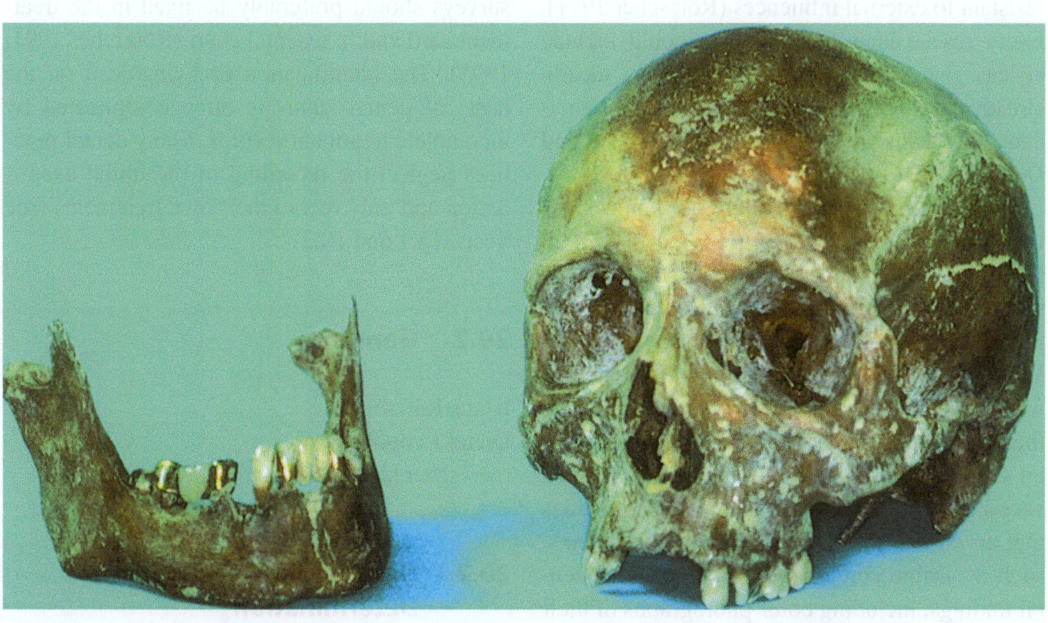

Fig. 20.8 Skull and mandible with a gold bridge on the *right* (Courtesy of Prof. Dr. W. Eisenmenger, Institute of Legal Medicine, University Munich. Released for publication by the public prosecutor in Frankfurt/Main, December 1999)

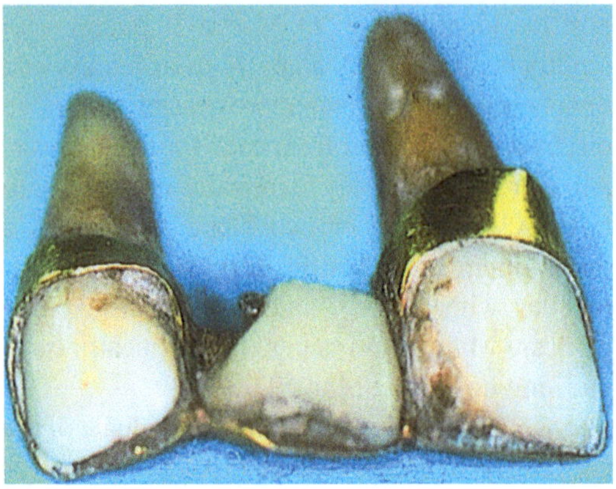

Fig. 20.9 Maxillary anterior bridge (teeth 12–21), no longer located in the jaw (Courtesy of Prof. Dr. W. Eisenmenger, Institute of Legal Medicine, University Munich. Released for publication by the public prosecutor in Frankfurt/Main, December 1999)

Chart 20.1
Principle of odontostomatological registration (Fiala 1968; Griffiths and Bellamy 1993)

Objective	Subjective
(a) Measuring (numeric)	(g) Treatment card
(b) Impression (plastic)	(h) Anatomical chart
(c) Photography (with mirror)	(i) Testimony
(d) Marking of dentures	
(e) Palatoscopy	
(f) X-ray images	

A systematic interdisciplinary cooperation between the investigating authorities and the medical (anthropologists, biologists, radiologists, forensic medicine, serological) and dental experts (forensic odontologists) is required for a thorough identification. In particular, identification after fires, mining accidents, and plane crashes is accelerated or even made possible by dentition features. Furthermore, teeth are very resistant to external influences (Rötzscher 1971). Every rescue identification unit should include at least one forensically trained dentist, ideally already a part of the unit at the time of the incident (Benthaus and Endris 1999; Dittmer and Dumser 1999).

Possibilities of registration of dental findings according to Fiala (1968) are shown in Chart 20.1. An intact dentition shows many specific points of comparison. However, treatment records must be available for comparison. Without those records, an identification can take weeks or months. The military has recognized the value of current and accurate premortal dental status records, which must be accessible in a very short time. In civilian life, many companies that are afflicted with a high risk for accidents, such as airline companies, strictly require dental findings, including color photographs of their staff (Fig. 20.11) (Johanson and Lindenstam 1961).

In cases of flight accidents, it is much easier to identify the bodies of military or airline personnel because of the accessibility and accuracy of their dental records (Johanson and Lindenstam 1961). The investigative reports of dentists and their index cards (records), together with dental charts and X-ray images, are the most valuable indicators. If possible, a forensically experienced dentist should be consulted (Schneider and Wandelt 1984).

In determining the identity of an unknown or unrecognizable dead, the findings of the teeth and jaws are one of the most efficient methods. All surveys should preferably be fixed in the treatment card and in a dental chart (Rötzscher 1991, 1995). The identification of living/dead on the basis of dental status is often complicated by incomplete treatment records. Many dental practices neglect the recording of the initial examination and only record their own treatments (see Sects. 18.1 and 18.2).

20.2 Gender

Klaus Rötzscher
Dieter Leopold
roetzscher.klaus.dr@t-online.de

20.2.1 Odontometric Gender Determination

Skeleton parts that are useful for gender determination often are incomplete or poorly preserved. Therefore, teeth are particularly

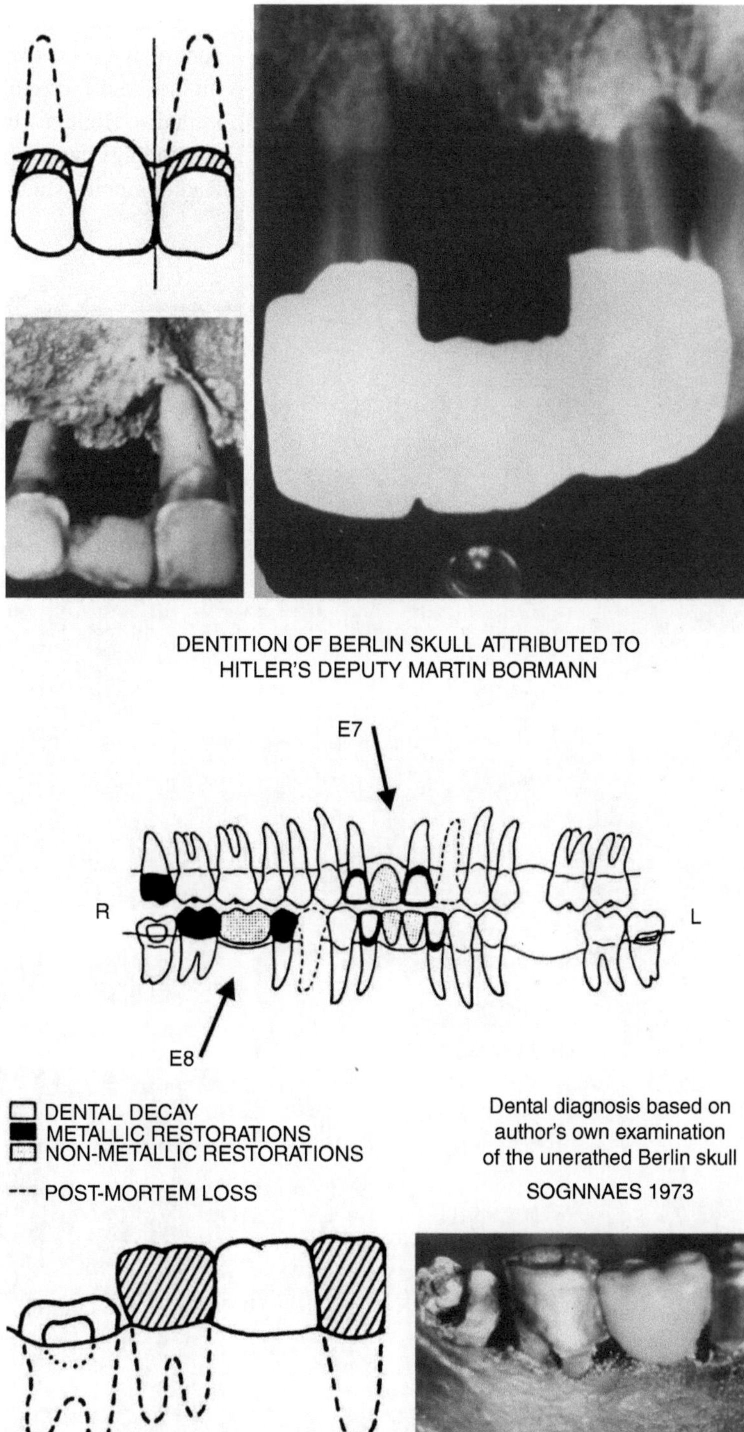

Fig. 20.10 Antemortem drawing by Dr. Blaschke. Bormann's maxillary bridge and mandibular bridge (see *arrow*) (Courtesy of W. B. Saunders Company, Philadelphia, PA, USA)

suitable for accurate and repeatable measurements. For these reasons, morphognostic and metric studies of gender characteristics are of high value (Albus 1998). Regarding the doctrine from 1964 that a gender determination by the aid of teeth and dentures is not possible (sexual dimorphism) or very doubtful (Schranz and Bartha 1964), recent studies have proven the opposite (Pilz 1974; Pilz and Krause 1980b).

Studies of front teeth by Schranz and Bartha (1964) showed that the crown width in males often, but not always, is larger than in females (Fig. 20.12). In female subjects, 2.42 % aplasia or hypoplasia of the maxillary lateral incisor was found, in males, it was only 0.58 %. Hyperodontia, mesiodens, gemination of the central incisors, two lateral incisors, three premolars, and four molars predominantly occurred in males. Both jaw halves must be examined and the findings must be completed by X-ray images. Radiographic studies showed that bifurcated

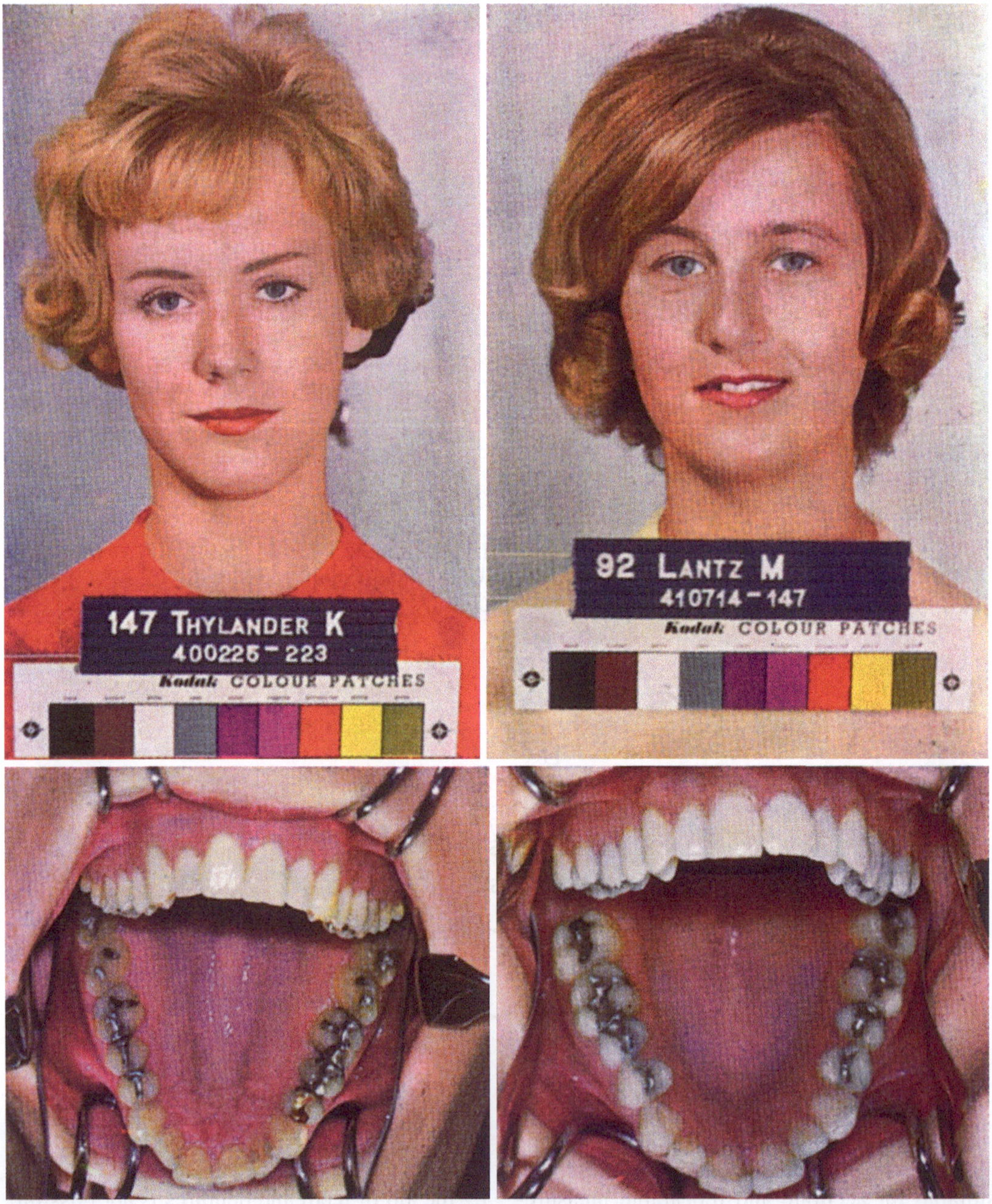

Fig. 20.11 Color photo, part of registration of airline personnel in Sweden (Courtesy of Prof. Dr. G. Johanson, Malmo, Sweden)

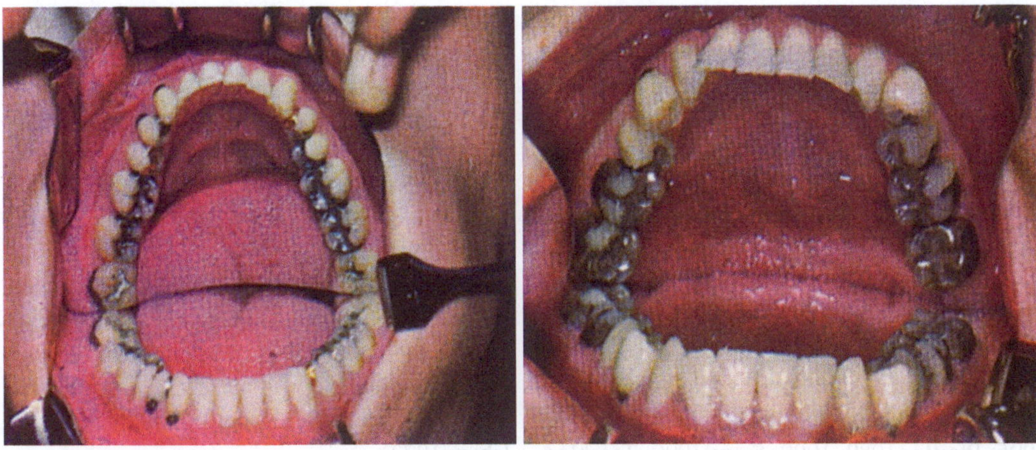

Fig. 20.11 (continued)

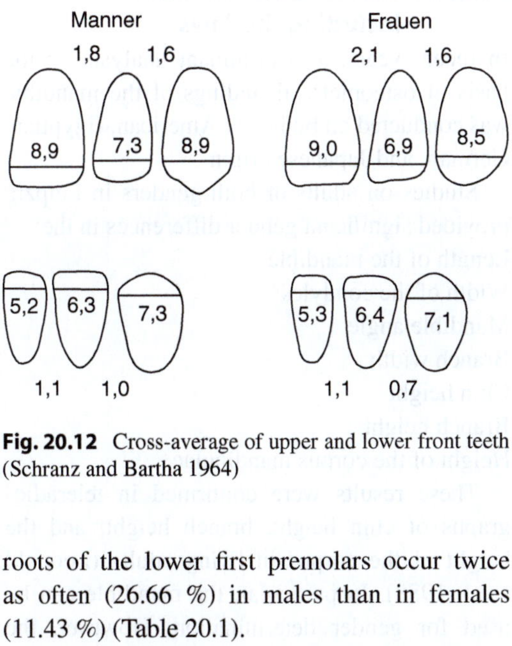

Fig. 20.12 Cross-average of upper and lower front teeth (Schranz and Bartha 1964)

roots of the lower first premolars occur twice as often (26.66 %) in males than in females (11.43 %) (Table 20.1).

Today, odontometric gender determination is an important feature for the identification of unknown skeleton remains as well as the treatment of skeleton remains from archaeological excavations. A detailed literature review on the research and method development about sexual dimorphism is presented by Albus (1998). Teeth currently provide the only basis for gender determination of children and adolescents (Reuling 1992). Preferred starting points are measurements of the crown diameter. Their mean values in boys are higher than in girls (Moorrees et al. 1963). Previous studies showed that sexual dimorphism in the deciduous dentition is significantly present, but less than in the permanent dentition. In 1978, for the first time, Black applied discriminant analysis of milk teeth for gender determination (he evaluated 64 white girls and 69 white boys from Ohio). His hit rate was relatively low

Table 20.1 Comparison of the particulars of the female and male dental morphological type with regard to gender characteristics (Schranz and Bartha 1964)

Female	Male
1. Minimum transverse diameter values exclusively in females	1. Maximum transverse diameter values are not gender dependent
2. The upper central incisor is wider than the canine	2. The upper central incisor and the canine have the same width
3. The difference in width between the upper central and lateral incisor is larger (2.1 mm)	3. The difference in width between the upper central and the lateral incisor is larger (2.1 mm)
4. The difference in width between the lower incisor and canine side is smaller (0.7 mm)	4. The difference in width between the middle incisor and the canine is bigger (1.0 mm)
5. Fusion of the roots of the lower 12-year molar is more common (30.9 %)	5. Fusion of the roots of the bottom 12-year molar is rare (22.0 %)
6. Aplasia (hypoplasia) of the teeth is more common	6. Supernumerary teeth (hyperodontia) are more common
7. The wisdom tooth often is missing	7. The wisdom tooth is missing less often

(63.9–67.7 %). Other researchers also studied the permanent teeth and attained much better results. evaluated 109 white boys and 95 white girls, with a hit rate of 86 %.

The single features of the teeth are not very significant in terms of gender specifics. Taken together with the indicators of the general skull and the mandible, the value of the dental characteristics for determination increases (Albus 1998). Gender determination by the quantitative analysis of the tooth width has gained a strong appreciation in recent years by applying the discriminant method (Alt and Vach 1995; Alt et al. 1995; Pfeiffer 1989, 1990; Starp 1990; Teschler-Nicola 1992).

New methods have also been developed for single teeth (Rao et al. 1989) and for the characteristics of the mandible (Pötsch-Schneider et al. 1985). Correlation analysis shows individual relationships between the widths of permanent teeth, i.e., in homologous neighboring teeth (central and lateral incisor, first and second premolar/molar) and the homologous antagonist (e.g., upper and lower right canine). In most cases, the gender determination was confirmed by the teeth sizes.

The canines are more resistant to periodontal disease and even to severe trauma than other teeth, and may therefore be best used to identify a person. Rao et al. (1989) propose a technique that is based on the evaluation of the Mandibular Canine Index (MCI), the relationship between two parameters of the permanent lower canine.

The mesiodistal crown diameter (MDKD) and the width of the canine–mandibular arch (WCMB) in millimeters is:

$$\mathrm{MCI} = \frac{\mathrm{MDKD}}{\mathrm{WCMB}}.$$

The mean MCI value is 0.296 (±0.016) for the male and 0.254 (±0.014) for the female gender. There is a significant difference between them.

The result is the standard value:

$$\begin{aligned}\mathrm{Standard-MCI} &= (\text{middle MCI} * M - X) \\ &\quad + (\text{mean MCI} * F + X) : 2\end{aligned}$$

$$\begin{aligned}\mathrm{Standard-MCI} &= (0.296 - 0.016) \\ &\quad + (0.254 + 0.014) = 0.274 : 2.\end{aligned}$$

All values above the standard characterize the female gender; all values under the standard characterize the male gender. The accuracy of the MCI method is 84.3 % in males and 87.5 % in females. The authors note that a more accurate assessment can only be made after further tests regarding the characteristics of the studied population.

The sole use of tooth size for gender diagnosis is limited and should only be applied in cases where other methods, such as chromatin examination or fluorescence of the Y chromosome from the pulp cells, are not possible (Seno and Ishizu 1973).

20.2.1.1 Gender Determination Including the Jaws

In recent years, a discriminant analysis on the basis of osteometrical findings of the mandible was conducted on bodies of American, Egyptian, German, and Japanese origin.

Studies on adults of both genders in Leipzig provided significant gender differences in the:

Length of the mandible
Width of the condyles
Mandible angle
Branch width
Chin height
Branch height
Height of the corpus mandibulae

These results were confirmed in teleradiographs of chin height, branch height, and the height of the corpus in living adults (Leopold et al. 1988). In particular, the mandible can be used for gender determination. However, the ethnic origin must be respected. The separation function of a discriminant analysis provides good results (Pfeiffer 1990); only three variables allow a significant determination:

Angular width
Branch height
Height of the mandibular foramen:

$$\begin{aligned}\mathrm{Y} = {} & \text{branch height } 0.9382 \\ & + \text{angle of the lower jaw } 1.025 \\ & + \text{level of the foramen mandibulae } 1.087; \\ & \text{mean value(male) } 1{,}946, \text{ cutpoint } 1.8375; \\ & \text{mean value(female) } 1.729.\end{aligned}$$

Table 20.2 Discriminant analysis to determine the gender of the mandible

Size (in cm)	Coefficient
Branch height	0.9382
Angular width	1.025
Height of the foramen mandibulae	1.087
Mean value in males	1.946
Cut point	1.8375
Mean value in females	1.729

The use of process analyses of complex three-dimensional structures, such as the examination of the palate and canines using "moiré topography" study (Takei 1985), will increase. The mesio-distal and bucco-lingual crown diameters are the most important parameters for odontometric investigation (Alt et al. 1995; Alt and Vach 1995).

One problem of tooth width measurements is differences between left and right sides. Opposite teeth of a jaw are approximately equal. The analysis of the data was performed using univariate statistical methods. The arithmetic mean value, the standard deviation, and the coefficient of variation of each tooth diameter, separated by gender, were determined. Almost all mean values of females are below those of males; the differences are between 0.64 mm OKBL3 (upper jaw width-length canine) and −0.3 mm OKMD8 (upper jaw-mesio-distal-tooth 8). The differences in the canines are particularly significant.

The method of discriminant analysis is an obvious choice. The principle of discriminant analysis is based on the selection of an optimal set of variables, i.e., a combination of features that ensures a maximum degree of separation between the sexes and the indication of a rule based on these variables, which allows a gender determination (Table 20.2). The assessment of the discriminant value requires mathematical knowledge (Langenscheidt 1983; van Vark 1976).

20.2.2 Morphological Relatedness

The need for interdisciplinary cooperation between forensic medicine, forensic odontology, and anthropology is is undisputed. In addition to dental charts, morphological tooth characteristics (such as accessory cusp/roots), and dental anomalies (such as congenital aplasia of teeth), familial comparisons (kinship analysis) may provide important additional information. Genetic aspects are of great value for the consideration of the development processes of the tooth, jaw, and face area. Teeth primarily are polygenic inheritance, with modifying exogenous factors. In order to examine the genetic and environmental influence on a characteristic, an estimation of the heritability by twin, family, and kinship studies can be made (Alt 1997b; Schulze 1982). For the affinity analysis, 137 dental characteristics, divided into 15 groups, were examined (Alt 1997b).

Basically, there are four types of characteristics:

1. Variations of the tooth crown and root
2. Odontogenic disturbances of the form, number, size, structure, and function
3. Selected and well-known irregular skull and jaw features
4. Congenital anomalies and syndromes of jaw and teeth

If dental records are not available, the comparison of tooth morphologic features can be a reliable contribution (Alt et al. 1995; Alt and Türp 1998; Alt and Vach 1995).

Gender in bodies or juvenile skeletons can be determined relatively easy with molecular genetic methods. A gender determination can be performed by amplification of a segment of the XY homologous gene *Amelogenin* and with fast and quantitative DNA testing. Using a single primer pair that spans a portion of the first intron, PCR products of 106 and 112 bp were generated (Mannucci et al. 1994) by the homologous portions of the X and Y chromosomes, which were separated using agarose gel electrophoresis. This test made it possible for even quantities as small as 20 pg of DNA amplified from degraded bones to be typed in a single reaction.

Because of the use of dye-labeled primers, it was also possible to quantify the relative yield of X- and Y-specific PCR products by automated fluorescence detection. The versatility of this assay was also demonstrated by the fact that a co-amplification with the HLA-DQA1 "Amplitype" kit in a combined sex determination and identification DNA test was possible (Mannucci et al. 1994).

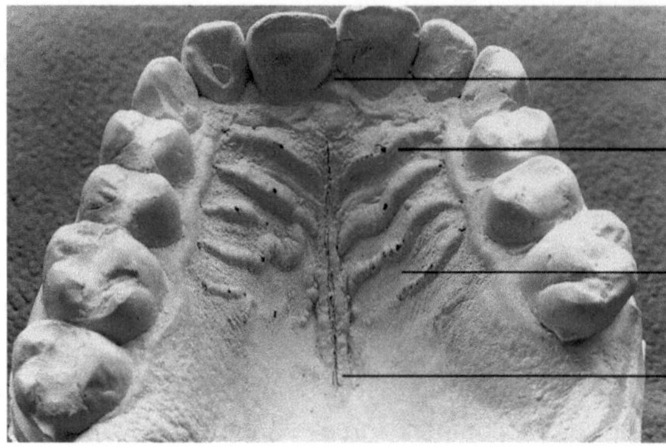

Fig. 20.13 Model with median palatine raphe and the medium and vertices marked (Wutzler 1991)

20.2.3 Palatoscopy

Planning models, impressions for dentures, orthodontics, etc. are accurate representations of a patient's teeth and and invaluable for comparison with postmortem remains. Even models of edentulous patients (for complete dentures) can be compared postmortem with remains, such as the contour of the alveolar ridge, size, and configuration of the palatal folds (rugae palatal). Rugae are irregular ridges in the hard palate of the maxillary mucosa behind the incisors (Fig. 20.13). Wutzler and Leopold (1995) distinguish the rugae according to the anatomical location toward the median palatine raphe (Table 20.3). The average length of the main folds in women are 11.7 mm (right side) and 12.3 mm (left side). The range of variation (Table 20.4) varies between 7.2 mm (men) and 6.6 mm (women) and 22 mm. In the left half of the palate, the extra folds are a little shorter, the average value is 14 mm (Wutzler 1991). The characteristics of the face are significant, because their shape is inseparable from the bony substructure, such as the maxillary complex, with the palate. Although the anatomy and histology of the palatal folds are known, measurements of gender-specific height and width development are not available (Brückner 1993; Wutzler 1991; Wutzler and Leopold 1995). The palatal vault is divided into four categories (Fig. 20.14) (Brückner 1995).

The average number of folds on the palate relief is four for both sexes, with a maximum of seven folds in individual cases. Of all examined subjects, 50 % had a side fold, and 30 % had an extra fold. The fold curve is very different and also very variable within the age groups. The basic pattern type, according to Murakami (1931), was modified and rescaled (Wutzler 1991). If <100 %, but at least >75 % of all folds have the same direction, it is the basic type A1, B1, C1. If at least 50 % of the folds but <75 % have the same direction, it is the basic type A2, B2, C2.

Table 20.3 Division of the existing rugae to their anatomical location for the median palatine raphe (Wutzler and Leopold 1995)

	Main fold	Extra fold	Additional fold
Beginning	of raphe	of raphe	
Length (mm)	12	14	8
Height (mm)	0.6	0.5	0.2

Table 20.4 The gender difference (average) in millimeters, statistically significant, probability of error 1 % (Wutzler 1991)

Extra palatal fold		Side palatal fold		Range of variation	
Male	Female	Male	Female	Male	Female
15.1	12.9	8.8	8.2	3–16.5	3–14

20.2.3.1 Gender Differences

1. Males have higher overall folding, main folds on two sides, wider and more frequently fragments, and more frequently have papillary folds
2. Major folds in males are only higher at the left side
3. Males often have three major folds at the left side

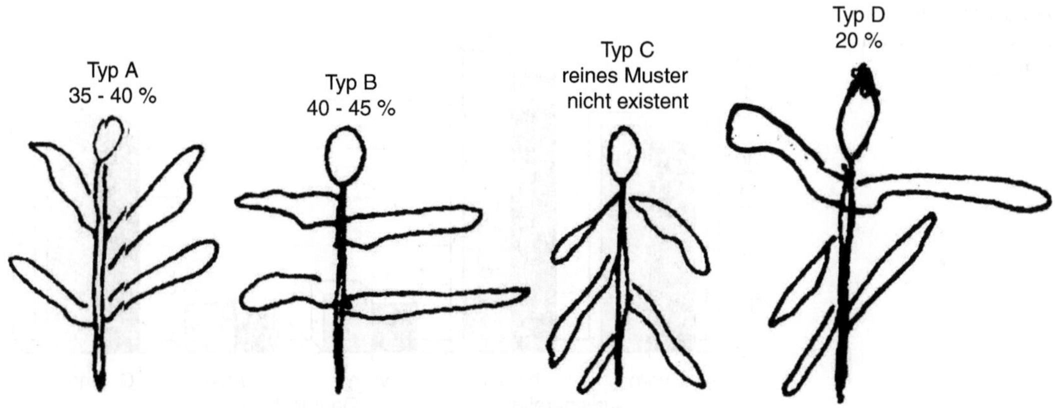

Fig. 20.14 Classification of the palatal vault (Brückner 1993)

Table 20.5 Palatal dimensions in males and females (Brückner 1993)

Palate width (mean) (mm)			Height volume		Length	Volume (cm³)
	Frontal	Back	Frontal	Back		
F	31.9	39.2	14.9	13.9	32.8	9.4
M	33.7	41.5	15.8	14.9	34.3	11.2

4. Females have an even more progressive form of the folds at the left
5. The feature "branching" at the left is significantly more common in men
6. The extra folds at the right in males are longer and the major and minor folds are significantly wider

Most common on the level:

Parabolic, 38 %

Keystone (horizontal), 42 %

Concave increase (longitudinal), 46 %

Top view supervision, *cross* crossways:

Arched, trapezoid, 15 %

Parabolic, trapezoid, 14 %

And in three levels:

1. Parabolic-Romanesque arch-concave increase of 3.9 %
2. Least often: horseshoe, 25 %
3. Gothic arch (horizontal), 23 %

Convex increase (longitudinal) and 21 % for supervision and cross gothic/horseshoe-Roman and 5 % each in three levels:

Horseshoe-Romanesque arch: 0.38 %

All palatal measurements show significant gender differences (chi-square test) (Brückner 1993). An anthropological survey of 258 palatal vaults confirmed that all palatal sizes in males are larger than in females (Table 20.5).

With advancing age, the palate as well as the facial bones increase in width (this is especially evident in male subjects). The palatal height tends to decrease with age, possibly because of age-related atrophy of alveolar horizontalis. The palatal height is more affected by periodontal disease than the other palatal dimensions (Figs. 20.15 and 20.16) (Brückner 1995).

20.3 Validation of Genetic Characteristics

20.3.1 Classic Conventional Individualization of Hemogenetic Features (Non-DNA Investigations)

The pulp cavity is generally well protected against external influences, as long as the tooth is firmly anchored in the gums and jaw bones. In cases in which (because of external factors such as autolysis, heat, or trauma) routine material (blood) for the detection of genetic features is

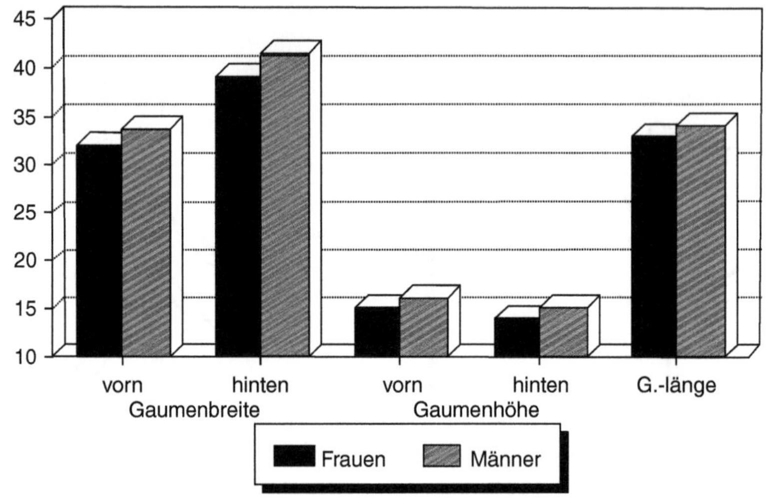

Fig. 20.15 Anthropological, gender-specific palatal dimensions

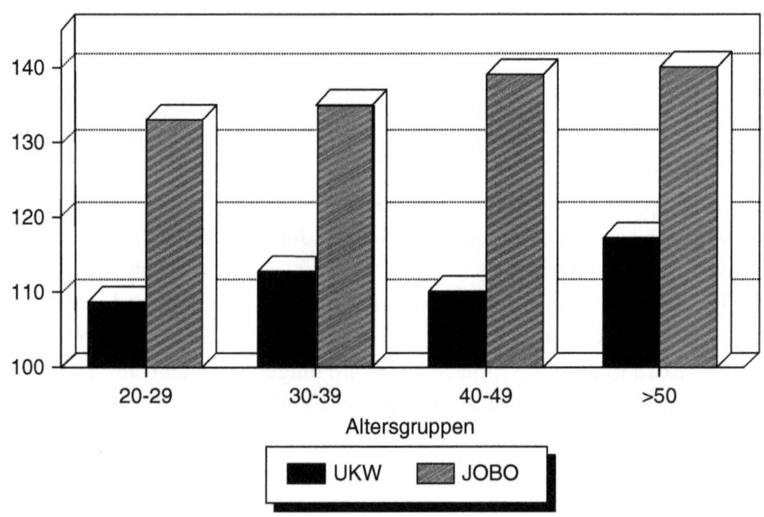

Fig. 20.16 Angle of the mandible and zygomatic width, depending on age (in millimeters) (Brückner 1995)

not available in sufficient quality or quantity, the dental pulp has been established as an acceptable research material. The successful morphological determination of gender has been described by several authors (Brinkmann and Jobst 1973; Duffy et al. 1991; Pötsch et al. 1991; Seno 1977; Thomsen 1977; Whittaker et al. 1975).

In addition to the blood group determination according to the ABO system, using the absorption-elution technique with pulpal tissue (the use of enamel from dentin is questionable (Smeets et al. 1991; Xingzhi et al. 1993)) and the detection of many enzyme polymorphisms, the following serum proteins are provable by electrophoresis: Gm, Km, Gc, and eight polymorphic enzymes (PGM, PGD, ADA, AK, ESD, Fuc, DiA3, and transferrin C) (Aitchinson 1964; Kido et al. 1993; Pötsch et al. 1992a, b). Lopez-Abadia and Ruiz de la Cuesta (1993) developed a simplified method of presentation of the alpha$_2$-HS glycoprotein in the serum, blood stains, and the pulpal tissue by means of electrophoresis.

20.3.2 Individualized Studies at the DNA Level

DNA analysis is a safe procedure, recognized in civil and criminal law, if the tests are performed according to the state of the art by personnel trained in molecular biology. All nucleated cells of human tissue (including the teeth) contain DNA. In addition to the genomic DNA (localized in the nucleus), there are also plasma or mtDNA groups in the mitochondria.

In cases of severe tissue destruction (fire victims, mass disasters, etc.), the teeth are a good source of nuclear and mitochondrial DNA (Ginther et al. 1992; Pötsch et al. 1992a). Teeth are a "dense tissue" that is difficult for secondary materials (e.g., microorganisms) to infiltrate. As long as the teeth are anchored in the alveolar bone, the dental pulp, which consists of blood, lymph, and nerve cells, is relatively well protected from necrosis and decay. Individualized studies at the DNA level can be successfully performed even after a long time. The conditions in which the teeth were preserved have a decisive influence on the quality and quantity of the DNA.

At room temperature, the pulp tissue rapidly dries, which explains the good condition of the DNA. Contamination of the freshly extracted soft tissues with other DNA is ruled according to. Experimental investigations regarding different storage conditions (soil, water, heat, cold, etc.) confirmed that environment influences have a crucial impact on the successful DNA analysis of the dental pulp (Alvarez-Garcia et al. 1996; Gill et al. 1994).

With the introduction of molecular biological technologies into forensic practice, the dental pulp was used for identification purposes (Alvarez-Garcia et al. 1996; Pötsch et al. 1992a; Rötzscher 1971; Schwartz et al. 1991; Smith et al. 1993; Woodward et al. 1994; Yamada et al. 1989). Restriction fragment length polymorphism (RFLP) can only be displayed by high molecular weight DNA (Schwartz et al. 1991). With the introduction of polymerase chain reaction (PCR) (Saiki et al. 1989) and the establishment of the amplifiable fragment length polymorphism (AmpFLs) and the short tandem repeat (STR) systems in the forensic diagnosis, the success rate of the examinations significantly increased.

Alvarez-Garcia et al. (1996) and Pfeiffer et al. (1999) showed that the gender system amelogenin (106, 112 bp) and the STR systems TH01, VWA, and FES/FPS can provide better amplification results at different storage conditions and times than the AmFLP System D1S80 and the PCR polymorphism HLA DQA. They explained this phenomenon by the small fragment lengths of the STR systems as well as the detection method of PCR products.

For further individualization, investigation of suitable reference material is necessary. For this survey, cell-containing biological materials (e.g., blood, saliva, hair roots) are investigated in terms of which DNA characteristics are identified and unambiguously assigned to a certain individual. If no reference material is available, the molecular biological material of family members can also be tested.

In addition to the study of so-called PCR—variable number of tandem repeat (VNTR) systems, including AmpFLP and STR, the examination of uniparental, exclusively maternally inherited, mitochondrial human mtDNA is important. Sequence polymorphisms in the displacement loop (D-loop) region with the highest variability within the mtDNA are decisive.

Because of the high copy numbers of mtDNA within a cell (100–10,000 copies/cell) and the small size of the mitochondrial genome (16,600 bp), DNA analysis is the most sensitive method in forensic DNA analysis and is used in the most difficult identification cases (e.g., for the analysis of exhumed corpse material, mummified or skeletonized bodies) (Hagelberg et al. 1991; Holland et al. 1993; Jeffreys et al. 1992; Lutz et al. 1996). MtDNA analysis is particularly successful for the analysis of older bone material (Berg et al. 1981; Gill et al. 1994), but also for mummified soft tissues (Pääbo et al. 1988) and for stored teeth (3 months–20 years). MtDNA analysis seems to be the most efficient identification method (Ginther et al. 1992; Pfeiffer et al. 1999).

Further development in molecular biological research, not only on teeth, will increasingly concentrate on the validation of STR-focusing systems with shorter fragment length (to increase the sensitivity) and the establishment of the analysis of human mtDNA.

Uniparental inheritance of mtDNA, which is exclusively maternally inherited (*Mater* line), is of major importance. Uniparental inheritance allows the use of material from relatives in the maternal line to determine the identity of an unknown dead person. Analogous to mtDNA, Y-localized systems (*Padre* line) also have uniparental inheritance, which means that all male relatives of an unknown dead person have the same Y-chromosomal heritage, independent of the degree of relationship or the generation.

20.3.3 Specific Population Characteristics

Features of ethnic origin can also be found in the orofacial area. In a corpse discovery, the ethnic origin must be examined, ideally by an anthropologist and a forensic odontologist. Often, the examined details are not obvious. A literature review for teeth is available (Haines 1972). For small and relatively homogeneous populations, such as the Laplanders, Icelanders, and the Australian Aborigines, good descriptions are available, but the major races and subgroups display many differences (Lasker and Lee 1957).

Discriminant analysis on the basis of skeletal measurements represents an objective method to distinguish between ethnic populations. Forensic determination of ethnic-specific features can be performed with the aid of the teeth, the bite, the jaw, and also the whole cranium (Aitchinson 1964). Major ethnic characteristics can also be detected with the form of the tooth and individual dental features. Tooth size was used to determine the ethnic origin by means of canonical discriminant analysis, with the result that Americans of color have teeth that are more robust than other groups. Dental restorations can allow conclusions regarding the homeland of the unknown living and/or dead person(s).

A narrow palate arch is characteristic for Europeans. The lateral incisor in the upper jaw is small in some individuals and degenerated to a tap tooth. The maxillary incisors are chisel-shaped and not shovel-shaped. The second molar has only four chew humps and many individuals have a Carabelli tubercle. In contrast, people of color have larger jaw arches with proclined incisors. The lower first premolar often has two lingual chew humps and the third molar is always present. People of color do not have shovel-shaped incisors and no Carabelli's tubercle. The teeth are smaller and therefore there are fewer space problems. Asians have a flat front upper jaw, which shapes the concave Mongolian face. Many Asians have a symmetrical hyperostosis on the inside of the horizontal ramus above the mylohyoid line (*torus mandibularis*), mainly in Eskimos and Laplanders. Mongolian Asians have larger teeth, the upper incisors are shovel-shaped (the tuberculum Carabelli is missing) and the third molar is often lacking or impacted. In the lower jaw, three-rooted molars are frequently observed Haines (1972).

20.4 Postmortem Changes

Under normal conditions, teeth can reach an infinite age. Young intact teeth are the most resistant. The pulp is putrefactive. Through decay of the periodontium, the tooth loses its strength in the alveolus. If a corpse is not putrid yet, an examination of the socket may reveal whether missing teeth were lost postmortem or antemortem (Zichel 1933).

20.4.1 Thermic Influences

The degree of destruction of the teeth and dental materials (Tables 20.6 and 20.7) is dependent on the duration and amount of the applied temperature (Andersen et al. 1995; Gebhardt 1923; Günther and Schmidt 1953; Komori 1960; von Lepkowski and Wachholz 1903; Müller 1938). Studies on isolated teeth and in situ showed no significant qualitative differences in the destruction process; its temporal order is dependent on the soft tissues. Because of their chemical composition, teeth resist even longer and hotter heat. Milk teeth are more flame-resistant than permanent teeth. Dental hard tissues do discolor, char, and calcify under heat influence (Günther and Schmidt 1953). The severity of thermic

Table 20.6 Influence of heat duration and temperature (Günther and Schmidt 1953)

Exposure time (in min)	Temperature (in °C)	Changes
5	400	The front teeth display considerable longitudinal columns in the crown with a partial loss of continuity and black and shiny surface "metallic luster"
15	400	Pitch-black "charcoal"-like gloss, front teeth badly damaged, although calcination is not visible. Exposed dentin fragmented. Amalgam fillings vesicularly distended, still located in the cavity
30	400	Front teeth completely destroyed. Enamel broken in pieces, already calcinated. Dentin stump turns black (charcoal), calcinated is white. Molars have low melting enamel crevices. Amalgam fillings are still located in the cavities. Pulp remains; white ash in the *cavum dentis*
60	400	Roots have deep longitudinal cracks. Spongiosa is darker than compacta. Teeth are broken and fall out of the alveola or been broken off the neck of the tooth, enamel "thimble-like" can be lifted
45–70	1,000–1,100	Teeth completely turned to ash. Cement panels are increasing in hardness. Silver amalgam has amalgamated gold fillings. Silver and silver amalgam turned to small balls. Phosphate cement fillings turned dazzling white

Table 20.7 Changes of dental materials caused by postmortem heat (1,000–1,100 °C) (Günther and Schmidt 1953)

Exposure time (in min)				
Material	Minutes			
	8–10	13–16	20–25	45–75
Temporary filling materials	Front teeth dropped	General information not found	–	–
Filling cements	Same	Front teeth dropped	Existing as under filling in posterior teeth	Ashed (white and hard)
Amalgam	Traces of mercury in the anterior area	Gold and silver amalgam intact in the molars, copper amalgam yellow-brownish	Generally not found	–
Casting filling materials	Loosening in cavity	Dropped in the anterior region	Generally dropped	Metal balls in the ashes
Metal crowns	–	Gold is reddish, Silver-Pd is yellow-red	Melting traces at the edges; Solderings no longer anchored; Silver-Pd is rough and dark gray	Gold turns to balls, Silver-Pd conserved
Ceramic crowns	Cracked or dropped	Fragmented, compact teeth conserved	–	Solid crowns and facets conserved
Plastics	Front teeth burned	Teeth burned up to the premolar teeth, charred anterior denture base	–	Completely burned

influences on the orofacial system (six categories) according to Andersen et al. (1995) is given in Table 20.8.

Griffiths and Bellamy describe how the fragile human skull can be stabilized and protected from massive heat and present a method for X-rays of the heat-affected tooth and bone material (1993). The morphological changes of enamel prisms in humans and animals after heat exposure were evaluated by Yamamoto et al. (1990). The enamel rods of monkey teeth are less heat-resistant than those of humans. At 600 °C, cracks occur frequently and the deformation of the arcades begins. After 5 min at 800 °C, the structures become unclear. In the oven, the morphological characteristics are destroyed, and a distinction between human and animal material is impossible.

20.4.2 Chemical Effects

In homicide cases, the removal of evidence with the aid of strong acids is possible. Organic material (muscle tissue) as well as bones will be completely solubilized by strong acids (hydrochloric acid, nitric acid). The effect of concentrated nitric acid on the bone results in oxidative destruction. Nitric acid and hydrochloric acid (*aqua regia*) cause bone destruction by chlorine formation (Endris 1980; Rötzscher and Reimann 1975).

Contrary to bones, teeth and dentures resist the effect of concentrated mineral acids (hydrochloric acid, sulfuric acid, and nitric acid) for a long time and therefore may still be subject to an assessment (Table 20.9). Hydrofluoric acid solubilizes porcelain teeth, hydrochloric acid (37 %) solubilizes metal prostheses, and *aqua regia* solubilizes gold alloys. A suitable combination and concentration of reagents may completely solubilize a human body (including denture material) (Endris 1980).

Table 20.8 Classification of the severity of thermic influences on the orofacial system of fire victims (six categories) (Andersen et al. 1995)

Grade 0	No damage
Grade 1	Damage to the front teeth (one or both jaws)
Grade 2	Damage to the anterior and posterior teeth, unilateral (one or both jaws)
Grade 3	Damage to the anterior and posterior teeth, bilateral (one or both jaws)
Grade 4	Fragments of jawbones, teeth and/or roots included conserved
Grade 5	No tooth remained

20.5 Marking of Identifying Characteristics

The number of persons with dentures is increasing worldwide, although with national and regional variations. After aircraft, ship, or natural disasters, victim identification by the aid of dentures is an established method. Thus, there is a need for marking of dentures (Zarb et al. 1990). A marking would also make sense for dentures of patients in retirement homes or hospitals, where dentures are easily lost or changed, either by inattentive behavior of the patients themselves or by nursing personnel. However, in all other cases where a person needs to be identified, the marking of dentures would also be extremely helpful.

In 1972, the 60th Annual World Congress of the Fédération Dentaire Internationale (FDI) recommended the marking of dentures. The Working Group for Forensic Odonto-Stomatology (AKFOS) raised this concern in 1977 as one of the main tasks (Rötzscher 1998b).

The United States has enacted laws or regulations regarding the marking of dentures for home residents and for identification purpose in mass disasters, usually with the patient's name, initials, or social security number. In 21 states, dentists are requested to mark dentures (Chart 20.2). In addition, New York recommends marking the prosthesis component when requested by the patient. Some other states in the USA expect dentures to be marked.

Table 20.9 The action of concentrated mineral acids on the human tooth, the dental prosthesis, and the bone tissue (Endris 1980; Rötzscher and Reimann 1975)

Material	Hydrochloric acid	Sulfuric acid	Nitric acid
Tooth	Solubilization after 3–4 days	Solubilization after 14–18 days	Solubilization within 18 h
Acrylic	See above	Dissolution after 14 days	See above
Rubber	See above	Porous within 7 days	Solubilization within 3–4 h
Porcelain	See above	See above	See above
Bone	Solubilization within 12 h	See above	Solubilization within 4 h

Chart 20.2
The 21 states in the USA where dentists are requested to mark dentures

Alaska	Maine	New Jersey	California	Massachusetts
North Dakota	Georgia	Michigan	Ohio	Illinois
Minnesota	Texas	Indiana	Missouri	Washington
Kansas	Montana	West Virginia	Louisiana	Nevada
Wisconsin				

Australia has no legal obligation for marking dentures (Thomas et al. 1995). The technical procedures are too difficult or expensive, thus, are not very promising (Gladfelter and Smith 1980). In South Africa, Bernitz and Blignaut (1998) tested a simple method using a P-touch 300 electronic lettering system with a 13-digit patient identification number plus an additional "ZA" (international code for South Africa) in 2-mm-large letters on a transparent tape that is embedded in the denture (the tape is 103-µm thick and resists temperatures up to 365 °C). The Swedish health ministry recommends marking, but without legal obligation (Borrman et al. 1995; Pilz and Krause 1980a).

A study by Teivens and Mörnstad (1992) evaluated more than 1,400 forensic odontological cases in which 19 % of the prostheses were marked. A study with long-term patients in Gothenburg (Olsson et al. 1993) showed that 64 % had no teeth and 43 % of the dentures were correctly marked. Initially the prostheses were marked (Engström et al. 1994; Johanson and Ekman 1984) with a thin stainless tape (because of possible nickel allergies), and later by a nickel-free steel tape (ID band Remanit, SDI AB, Prod. No. 1370) with the typed patient's name and the Swedish Personal identity number (Fig. 20.17). For this purpose (Prod. No. 1371), a recess is cut (by an acrylic fraise) into the denture. It can resist 800 °C for 10 min (Engström et al. 1994). Transparent bonding covers the plates and protects them from saliva contamination, so the indices are not changed. Nordell et al. (1997) used an ID tape containing a nickel–aluminum-rich alloy (Al_2O_3, $NiAl_2O_3$) that can withstand a temperature of 1,300 °C for 10 min and does not cause allergies in the denture resin. In a study of 568 patients, Görlach and Görlach (1982) used a 0.03-mm-thick stainless sheet labeled by typewriter as an information carrier. In the follow-up (4 weeks to 1 year) deposits (calculus and/or smoking lining) were found in only 10 %. The marking has the advantage of being protected by the prosthesis and the surrounding soft tissues from external influences.

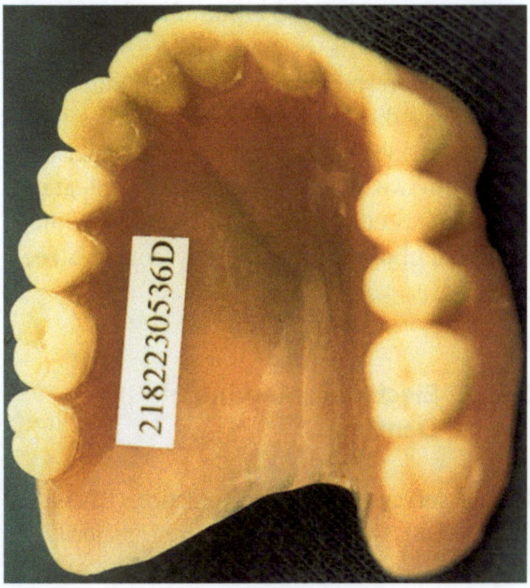

Fig. 20.17 ID tape (demonstration model)

A denture marking should resist high temperatures and should be biocompatible, easy to implant, easily detectable in case of accident and inexpensive (Nordell et al. 1997). Because the back section of the palate is very well protected from heat influence, the marking will remain readable, even if it is not fire resistant (Thomas et al. 1995).

Perenack (1980) reports a probably very rare case:

A male patient (diabetes mellitus, Alzheimer's disease) swallowed his lower jaw full denture and came to the clinic without significant symptoms. The radiograph of the chest did not show the swallowed denture, since it was made of plastic. If the denture would have been marked, the radiopaque plates would have been detected on the X-ray image. The position of the prosthesis could be located by palpation and were surgically removed.

Jacobs (1980) reported another case in which a 62-year-old woman with organic brain damage was referred to the clinic for removal of a foreign body in the esophagus. The day before, she had had respiratory problems and the X-ray of the chest displayed two foreign bodies in the cervical esophagus. It was a partial upper denture with two plastic teeth and an integrated clip that was embedded in the mucosa. Without the metal clip, this denture may not have been detected.

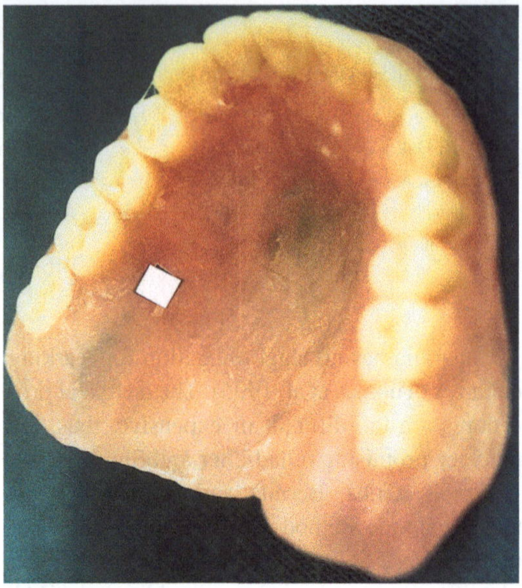

Fig. 20.18 Microchip in denture base (demonstration model)

20.5.1 Electronic Marking of Dentures

Patient surveys in my own practice (Rötzscher 1977–1998) showed that the vast majority of respondents refused the marking of prostheses (e.g., by means of personal identification number). The respondents felt stigmatized. However, microchips on the prosthesis and the storage of personal data that is accessible only to entitled persons found acceptance. From the viewpoint of data privacy, the recording of patient's name and insurance number on the denture is also not problematic (Rötzscher et al. 1997).

For electronic marking of prostheses (Rötzscher et al. 1998), a memory chip (micro-Sensysâ) with wirelessly storable and readable information (ILD-2000) of the size of $4 \times 4 \times 1$ mm^3 that is permanently embedded in the denture base is recommended (Fig. 20.18).

1. System Description
   - 1.1 Hardware
     Reading pen (PEN 232standard) and "handheld PSION Workabout" (128 K Flash SSD with software, 2 batteries R6 1.5 V or Ni-Cd batteries R6 V/700 1.2 mAh) and a computer memory chip.
   - 1.2 Software
     The main program PROTHE1.OPO is on the internal RAM drive of the mobile hand-held device as well as the database file PROTHE1.DBF for detecting the initialization data with backup copies of both program tools (on a 128 k flash ROM), which can be copied if needed to the internal drive. To avoid data loss, a frequent backup of the file PROTHE1.DBF is recommended.
2. Application technology
   In full or partial dentures made of plastic, a chip tray is created or subsequently milled, and the chip is fitted and sealed with clear plastic. The data is transferred by read/write pin. The data is stored in the PC, laptop, or handheld device (network-capable database system).
3. Data Management
   - 3.1 Patient Information
     Patient name, first name, insurance number.
4. Data Security
   Password protection, information crypto chromatographed, private or legal key code, unique chip identification (ID) number.

5. Conditions for the application
   5.1 The patient must give consent for the electronic storage.
   5.2 Cost assumed by the patient as a private service.

A survey of the Institute for Medical Statistics and Documentation in Mainz of 1,200 dentists and 639 patients about their attitude to the marking of prostheses (Wehr 1970) had the following result:

> 67 percent of the surveyed dentists had no concerns, 24 percent had the following concerns:
>
> > difficulties in the technical implementation, the patient's consent misuse by unauthorized persons
> > only nine percent of the dentists were against a marking (too much bureaucracy, confusion within the practice, benefits are not in relation to the effort).

The survey also included questions for the patients:

1. Would you agree with the marking of your dentures?
2. Would you be willing to participate in the resulting costs?

The result was that 92 % of patients agreed with the marking and 64 % were willing to participate in the costs.

The survey was repeated a year later:

Of the dentists, 80 % agreed without restrictions and 17 % agreed with concerns and only 3 % were opposed to marking. Of the patients, 94 % (!) agreed with a marking (only 6 % were opposed), and 67 % were willing to participate in the resulting costs.

Borrman et al. (1997) conducted a survey of 114 dentists and 204 patients in Sweden, of whom the majority agreed with a marking of prostheses. The authors proposed an international cooperation to consider different opinions and national features and ethical principles (Rötzscher 1998b).

20.5.2 Marking of Dentures

In 283 patients with prosthetic teeth, the teeth were marked by using a nonvisible Rheotan-130 film, which was introduced into the apical cavity of the denture tooth (time exposure 5 min, laboratory error 6 %) (Görlach and Görlach 1982). Hansen (1991) labeled plates of plastic or stainless metal (2.5×5 mm^2) with the ID number (letters 0.3 mm) and placed them into the buccal enamel surface of the first permanent or second deciduous molars. A conventional etch and bonding technique (intraoral microidentification and computer-readable discs) was used. The metal was photochemically etched or typed with a computer-driven YAG laser.

20.6 Studies of Dental Alloys

Each person has a kind of national flag in the teeth if the type, quality, and material of dental work is considered (Keiser-Nielsen 1965). The analysis of alloy components is possible with fixed and with removable dentures in vitro and in vivo.

Opportunities for the study of dental alloys that allow a nondestructive editing of the tracks include wet-chemical analysis, instrumental neutron activation analysis (INAA), solid-atomic emission spectrometry (AAS), plasma-atomic emission spectrometry (ICP-OES), inductively coupled plasma–mass spectrometry (ICP-MS), and energy dispersive (EDX) and wavelength dispersive (WDS) X-ray analysis (Kollmannsperger and Helfmeier 1983; Lindemaier et al. 1993; Reuling 1992; Stöppler and Nürnberg 1984; Wirz et al. 1992).

20.6.1 Neutron Activation Analysis (NAA)

In cases of complicated identifications, neutron activation analysis (NAA) is useful for dental alloys, although it is complicated and expensive (Fig. 20.19). NAA is based on the analysis of the alloy without destruction of the track (Figs. 20.20, 20.21, and 20.22). The elements are listed in a comparison of Laser and Pfeilsticker. Identification would be much easier if pilot elements were introduced by the manufacturer (Rötzscher et al. 1973).

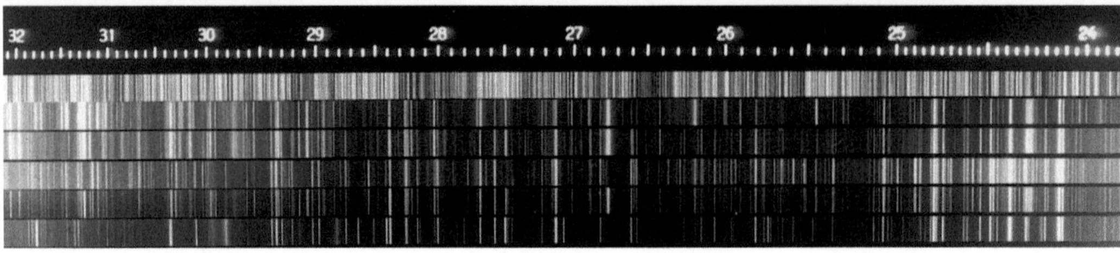

Fig. 20.19 Spectra using Carbon Electrode Spectral Analyser (Pfeilsticker Abreissbogengerät, Carl Zeiss, Jena)

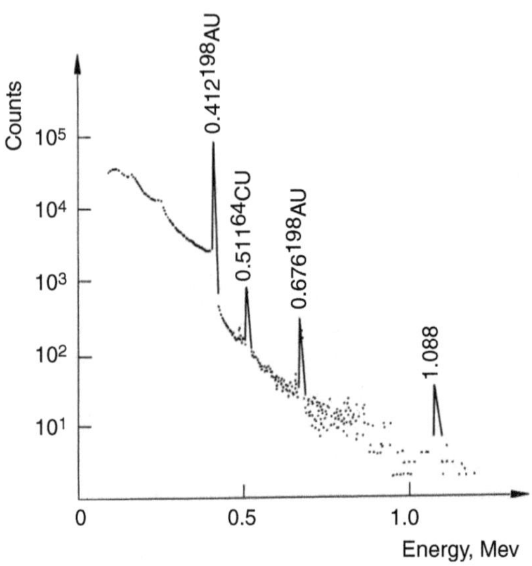

Fig. 20.20 Gamma-ray spectrum (Gopal, Halsbruecke, Freiberg)

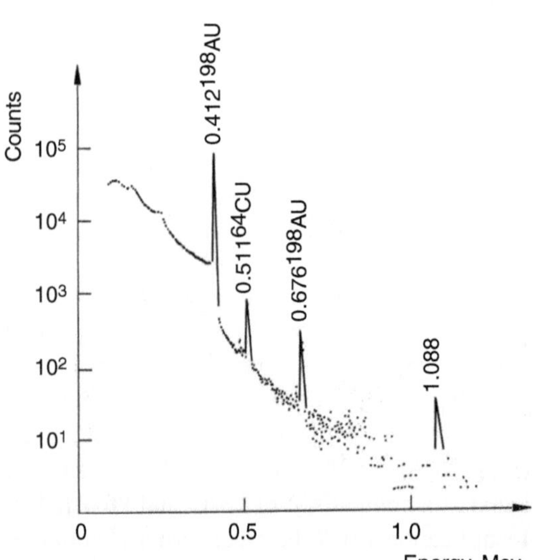

Fig. 20.21 Gamma-steel range (Godent, Halsbruecke, Freiberg)

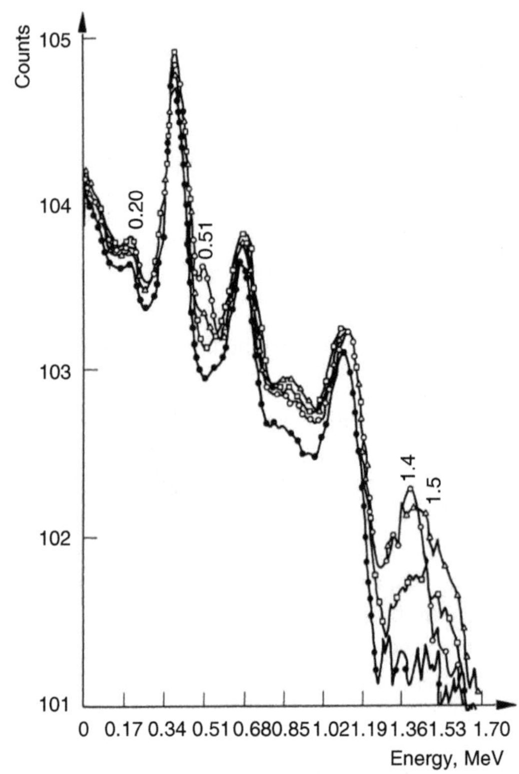

Fig. 20.22 Gamma-ray spectrum (Godent 181 Goplat 187, Gopal 567, gold standard, Halsbruecke, Freiberg)

20.6.2 Scanning Electron Microscope (SEM) Identification

The scanning electron microscopic structure analysis of dental alloys provides information about the nature and structure of the prosthesis.

20.6.3 Energy-Dispersive X-Ray Analysis (EDX)

Energy dispersive X-ray analysis (EDX, previously used as a standard) allows the quantitative

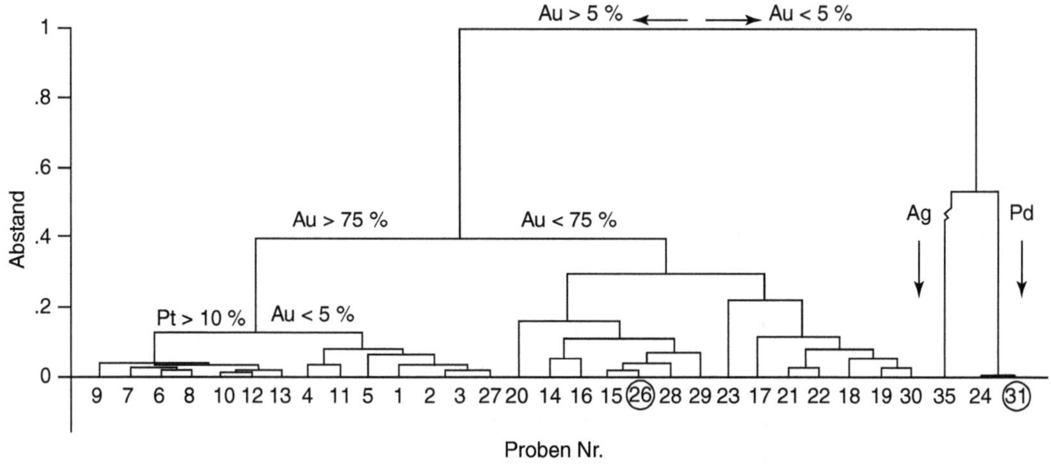

Fig. 20.23 Dendrogram of hierarchical cluster analysis of a data set (noble metal) = 26.31 dental materials (Lindemaier et al. 1993)

determination of the composition of dental materials (Kollmannsperger and Helfmeier 1983; Wirz et al. 1992). In this method, a focused high-energy electron beam induces a surface X-ray emission on the object. The element concentration in the target point is determined by X-ray spectrometry (Stöppler and Nürnberg 1984). The combination of EDX with mathematical pattern recognition techniques (hierarchical cluster analysis, factor analysis) allows nondestructive analysis of the evidence (Fig. 20.23). Evidence can be kept for further investigations. A comprehensive reference file, which takes into account the regional or manufacturer-characteristic differences in the composition of dental materials, is required (Lindemaier et al. 1993).

20.6.4 Inductively Coupled Plasma–Mass Spectrometry (ICP–MS)

Although EDX analysis identifies seven of the nine elements (according to the manufacturer), ICP-MS analysis is able to reproducibly detect six additional existing elements, some only in traces. Because of the possibility of simultaneous multielement detection of even very low traces (detection accuracy up to 0.1 μg/g), ICP-MS is used for routine clinical alloy analysis, especially if an element identification of minimum amounts of material or organic tissue must be performed (Artelt 1993; Markert et al. 1996; Nuttall et al. 1995; Vanhoe 1993). After the wet chemical outcrop of the samples, the atomization happens in an argon plasma flame. The energy-focusing mass ionized element components can be composed and electrometrically determined in a magnetic field (Artelt 1993).

A practical method has been developed for easy and contamination-free material removal. Sample taking is routinely used in dental practice and dental laboratories with low costs (Wichmann et al. 1999).

20.7 Missing Person Bulletins

The number of unknown persons that need to be identified grows increasingly (Riepert and Rittner 1989). If identification is not successful within 4 weeks, search announcements in dental bulletins are published in order to receive relevant information. The entire dental profession is asked (in the bulletins of the chambers, such as the dental releases (ZM) of the Federal Chamber of Dentists (BZÄK) or the National Association of Panel Dentists) to participate in the identification (Figs. 20.24 and 20.25).

The search in print media takes a relatively large amount of time and is often a "last chance" effort to identify an unknown dead person (Grundmann 1996, 1997; Walz 1997). A study of the relevance of search announcements in print

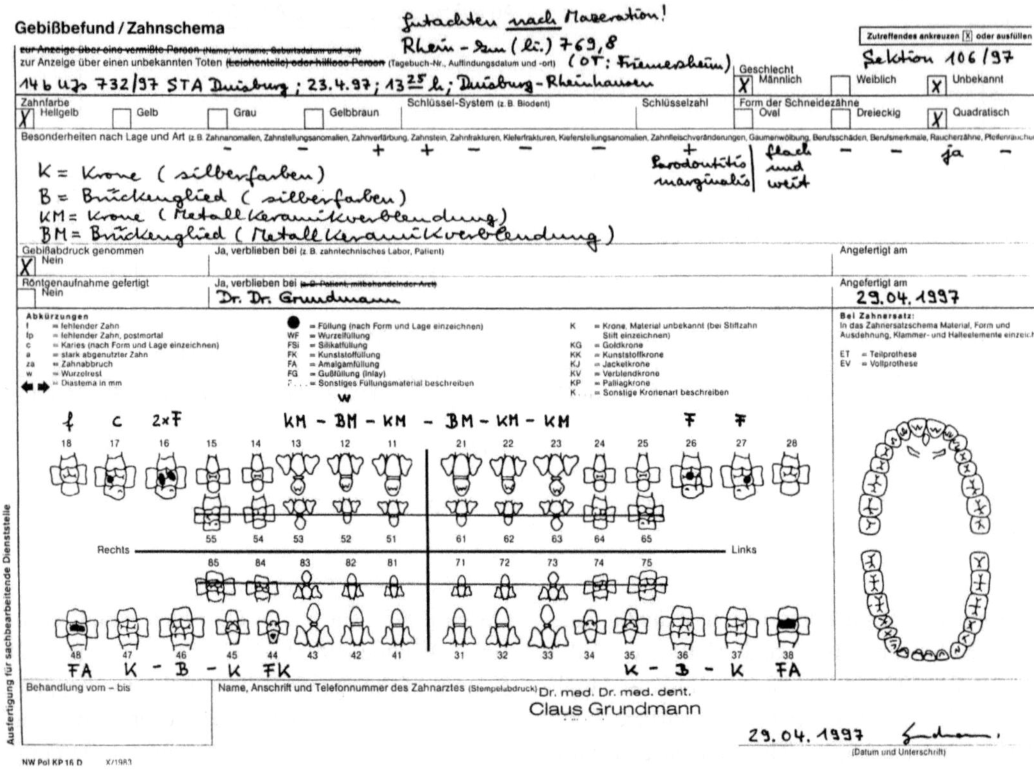
Gebißbefund / Zahnschema
Gutachten nach Mazeration!
~~zur Anzeige über eine vermißte Person~~ (Name, Vorname, Geburtsdatum und -ort)
zur Anzeige über einen unbekannten Toten ~~(Leichenteile) oder hilflose Person~~ (Tagebuch-Nr., Auffindungsdatum und -ort)
Rhein - km (li.) 769,8 (OT: Friemersheim)
Zutreffendes ankreuzen [X] oder ausfüllen
Sektion 106/97
14 b UJs 732/97 STA Duisburg; 23.4.97; 13²⁵ h; Duisburg-Rheinhausen
Geschlecht: [X] Männlich [ ] Weiblich [X] Unbekannt
Zahnfarbe: [X] Hellgelb [ ] Gelb [ ] Grau [ ] Gelbbraun
Schlüssel-System (z. B. Biodent) | Schlüsselzahl
Form der Schneidezähne: [ ] Oval [ ] Dreieckig [X] Quadratisch
Besonderheiten nach Lage und Art (z. B. Zahnanomalien, Zahnstellungsanomalien, Zahnverfärbung, Zahnstein, Zahnfrakturen, Kieferfrakturen, Kieferstellungsanomalien, Zahnfleischveränderungen, Gaumenwölbung, Berufsschäden, Berufsmerkmale, Raucherzähne, Pfeifenraucher)
- - + + - - - + Parodontitis marginalis | flach und weit | - - ja -
K = Krone (silberfarben)
B = Brückenglied (silberfarben)
KM = Krone (Metallkeramikverblendung)
BM = Brückenglied (Metallkeramikverblendung)
Gebißabdruck genommen: [X] Nein | Ja, verblieben bei (z. B. zahntechnisches Labor, Patient) | Angefertigt am
Röntgenaufnahme gefertigt: [ ] Nein | Ja, verblieben bei ~~(z. B. Patient, mitbehandelnder Arzt)~~ Dr. Dr. Grundmann | Angefertigt am 29.04.1997
Abkürzungen
f = fehlender Zahn
fp = fehlender Zahn, postmortal
c = Karies (nach Form und Lage einzeichnen)
a = stark abgenutzter Zahn
za = Zahnabbruch
w = Wurzelrest
⬅➡ = Diastema in mm
● = Füllung (nach Form und Lage einzeichnen)
WF = Wurzelfüllung
FSi = Silikatfüllung
FK = Kunststoffüllung
FA = Amalgamfüllung
FG = Gußfüllung (Inlay)
F... = Sonstiges Füllungsmaterial beschreiben
K = Krone, Material unbekannt (bei Stiftzahn Stift einzeichnen)
KG = Goldkrone
KK = Kunststoffkrone
KJ = Jacketkrone
KV = Verblendkrone
KP = Palliagkrone
K... = Sonstige Kronenart beschreiben
Bei Zahnersatz: In das Zahnersatzschema Material, Form und Ausdehnung, Klammer- und Halteelemente einzeichnen
ET = Teilprothese
EV = Vollprothese
f c 2×F KM - BM - KM - BM - KM - KM F F
18 17 16 15 14 13 12 11 21 22 23 24 25 26 27 28
55 54 53 52 51 61 62 63 64 65
Rechts Links
85 84 83 82 81 71 72 73 74 75
48 47 46 45 44 43 42 41 31 32 33 34 35 36 37 38
FA K - B - K FK K - B - K FA
Behandlung vom - bis | Name, Anschrift und Telefonnummer des Zahnarztes (Stempelabdruck) Dr. med. Dr. med. dent. Claus Grundmann
29.04.1997 (Datum und Unterschrift)
Ausfertigung für sachbearbeitende Dienststelle
NW Pol KP 16 D X/1983

Fig. 20.24 NW Pol KP 16 D Dental finding (semianatomic dental chart) of an unknown dead person (Courtesy of Dr. Claus Grundmann, Moers)

media (Alt and Walz 1997a, b) in 177 cases from the years 1975–1995 concluded that, in 48 cases out of 55 that were not identified by a search announcement, the following content requirements for a search announcement are optimal:

Meaningful pictures of the teeth, jaws, and photo of the dead body (visual information)
- Listing of related places
- Precise description of the dental restoration work

In contrast, the number of cases that were identified by a search announcement was so small that no conclusions could be drawn regarding which specific information is useful in a search announcement. The accompanying text of a search announcement awakened only low interest in the readers. Visual information generally offers a high recognition value (Figs. 20.26, 20.27, 20.28, and 20.29) and should therefore (see Fig. 20.25) be part of any search announcement (Grundmann 1996).

Attention should be taken to ensure that all displayed details are of good quality. The postmortem (PM) dental status should be reviewed by dental specialists before being published in dental bulletins (Benthaus 1998; Wetzel and Ferchland 1997). In a study of 77 criminal search announcements in the "dental messages," Wetzel and Ferchland (1997) detected that 23.4 % of the announcements were faulty, e.g., prostheses facets were described as crowns and denture teeth as bridge members. The text should be short, unambiguous, informative, and not be wordy. The title should always include the location, because this information first awakes interest (Alt 1997a, b).

A crucial element for successful dental identification is accurate and comprehensive antemortem (AM) findings. In the Federal Republic of Germany, a total of 76,766 dentists and dental surgeons is practicing, 52,116 in their own practices.

Seite 66 · **Rheinisches Zahnärzteblatt** · 6/1997

Die Kriminalpolizei bittet um Mithilfe

Identifizierung einer Leiche

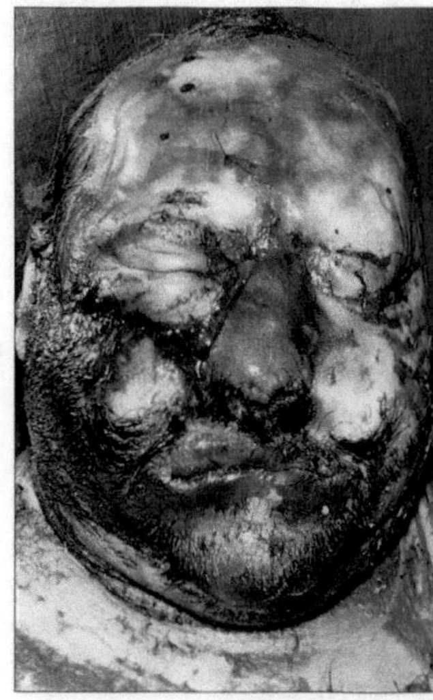

Am 23. April 1997 wurde im Rhein (Strom-km 770, Höhe Duisburg-Rheinhausen) treibend der Leichnam einer männlichen Person vorgefunden. Der Leichnam war noch vollständig erhalten und dürfte ca. acht bis zehn Tage im Wasser gelegen haben.

Die Leiche war, bis auf einen braunen Socken am rechten Fuß, unbekleidet.

Die bislang durchgeführten Ermittlungen zur Identifizierung der Leiche verliefen negativ.

Die Person kann wie folgt beschrieben werden:

Alter ca. 30 bis 40 Jahre
Größe: 1,77 m
Dunkelblonde, nackenlange Haare

Körperliche Merkmale: am rechten Handgelenk schräg von der Daumenseite in Richtung Handrücken verlaufende Narbenbildung von etwa 10 cm Länge. An der rechten Brustkorbseite eine horizontal verlaufende, querfingerbreit unterhalb der Brustwarze liegende Narbe von ca. 28 cm Länge.

Bei der Obduktion der Leiche ergaben sich keine Hinweise auf einen gewaltsamen Tod. Durch die Rechtsmedizin Duisburg wurde ein zahnärztliches Gutachten über das extrahierte Gebiß mit folgenden Ergebnis erstellt:

1. Das Gebiß macht insgesamt einen ungepflegten Eindruck.
2. Ausgeprägte Zahnsteinbildung an den Unterkieferfrontzähnen 31, 32, 33, 41, 42.
3. Chronische Zahnfleischentzündung mit subgingivaler Konkrementbildung an allen Zähnen.
4. Keramikbrücke im Oberkiefer vom rechten bis zum linken Eckzahn. Auffallend ist der Zahnwurzelrest unter dem Brückenglied 12.
5. Silberfarbene Brücken im rechten und linken Unterkiefer. Keine Verblendungen.
6. Zahn 18 fehlt. Eine Verlagerung des Weisheitszahnes liegt nicht vor, wie das angefertigte Röntgenbild zeigt.
7. Zahn 28 in leichter Bukkalposition.
8. Zahn 38 mesial gekippt. Interdental angeschliffen bei der Präparation des Zahnes 37.
9. Exostosen (palatinal) im Bereich der Zähne 17, 18, 27, 28.
10. Schliffacetten insbesondere an den Zähnen 32 und 33.
11. Beim Füllungsmaterial der Zähne 16, 26 und 27 könnte es sich um Glasionomerzemente handeln.
12. Ausgeprägte Zahnsteinbildung an den Bukkalseiten der Zähne 15, 16, 25 und 26.

Sollten Sie feststellen, daß Sie an den abgebildeten Zähnen Behandlungen vorgenommen haben, bitten wir um Nachricht an das
Polizeipräsidium Duisburg
Kriminalkommissariat 11
Düsseldorfer Straße 161–163
47053 Duisburg
Telefon (02 03) 2 80-41 14

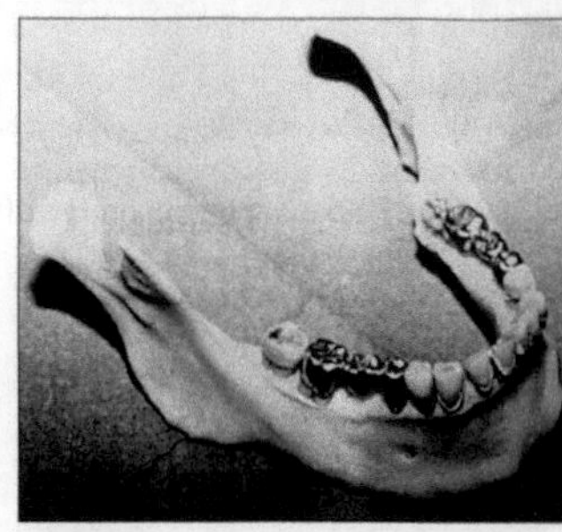

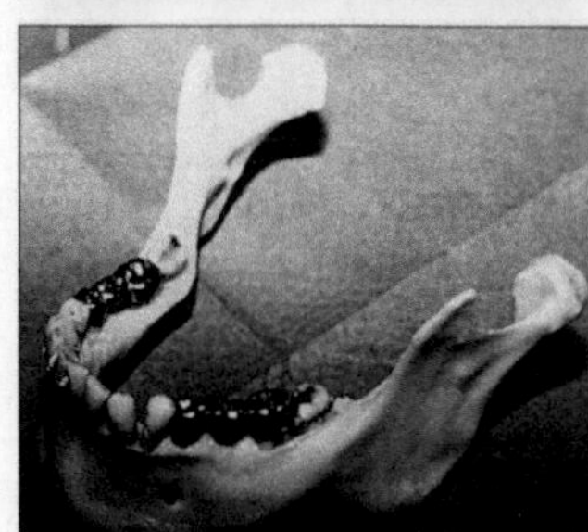

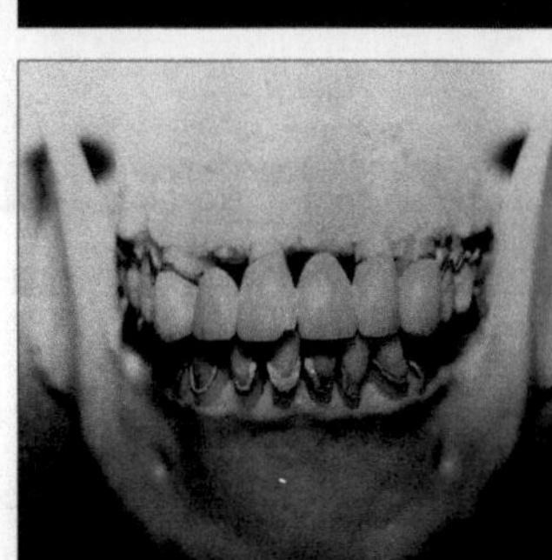

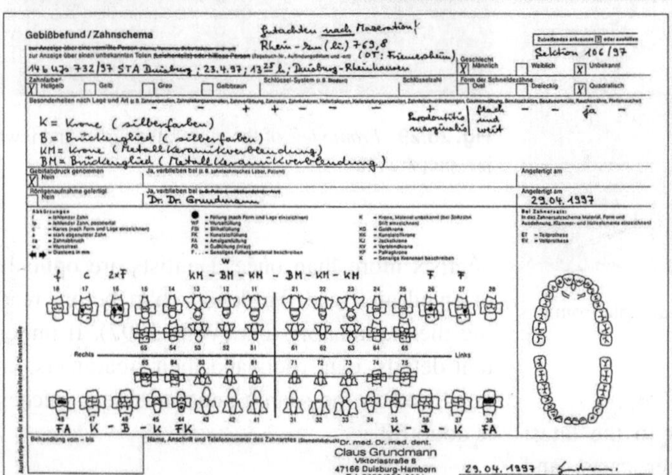

Fig. 20.25 Search display (Grundmann 1997) (Courtesy of Dr. Claus Grundmann, Moers)

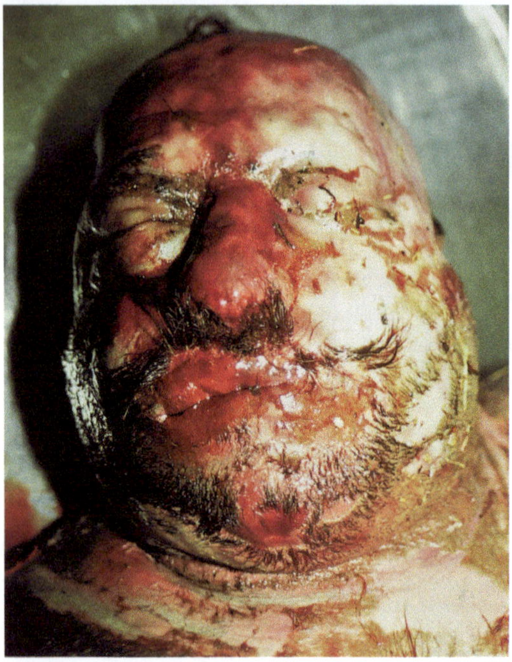

Fig. 20.26 Head of a male body (after ~8–10 days in water)

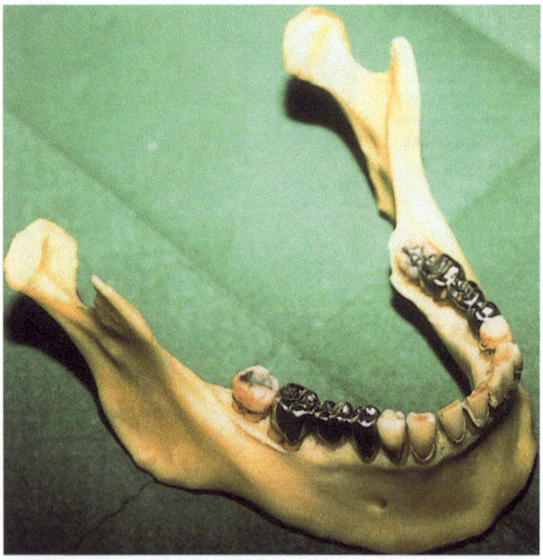

Fig. 20.27 *Top view* of the macerated mandible from the right side

The dental status with respect to the latest changes, the x-ray images, plaster casts, and additional notes is relevant for an identification (Andersen et al. 1995). Unfortunately, these data are very often incorrect and incomplete and without consideration of the work of the predecessor. It is common for patients to change

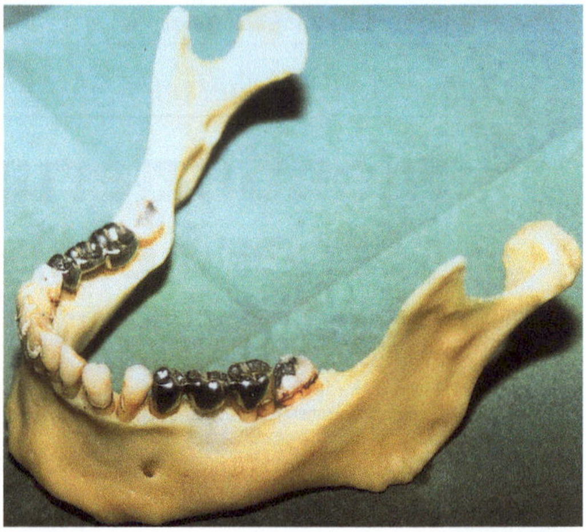

Fig. 20.28 *Top view* of the macerated mandible from the left side

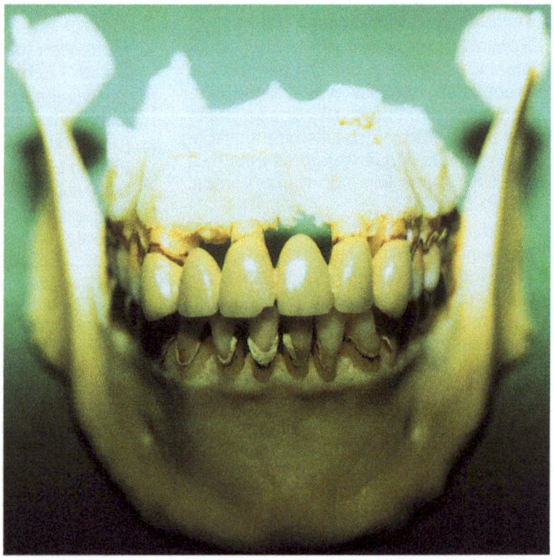

Fig. 20.29 *Front view* of the macerated upper and lower jaw preparation

dentists more than once. Dentists are optically oriented and read the dental chart before reading the explanatory text (Walz 1997). If important details, e.g., roots and their treatments, are not listed in the search announcement, success is doubtful.

20.7.1 Identifying a Missing Person

Each case bears a private, social, or legal interest for successful identification, e.g., in an inheritance matter, damage claim, or pension claim. All of these cases cannot be finally processed without a definitive identification.

References

Aitchinson J (1964) Some racial differences in human skulls and jaws. Br Dent J 116:25–33

Albus M (1998) Morphognostische und metrische Zahnuntersuchungen. Inaug. Med. Diss. Bonn 52–86

Alt KW (1997a) "Dental Fingerprinting"-Zähne und Rechtsmedizin. Quintessenz 48(10):1411–1424

Alt KW (1997b) Odontologische Verwandschaftsanalyse. Individuelle Charakteristika der Zähne in ihrer Bedeutung für Anthropologie, Archäologie und Rechtsmedizin. G Fischer, Stuttgart/Jena/Lübeck/Ulm, pp 17–19

Alt KW, Türp JC (1998) Hereditary dental anomalies. In: Alt KW, Rösing FW, Teschler-Nicola M (eds) Dental anthropology. Fundamentals, limits, and prospects. Springer, Wien/New York, pp 96–128

Alt KW, Vach W (1995) Odontologic kinship analysis in skeletal remains – concepts, methods and results. Forensic Sci Int 74:99–113

Alt KW, Walz M (1997a) Zur Valenz polizeilicher Suchanzeigen in zahnärztlichen Printmedien. Rechtsmedizin 8(1):17–21

Alt KW, Walz M (1997b) Zur odontologischen Identifizierung unbekannter Toter. Kriminalistik 10:669–672

Alt KW, Rieger S, Vach W, Krekeler G (1995) Odontometrische Geschlechtsbestimmung. Evaluierung frühmittelalterlicher Bestattungen. Rechtsmedizin 5:82–87

Alvarez-Garcia A, Munoz I, Pestoni C, Lareu MV, Rodriguez-Calvo MS, Carracedo A (1996) Effect on environmental factors on PCR-DNA analysis from dental pulp. Int J Legal Med 109:125–129

Amoëdo O (1897) Le rôle des dentistes dans l'identification des victims de la catastrophe du bazar de la Charité, Paris, 4 Mai 1897. Dtsch Mschr Zahnheilk Oktober 1897, pp 550–552

Amoëdo O (1900) Die Zahnheilkunde in der gerichtlichen Medizin. Aus dem Französischen übersetzt von G Port. A. Felix, Leipzig

Andersen L, Juhl M, Solheim T, Borrman H (1995) Odontological identification of fire victims – potentialities and limitations. Int J Leg Med 107: 229–234

Artelt S (1993) Bestimmung von Platin in katalysiertem Autoabgas mittels ICP-MS. Dissertation, Universität Hannover

Benthaus S (1998) Forensische Odontologie in Deutschland – eine Fachdisziplin für den Spezialisten? Quintessenz 49:411–416

Benthaus S, Endris R (1999) Katastrophe in Eschede – Hier waren auch Zahnärzte gefordert. Zahnärztl Mitt 89(59):52–55

Berg S, Ladiges ML, Ladiges O (1981) Der Einfluß von Blutproben- und Spurenalterung auf das PGMI- und GC-Subtypenmuster. Z Rechtsmedizin 87:85–94

Bernitz H, Blignaut J (1998) An inclusion technique for marking dentures. J Forensic Odontostomatol 16(1):14–16

Bezymenski LA (1968) Der Tod des Adolf Hitler. Unbekannte Dokumente aus Moskauer Archiven. Christian Wegner Verlag, Hamburg, pp 64–77

Borrman H, Thomas CJ, Engström EU (1995) Denture marking. Clinical and technical aspects. J Forensic Odontostomatol 13(1):14–17

Borrman H, René N, Wasén J (1997) Denture marking: a questionnaire for patients and dentists. J Forensic Odontostomatol 15(1):30–36

Brinkmann B, Jobst U (1973) Bestimmung des Kerngeschlechts an biologischen Spuren. Z Rechtsmed 73:1–6

Brückner K (1993) Alters- und Geschlechtsbestimmungen an Gaumenformen und -maßen. Med. Dissertation, Med. Akademie Erfurt

Brückner K (1995) Age and sex determination by palatine form measurements. In: Alt KW, Pieper P (eds) Forensic odontology and anthropology, Jacob B, Bonte W (eds) Advances in forensic sciences. Köster, Berlin, p 302

Dittmer M, Dumser T (1999) Zahnärztliche Identifizierungsgrundlagen. Zahnärztl Mitt 89(4): 54–57

Duffy JB, Waterfield JD, Skinner MF (1991) Isolation of tooth pulp cells for sex chromatin studies in experimental dehydrated and cremated remains. Forensic Sci Int 49:127–141

Endris R (1980) Odontologische Identifizierung nach versuchter chemischer Leichenbeseitigung. Dtsch Zahnarztl Z 35:248

Engström EU, Borrman H, Wasén J (1994) Prothesen-Identifikations-Markierungen – Wie müssen sie beschaffen sein? Vortrag: XII Nordiske Mote I Rettsmedisin, Lillehammer, August 1994

Fiala B (1968) Identifikace osob podle chrupu – Forensni stomatologie (Identifikation anhand des Gebisses – Forensische Stomatologie). Státní Zdravotnické Nakladelství, Praha, p 43

Gebhardt H (1923) Verbrennungserscheinungen an Zähnen und Zahnersatz und ihre gerichtsärztliche Bedeutung für die Identifizierung verbrannter Leichen. Dtsch Z Gerichtl Med 2:191

Gill P, Ivanov PL, Kimpton C, Piercy R, Benson N, Tully G, Evett I, Hagelberg E, Sullivan K (1994) Identification of the remains of the Romanov family by DNA analysis. Nat Genet 6:130–135

Ginther C, Issel-Tarver L, King MC (1992) Identifying individuals by sequencing mitochondrial DNA from teeth. Nat Genet 2:135–138

Gladfelter I, Smith B (1980) An evaluation of microdisks for dental identification. J Prosthet Dent 62(3):352–355

Görlach M, Görlach M (1982) Historischer Abriß der Entwicklung der Methoden zur Prothesenmarkierung seit 1931. Med. Dissertation, Med. Akademie Dresden

Griffiths CJ, Bellamy GD (1993) Protection and radiography of heat affected teeth. Forensic Sci Int 60(1–2):57–60

Grundmann C (1996) Differenzen zwischen ante-mortem- und post-mortem-Befunden bei zahnärztlichen Maßnahmen zur Identifizierung von unbekannten verstorbenen Personen. Med. Dissertation, Heinrich-Heine-Universität Düsseldorf

Grundmann C (1997) Identifizierung einer Leiche. Suchanzeige. Rheinisches Zahnärztebl 6:66

Günther H, Schmidt O (1953) Die Zerstörung des menschlichen Gebisses im Verlaufe der Einwirkung hoher Temperaturen. Dtsch Z Ges Gerichtl Med 42:180–188

Hagelberg E, Bell LS, Allen T, Boyde A, Jones SJ, Clegg JB (1991) Analysis of ancient bone DNA: techniques and applications. Phil Trans R Soc Lond B 333:399–407

Haines DH (1972) Racial characteristics in forensic dentistry. Med Sci Law 12:131

Hansen RW (1991) Intraoral micro-identification discs. J Forensic Odontostomatol 9(2):76–85

Holland MM, Fisher DL, Mitchell LG, Rodriguez WC, Canik JJ, Merril CR, Weedn VW (1993) Mitochondrial DNA sequence analysis of human skeletal remains: Identification of remains from the Vietnam war. J Forensic Sci 38:542–553

Hutt JM (1998) L'Association Française d'Identification Odontologique. Ein Bericht. Teil 2. AKFOS Newsl Jg 5(3):71–73

Jacobs LI (1980) Ingestion of partial denture. J Am Dent Assoc 101:801

Jeffreys AJ, Allen MJ, Hagelberg E, Sonnberg A (1992) Identification of the skeletal remains of Josef Mengele by DNA analysis. Forensic Sci Int 56:65–76

Johanson G, Ekman B (1984) Denture marking. J Am Dent Assoc 108:347–350

Johanson G, Lindenstam B (1961) Dental evidence in identification. Photographic registration of the dentition and a method for rapid identification. Acta odontol Scand 19:101–119

Keiser-Nielsen S (1965) Geographic factors in forensic odontology. Int Dent J 15:343–347

Kido A, Kimura Y, Oya M (1993) Transferrin subtyping in dental pulps. J Forensic Sci 38(5):1063–1067

Kollmannsperger P, Helfmeier H (1983) Zur Analyse von Edelmetall-Dentallegierungen. Dtsch Zahnarztl Z 38:1040

Komori H (1960) On the changes of the hard tissues of extracted human teeth under high temperature. Jpn J Leg Med 14:558

Langenscheidt F (1983) Diskriminanzanalytische Geschlechtsbestimmung anhand von Zahnmaßen unter Verwendung von Verfahren zur annähernd unverzerrten Schätzung der Trennstärke. Homo 34:22–27

Lasker GW, Lee MMC (1957) Racial traits in the human teeth. J Forensic Sci 2:401–419

Leopold D, Pfeiffer H, Beckert G (1988) Neuere Untersuchungen zur Geschlechtsdiagnostik an der Mandibula. Kriminalistik Forensic Wiss 71(72):111–114

Levine PH (1995) Investigation for identification denture marking, educational conference. ASFO News, Spring, p 7

Lindemaier G, von Czarnecki J, Loipführer C (1993) Mustererkennung zur Identifizierung von Zahnersatz im Rahmen der Forensischen Odontologie. Rechtsmed 4:19–25

Lopez-Abadia I, Ruiz de la Cuesta JM (1993) A simplified method for phenotyping alpha-2-HS-glycoprotein. J Forensic Sci 38(5):1183–1186

Lutz S, Weisser HJ, Heizmann J, Pollak S (1996) MtDNA as a tool for identification of human remains. Identification using mtDNA. Int J Legal Med 109:205–209

Mannucci A, Sullivan KM, Ivanov PL, Gill P (1994) Forensic application of a rapid and quantitative DNA sex test by amplification of the X-Y homologous gene amelogenin. Int J Leg Med 106:190–193

Markert B, Herpin U, Siewers U, Berlekamp J, Lieth H (1996) The German heavy metal survey by means of mosses. Sci Total Environ 182:159

Matsikidis G, Schulz P (1982) Altersbestimmung nach dem Gebiß mit Hilfe des Zahnfilms. Zahnarztl Mitt 72:2524–2528

Moorrees CFA, Fanning EA, Hunt EE Jr (1963) Age variation of formation stages for ten permanent teeth. J Dent Res 42:1490–1502

Müller M (1938) La calcination du foetus en médecine legale. Verh.1.int.Kongreß gerichtl u soz Med, p 483

Murakami K (1931) Die Gaumenleisten der Japaner. Arb Anat Inst Sendai 14:1–16

Nordell H, Wasén J, Borrman HIM (1997) Denture identification: a new band material and the Swedish ID-band revisited. J Forensic Odontostomatol 15:23–25

Nuttall KL, Gordon WH, Ash KO (1995) Inductively coupled plasma mass spectrometry for trace element analysis in the clinical laboratory. Ann Clin Lab Sci 25:261

Olsson T, Thuresson P, Borrman H (1993) Denture marking – a study of temperature resistance of different metal bands for ID-marking. J Forensic Odontostomatol 11:37–44

Pääbo S, Gifford JA, Wilson AC (1988) Mitochondrial DNA sequences from a 7000-year-old brain. Nucleic Acids Res 16:1775–1787

Perenack DM (1980) Ingestion of mandibular complete denture. J Am Dent Assoc 101:802

Pfeiffer H (1989) Geschlechtsbestimmungen an der Mandibula. Verh Anat Ges 82(Anat Anz Suppl 164):759–760

Pfeiffer H (1990) Geschlechtsdimorphismus an der Mandibula. Kriminal Forensic Wiss 75(76):93–105

Pfeiffer H, Hühne J, Seitz B, Brinkmann B (1999) Influence of soil storage and exposure period on DNA recovery from teeth. Int J Legal Med 112:142–144

Pilz W (1974) Forensische Stomatologie. J.A. Barth, Leipzig

Pilz W, Krause D (1980a) 5. Identifizierung, 5.1.4. Prothesenmarkierungen. In: Pilz W, Reimann W, Krause D (Hrsg) Gerichtliche Medizin für Stomatologen. JA Barth, Leipzig, pp 110–113

Pilz W, Krause D (1980b) Zum Geschlechtsdimorphismus der Zähne und des Gebisses. In: Pilz W, Reimann

W, Krause D (Hrsg.) Gerichtliche Medizin für Stomatologen. JA Barth, Leipzig, pp 134–136

Pötsch L, Prager-Eberle M, Penzes L, Rittner CH (1991) Bestimmung von Identitätsmerkmalen an der Zahnpulpa. Int Symposium über Massenkatastrophen, Lausanne. Zbl Rechtsmed 3, p 224

Pötsch L, Meyer U, Rothschild S, Schneider PM, Rittner CH (1992a) Application of DNA techniques for identification using human dental pulp as a source of DNA. Int J Legal Med 105:139–143

Pötsch L, Penzes L, Rittner CH (1992b) GC-Subtypisierung an der menschlichen Zahnpulpa durch isoelektrische Fokussierung in immobilisierten pH-Gradienten. Rechtsmedizin 2:67–70

Pötsch-Schneider L, Endris R, Schmidt H (1985) Diskriminanzanalyse zur Geschlechtsbestimmung am Unterkieferknochen. Z Rechtsmed 94:21–30

Rao NG, Rao NN, Pai ML, Kotian MS (1989) Mandibula canine index – a clue for establishing sex identity. Forensic Sci Int 42:249–254

Reuling N (1992) Biokompatibiltät dentaler Legierungen. Toxikologische, histopathologische und analytische Aspekte. Hanser, München

Riepert TH, Rittner CH (1989) Zur Röntgenidentifizierung unbekannter Leichen bei fortgeschrittenen postmortalen Veränderungen. Rechtsmed 102(11):207–216

Rötzscher K (1971) Die forensische Stomatologie – eine forensische Wissenschaft. III. Die Mitarbeit im Erkennungsdienst. Kriminal Forensic Wiss 6:171–175

Rötzscher K (1991) Die internationale und interdisziplinäre Zusammenarbeit auf dem Gebiet der Forensischen Odonto-Stomatologie. Die Erhebung des Zahnstatus bei Identifikationen. Vortrag S16, Internationales Symposium über Massenkatastrophen. 70. Jahrestagung Dtsch Ges Rechtsmedizin, Lausanne, 10–14 Sept 1991

Rötzscher K (1995) Organisation der Personenidentifikation mit dem BKA. AKFOS Newsl Jg 2(3):77–80

Rötzscher K (1998a) Gentest identifiziert Bormann-Skelett – Anmerkungen. AKFOS Newsl Jg 5(2):36

Rötzscher K (1998b) Prothesenmarkierung – Eine kurze Darstellung. AKFOS Newsl Jg 5(1):14–15

Rötzscher K, Reimann W (1975) Die forensische Stomatologie. In: Prokop O, Göhler W (Hrsg) Forensische Medizin 3. Aufl. Volk und Gesundheit, Berlin, pp 545–564

Rötzscher K, Mende S, Flachowski J, Geisler M, Wehran HJ (1973) Neutron activation analysis of dental metals with regard to forensic odontology (dental identification). J Radioanal Chem 15:317–328

Rötzscher K, Bedrich MR, Jurisch R, Peitsch P (1997) Electronic marking dentures – a study. IOFOS Newsl 19(4):6–7

Rötzscher K, Bedrich MR, Jurisch R, Peitsch P (1998) Die elektronische Kennzeichnung von Zahnprothesen – Ein Hilfsmittel zur Personenidentifikation. Electronic Denture Marking. An aid for identification. Rechtsmedizin 8:115–117

Saiki RK, Walsh PS, Levenson CH, Erlich HA (1989) Genetic analysis of amplified DNA with immobilized sequence-specific oligonucleotide probes. Proc Natl Acad Sci USA 86:6230

Schneider V, Wandelt S (1984) Die Bedeutung der Zahnheilkunde im Rahmen rechtsmedizinischer Fragestellungen. Kriminalistik 4:158–164

Schranz D, Bartha M (1964) Geschlechtsbestimmungen an Zähnen. Dtsch Z Gerichtl Med 54:10ff

Schulze C (1982) Lehrbuch der Kieferorthopädie. 3 Aufl Quintessenz, Berlin

Schwartz TR, Schwartz EA, Mieszerski L, McNally L, Kobilinsky L (1991) Characterization of desoxyribonucleic acid (DNA) obtained from teeth subjected to various environmental conditions. J Forensic Sci 36(4):979–990

Seno M (1977) Sex identification of the human tooth by Y-chromatin in the nucleus of dental pulp cells. Jpn J Leg Med 31:172–179

Seno M, Ishizu H (1973) Sex identification of a human tooth. Int J Forensic Dent 1:1

Smeets B, van de Vorde H, Hooft P (1991) ABO bloodgrouping on tooth material. Forensic Sci Int 50(2):277–284

Smith BC, Fisher DL, Weedn VW, Warnock GR, Holland MM (1993) A systematic approach to the sampling of dental DNA. J Forensic Sci 38:1194–1209

Sognnaes RF, Strøm F (1973) The odontological identification of Adolf Hitler. Definitve documentation by X-rays, interrogations and autopsy findings. Acta Odontol Scand 31:43–69

Starp SE (1990) Untersuchungen zur Geschlechtsbestimmung der Individuen zweier frühneolithischer Skelettserien aus Baden-Württemberg anhand der Zahnmaße. Med. Dissertation, Tübingen

Stöppler M, Nürnberg HW (1984) Analytik von Metallen und ihren Verbindungen. In: Merian E (Hrsg) Metalle in der Umwelt. Chemie, Weinheim

Takei T (1985) Application of moiré topography to forensic odontology. J Nihon Univ Sch Dent 27:87

Teivens A, Mörnstad H (1992) Ten years of forensic odontology – a report from the Department of Forensic Odontology in Stockholm, Sweden. J Forensic Odontostomatol 10:50–57

Teschler-Nicola M (1992) Sexualdimorphismus der Zahnkronendurchmesser: Ein Beitrag zur Sexualdiagnose subadulter Individuen anhand des frühbronzezeitlichen Gräberfeldes von Franzhausen. I Ann Naturhist Mus Wien 125–142

Thomas CJ, Mori T, Miyakawa O, Chung HG (1995) In search of a suitable denture marking. J Forensic Odontostomatol 13(1):9–13

Thomsen JL (1977) Sex determination of severely burned bodies. Forensic Sci Int 10:235–242

van Vark GN (1976) A critical evaluation of the application of multivariate statistical methods to the study of human population from their skeletal remains. Anthropol Anz 24:231–241

Vanhoe H (1993) A review of the capabilities of ICP-MS for trace element analysis in body fluids and tissues. J Trace Elem Electrolytes Health Dis 7:151

von Lepkowski V, Wachholz L (1903) Über Veränderungen natürlicher und künstlicher Gebisse durch extreme Temperatur und Fäulnis (Beitrag zur Identitätslehre). Ärztl Sachverst Z 9:119

Walz M (1997) Polizeiliche Suchanzeigen in zahnärztlichen Printm edien zur Identifizierung unbekannter Toter und ihre Valenz als forensisch-odontologisches Verfahren. Med. Dissertation, Universität Freiburg

Wehr H (1970) Möglichkeiten der Kennzeichnung von zahnärztlichen Arbeiten zum Zwecke der Identifikation. Inaug Dissertation, Mainz

Wetzel W, Ferchland U (1997) Zahnärztliche Mithilfe bei der Identifzierung unbekannter Toter. Zahnarztl Mitt 87:38–46

Whittaker DK, Llewelyn DR, Jones RW (1975) Sex determination from necrotic pulp tissue. Br Dent J 139:403–405

Wichmann M, Artelt S, Karau K, Kock H (1999) Quantitative Bestimmung von Legierungsbestandteilen – EDX- und ICP-MS – Analyse im Vergleich. Dtsch Zahnarztl Z 54(3):180–183

Wirz J, Schmidli F, Jäger K (1992) Splittertest. Quintessenz 43:1017

Woodward SR, King MJ, Chiu NM, Kuchar MJ, Griggs CW (1994) Amplification of ancient nuclear DNA from teeth and soft tissues. PCR Methods Appl 3:244–247

Wutzler A (1991) Alters- und Geschlechtsabhängigkeiten der Gaumenfalten beim Menschen. Med. Dissertation, Med. Akademie Erfurt

Wutzler A, Leopold D (1995) Die Analyse der Morphologie der Gaumenfalten. Advances in forensic sciences, vol 7. Köster, Berlin, p 300

Xingzhi X, Ji L, Hao F, Ming L, Zhuyao L (1993) ABO blood grouping on dental tissue. J Forensic Sci 38(4):956–960

Yamada Y, Yamamoto K, Yoshii T, Ishiyama I (1989) Analysis of DNA from tooth and application to forensic dental medicine. Nippon-Hoigaku-Zasshi 43(5):420–423

Yamamoto K, Ohtani S, Kato S, Sugimoto H, Miake K, Nakamura T (1990) Morphological changes in human and animal enamel roots with heading — especially limits in temperature allowing discrimination between human and animal teeth. Bull Kanagawa Dent Coll 18(1):55–61

Zarb GA, Hickey JC, Carlsson GE (1990) Bouchers prosthodontics treatment for edentulous patients, 10th edn. CV Mosby, St. Louis, p 4

Zichel G (1933) Gerichtlich-medizinische Untersuchungen an Zähnen, unter besonderer Berücksichtigung der quantitativen Bestimmung ihrer Luminescenz. Dtsch Z Gerichtl Med 21:278–290

21 Organization of Identification

Klaus Rötzscher and Eddy de Valck

21.1 Preliminary Comments

The organization of odontostomatological identification varies in each country. Most countries have only few or no forensic odontologists, and the quality standard of forensic odontologists is different from country to country. The need for forensic odontologists is often only recognized after a mass disaster has happened. Good cooperation between authorities and forensic odontologists usually develops after dealing with a mass disaster. By 1968, the Fédération Dentaire International (FDI) had already recommended that the subject Forensic Odontology should be included in the curricula of dental schools (Keiser-Nielsen 1980).

The identification of an unknown body lies within the mandate of the prosecutor (Unnatural death, corpse fund – Code of Criminal Procedure [CCP] § 159), who in turn asks the local police authority to perform the identification. CCP § 159 is also mandatory if a disaster victim cannot be immediately identified.

The appropriate police authority is charged with preserving any evidence (bodies and body parts) at the site. The question of identity should be clarified before the autopsy is performed (CCP § 88). For this purpose, photos, fingerprints, and other meaningful measurements are taken (CCP § 81b). The identification of an unknown corpse is frequently carried out in the outer and inner morgue. If necessary, the prosecutor or judge deposes the consultation with the physician (CCP § 87). The autopsy shall, as far as possible, always cover the opening of the head, chest, and abdominal cavities (CCP § 89).

In some cases, the responsibility for identification of the living and/or dead is given to the Institute of Legal Medicine. Examination of the dentition (Removal of body parts: Guidelines for criminal and administrative penalties – Ri StBV No.35) will be performed if the identification is not successful because of adverse conditions, such as:

- Fire exposure
- Adverse weather conditions
- Long stay in water
- Putrefaction
- Skeletonization

The head of the Institute of Legal Medicine decides on the deployment of personnel and the possible involvement of a forensic odontologist. Most institutes do not have a forensic odontologist, so they consult with a dentist from a university dental clinic or a practice. The local criminal investigation unit delivers the order to the forensic pathologist (possibly a forensic odontologist) and together they go to the crime scene or the person to be identified is brought to the Institute of Legal Medicine. Cells are removed and studied by molecular genetics to determine DNA patterns for identification (CCP § 81g).

K. Rötzscher, Dr. med. Dr. med. dent. (✉)
German Academy of Forensic Odontostomatology (AKFOS),
Wimphelingstraße 7, 67346 Speyer, Germany
e-mail: roetzscher.klaus.dr@t-online.de

E. de Valck, DDS
Forensic Odontologist, DVI Team Belgium,
Beigem, Belgium

K. Rötzscher (ed.), *Forensic and Legal Dentistry*,
DOI 10.1007/978-3-319-01330-5_21, © Springer International Publishing Switzerland 2014

Table 21.1 Natural and civil disasters

(a) *Natural disasters caused by*	(b) *Civil disasters caused by*
Thunderstorm, flood, snow, storm, earthquake, forest fire, fire in populated areas	Reactors, transport, industry (rail, plane, ship), explosions, failure of power, gas, water, failure of disposal (garbage, sewage)

Table 21.2 Measures before, during, and after a disaster

(a) *Preventive measures*	(b) *Immediate measures (during and after a disaster)*
Civil protection measures	Disaster management
Emergency response plans	Determining the scale of the disaster
Plan conferences	Providing of operational guidance to alert the emergency services
Organizational chart of the BKA IdKo	Issuing warnings
Assignment of legal physicians	Providing communication
Assignment of forensic odontologists	Assessing the situation
Emergency response drill	Action planning for security force for
Education of the population	search and rescue of people—triage

In case of a disaster (Table 21.1), the *Calendar Reference Book on Disaster* is a reference book used for the alert and performance of necessary measurements. This text helps the operation commanders (Technical Management) to find needed information for the fast and smooth cooperation of the relief forces.

The medical and forensic measures in case of a disaster are regulated by law (Table 21.2). In the Federal Republic of Germany, civil protection is legislated in the basic law (Rötzscher et al. 1998). The deployment of forces for the immediate defense of danger and rescue of people (including security service) is legislated in federal and state law.

21.1.1 Identification Commissions

The Federal Criminal Police (BKA) in Wiesbaden (decree from 01.15.1970 – OS I5 – 625400/7, Report BKA 1970) has had an Identification Commission since 1972 (IdKo) (Beyer et al. 1966; Endris 1982; Heidemann 1988; Rötzscher 1995). The Commission is associated with the Department OA 31 – *Capital crimes, missing and dead persons*.

Currently, 22 countries have identifying commissions (FBI 1961; Johnson 1995; Sperber 1979; Warnick 1995). These commissions (IdKo) are appointed by a department or organized by the police authority. They are deployed in disaster situations and under difficult conditions. Their composition varies depending on their underlying philosophies.

In France, the commission is the Service Central d'Identité Judiciaire (Hugret 1973). Surprisingly, some European countries, such as Austria and Italy, do not have an identifying commission (Rotondo 1967). In the USA, since 1940, the commission is the Disaster Identification Squad of the Federal Bureau of Investigation (FBI).

The Identifying Commission of the Federal Criminal Police (BKA) in Wiesbaden works with several forensic odontologists (Rötzscher 1992b). In case of an accident involving a German aircraft in countries that are members of the International Civil Aviation Organisation (ICAO), the Federal Aviation Authority (LBA) in Braunschweig (according to the Convention on International Civil Aviation) sends an air accident investigation team; the IdKo of the BKA may be part of this team. In all other cases, the LBA and BKA offer their help to the countries involved (Endris 1982).

People from different countries are affected in accidents with aircrafts or ships or in rail accidents. Since 1988, when INTERPOL was concerned with the exchange of information about missing and/or dead persons of unknown identity, the Federal Criminal Police Office established a working group "identification" to develop uniform documents for sampling of antemortem (AM) and postmortem (PM) data. They designed forms for identification including dental forms for AM and PM recording as well as comparison and conclusion forms. There is a guide for disaster victim identification (DVI) work and also a computer program, DVI International, from Plass Data® in Denmark. Nowadays, version 3.1 is available with the most recent design of the DVI forms (T. Solheim, IOFOS Newsletter 2011/1, pp 8ff.). In this group, forensic scientists and forensic odontologists work together as an expression of the interdisciplinary nature of the task. German forensic odontologists (members of the Federal Criminal IdKo) as members of the INTERPOL Standing Committee on DVI attend the annual meetings in part as needed.

21.2 Odontology in Relation to the INTERPOL Guidelines in the Disaster Victim Identification Process (DVI)

Eddy de Valck

21.2.1 Introduction

Globalization of the world results in an increasing travel pattern by more and more people. This will undoubtedly result in a higher probability that a disaster anywhere on earth, regardless of its nature, will result in the deaths of people from many different countries in the world. It is rarely possible to identify victims of major disasters such as airplane crashes, terrorist attacks, or earthquakes by visual recognition, and identification by visual recognition is not accepted in most countries because of legal considerations.

Comparisons of fingerprints, dental records, or DNA samples of the unknown victims with ones stored in databases or taken from victims' personal effects are often required to obtain a conclusive identification. These primary identification elements can guarantee a scientific proof of identity that can withstand the scrutiny of different international legal standards.

When a major disaster occurs, the affected country may not be able to handle the crisis in an adequate way for different reasons. The country may not have a properly trained and equipped DVI team or may not have sufficient resources to deal with the mass casualty. In some cases, the incident may have damaged or destroyed the country's existing emergency response infrastructure, making the task of victim identification even more difficult.

Member countries can, in these circumstances, call on INTERPOL for assistance in disaster victim identification (DVI) in the immediate aftermath of a disaster. The services offered by INTERPOL to its member countries include a wide range of support:

- A downloadable DVI guide
- Assistance from the Command and Coordination Centre at the INTERPOL General Secretariat in Lyon, France to send messages between National Central Bureaus 24 hours a day in Arabic, English, French, or Spanish
- An Incident Response Team to provide further assistance upon request, such as on-site investigative support or connection to INTERPOL's databases

Such a coordinated effort by the international DVI community can significantly speed up the victim recovery and identification process, enabling victims' families to begin the healing process and societies to rebuild, and, in the event of a terrorism incident, assisting investigators to identify possible attackers.

The DVI process is an intensive and demanding task requiring a multidimensional approach, involving well-trained specialists from various disciplines. INTERPOL's DVI activities are supported by a Steering Group and a Standing Committee on Disaster Victim Identification, both of which are made up of forensic and police experts. The Steering Group formulates INTERPOL DVI policy and strategic planning, whereas the Standing Committee meets annually at INTERPOL's Headquarters in Lyon to discuss improvements to procedures and standards in DVI matters.

In recent years, many disaster incidents have occurred that challenged the DVI team with various kinds of difficulties related to disaster management and different situations in each disaster. New technologies have been developed to make the working process faster and more effective and the different DVI protocols have been evaluated and improved.

Subsequently, policies and guidelines have been produced in the following areas and are backed up by training programs:

- Victim care and family support
- Occupational care for DVI teams

- Compliance with international standards and forensic quality assurance controls
- Information sharing and exchange
- Operational assistance to countries that lack DVI capacity

The forensic dentist (odontology being one of the primary identifiers) is one of the key persons who play important roles in the DVI human identification process.

21.2.2 INTERPOL Standing Committee on DVI (History)

The first INTERPOL DVI guide was published in 1984, revised in 1997, and updated in 2009 by the INTERPOL Standing Committee on Disaster Victim Identification. It provides guidelines for use by INTERPOL member countries in the identification of victims of disasters, and outlines how to set up a DVI team and how to manage DVI operations. It is designed to encourage the compatibility of procedures across international boundaries and can serve as a basis for INTERPOL Member States that do not have their own DVI teams or have never been confronted with such operational situations to set up a DVI team and to manage DVI operations. This DVI guide reflects the INTERPOL standard for DVI operations. It should be explicitly specified as the basis for DVI operations involving teams from different nations in advance of such operations. The current version is the result of the experience gained by the different international DVI teams over the years accrued through dealing with different kinds of disasters. It is designed to encourage the compatibility of procedures across international boundaries.

Of course, the recommendations cannot address every possible eventuality, but they give sound practical advice on major issues of victim identification. The emphasis is on the multidisciplinary approach of victim identification and the recommendations aim to stimulate DVI teams to apply "best practices" in order to obtain maximal results in DVI operations.

The most important requirement for victim identification work is the application of standards, across personal and national preferences, that are the common basis for the work in multinational DVI operations. For this reason, Standard Operation Protocols (SOP) for antemortem (AM) and postmortem (PM) procedures were established for fingerprinting, forensic pathology, forensic odontology, and DNA profiling. These protocols and standards were found to be crucial in the overall quality of the entire DVI process.

In order to establish, maintain, and review protocols and standards and promote effective international cooperation, INTERPOL calls upon each Member State to make preparations for DVI operations. If a disaster occurs in a country that does not have its own DVI team or if the disaster overpowers the country's capacities, support by other DVI teams can be requested by INTERPOL. This has shown to be advantageous when disaster victims of different nationalities are expected. The nation in charge should then do its utmost to secure participation from other nations, at least as liaison officers, definitely from the medical and dental specialties, but also from the police system, in order to facilitate the exchange of information (particularly AM information).

21.2.3 Proceedings in INTERPOL DVI Guide

The overall identification process involves recovery, AM, PM, reconciliation, and identification teams. It is clear that the actions and operation of these different teams should be active and well coordinated. Explicit descriptions of individual tasks involved in recovery, evidence collection, and victim identification are provided in the INTERPOL guide.

21.3 Recovery Team

The recovery of bodies/body parts and the preservation of evidence/personal effects found at the disaster site represent the first steps in the victim identification process. As a rule, the search for the bodies of victims of a disaster cannot begin until all have been rescued. In general, these operations are initially chaotic and disorganized.

The recovery team has the important tasks of collecting evidence, such as bodies and body parts and personal property, from the disaster scene and accurately recording the findings. This requires accurate mapping (photographic aerial overview or GPS mapping) of the disaster area, which allows the team to record from which part of the site the given evidence was recovered. Usually the incident site will be organized in a grid system. Body numbering is performed according to INTERPOL guidelines and has to be applied by all teams to avoid errors and the creation of even more chaos. The given body numbering system (international country telephone code, site number, and body number as applied in the Tsunami disaster (ex. 32-1-00596)) is the reference for future disasters. This unique body number has to stay with the body during the subsequent stages of the identification process and will be visible on all related documentation (forms and photographs).

It is recommended that a forensic odontologist be part of the recovery team because a trained specialist has a better eye for dental evidence. In some cases, such as with charred bodies, it might be necessary for the odontologist on the recovery team to consolidate or describe the dental evidence on site before it is removed to avoid destruction of the brittle dental substances during transportation to the mortuary.

The matching of separate body parts should be performed only by authorized forensic medical experts, and not by recovery personnel. More generally, each body part should be labeled. Medical and dental experts should be at the scene to assist the police in collecting body parts, particularly bones and teeth.

The Recovery and Evidence Collection Team performs the following tasks relating to the recovery of bodies:

- Localization of all bodies/body parts
- Exposure of the body, if necessary (with the aid of appropriate support personnel and suitable equipment)
- Marking of bodies/body parts with an evidence plate or numbered post on which the recovery number is clearly readable and cannot be erased
- Assignment of a separate, unique number to each body/body part
- Documentation of the discovery site (description, photos, sketch, or survey of the position of the body with the aid of GPS and/or crime scene surveying instrument)
- Photographic documentation of the body for recovery files and forensic medical examination
- Attachment of the recovery number to the body/body part. This number is used as the body reference number and remains affixed to the body/body part during the entire identification process
- Completion of the INTERPOL DVI Post Mortem Form (pink), Part Dental findings (83) in single cases recovery number.
- Placement of the body/body part in a body bag, attachment of the recovery number to the outside of the body bag, sealing of the body bag
- Removal of the body/body part and transport to the Recovery Command Center
- Preparation and compilation of recovery documents and submission of documentation to the Recovery Command Center; procurement of new recovery documents as needed
- Transfer of the body/body part and recovery documents to the Recovery Command Center

21.4 Methods of Identification

Victims of large-scale disasters should be identified by assessment of different elements. All possible elements available should be used, but the methods used should be reliable, scientifically sound, applicable under field conditions, and capable of being performed within a reasonable period of time.

The primary and most reliable methods of identification are fingerprint analysis, comparative dental analysis, and DNA analysis (Fig. 21.1). These methods match the requirements as mentioned earlier.

Secondary means of identification (Fig. 21.2) include personal description and medical findings as well as evidence from clothing and personal belongings found on the body. This is considered circumstantial evidence that serves to support identification by other means but is mostly not sufficient as a sole element for identification.

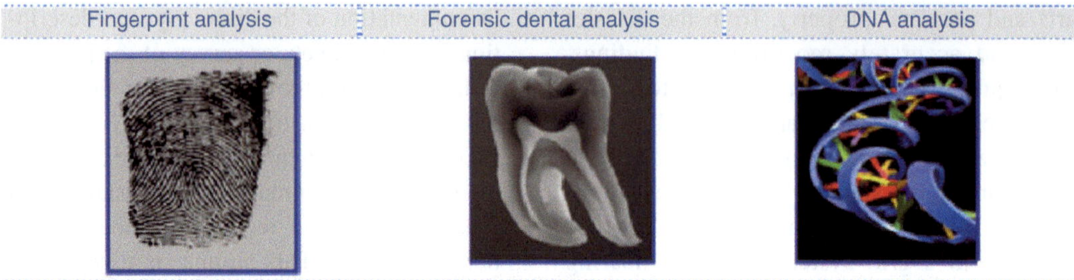

Fig. 21.1 The primary and most reliable methods of identification

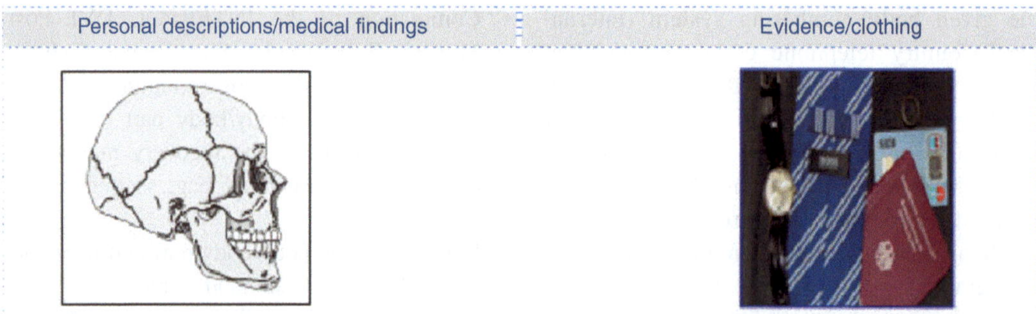

Fig. 21.2 The secondary means of identification

All PM data obtained from the unknown body will be compared with information gathered on missing persons. Because it is impossible to know which kind of information will be available, all possible information (AM and PM) must be collected and documented.

21.5 AM Team

The work of the AM team starts with eliciting a missing persons list and entering this information into a missing persons database. The AM team should however not begin collecting AM data from relatives, friends, etc. until a reliable list of actual victims is available. All of this information is collected solely on the basis of the INTERPOL yellow AM forms. From that point on, the AM information of the reported missing people is obtained through family members, who provide names of health care providers where medical/ dental records or information can be obtained. After the missing persons dentist(s) has been contacted by the police, a forensic odontologist should allocate the AM dental data and materials. Other agencies such as dental hospitals, specialists, health insurance companies, school dental services, correctional facilities, and military organizations should be contacted to obtain additional AM information. The non-availability of AM data must also be documented on the yellow AM forms.

All available dental information (original dental records, X-ray images, dental scans, dental models, full-face photographs, retainers, mouth guards, bleaching trays, and dentures) should be collected and recorded with respect to the patient's right of medical privacy. It is essential that all available information be labeled with the patient's name and date of birth and the dentist's contact information. AM records are to be forwarded to the AM DVI center, where the source and content of the original dental AM records will be carefully examined, analyzed and transcribed into the AM F1/ F2 yellow files. In any cases of doubt, the forensic odontologist on the AM team should contact the treating dentist and discuss and clarify all uncertainties.

It is common for dentists to not want to release the originals of the patient's records, but, because this is mandatory for DVI efforts, it is appropriate to suggest that the dentist makes duplicates and releases the originals. All of this is needed to ensure that the complete AM dental status of the missing person is reconstructed. Speed in acquiring the AM records is important, but not at the expense of receiving all of the best original records.

The quantity and quality of AM dental records is extremely variable across the world and often even in the same country. This is mainly because of differences in legislation in the way dental records are compiled and need to be kept, their content, and the legally required retention periods. Managing this AM information (searching, collecting, receiving, quality assurance, transcribing, tasking, and analyzing) from all countries is a crucial step in the quality system of a DVI process. The importance of producing proper (complete and accurate) dental records should be emphasized to all dentists and dental and health organizations throughout the world.

The records (personal, medical, dental, DNA, and fingerprints) forwarded by the specialists of countries with missing citizens will be entered into a central computer system—DVI System International (Plass Data®) or WinID® or DAVID® or other software available—by trained and experienced forensic odontologists. When AM fingerprint records are received with these records, they are scanned into a separate computer system called the Automated Fingerprint Identification System (AFIS).

The INTERPOL DVI community uses the DVI System International from Plass Data®. This program uses the INTERPOL DVI forms and all information is entered in a similar way as on the paper forms. The dental part requires specific abbreviations and codes that are agreed upon by the Forensic Odontology working group of the INTERPOL DVI Standing Committee. See Annexes 21.1 and 21.2, INTERPOL Disaster Identification (DVI) form (F1/F2) for missing persons (yellow); and Annexes 21.3 and 21.4 INTERPOL Disaster Victim Identification (DVI) form (F1/F2) for unknown corpses found (pink).

21.5.1 General Information (update)

International forensic and law enforcement experts gathered at INTERPOL's General Secretariat to enhance international victim identification standards in Lyon, France (May 28–30, 2013) to review international victim identification methods and discuss new technologies and other ways to improve identification efforts. Bringing together some 155 representatives from some 50 member countries, international organizations, and private sector partners, including the International Commission on Missing Persons (ICMP) and the International Committee of the Red Cross, the 24th meeting of the INTERPOL Standing Committee on Disaster Victim Identification (May 2013) highlighted the importance of a global response using INTERPOL's internationally recognized DVI standards. In his opening remarks, INTERPOL's Executive Director of Police Services, Jean-Michel Louboutin, said that greater communication and information sharing is key to improving the speed and efficiency of future international DVI efforts.

Discussions during the meeting focused on the latest methods and tools available to enhance the identification of victims following natural or manmade disasters, including virtual autopsy techniques, CT imaging, forensic dentistry, and the use of INTERPOL's DVI forms. The newly adopted INTERPOL DVI forms were presented to the group. The dental pages will no longer be marked as "F" pages but will be under the 600s series (see Annex 21.8–21.11). Much of the information that was available on the old F pages will, in the new forms, have to be written on the free pages in the 700s series (see Annex 21.12 ff). All present agreed that there had been too many dental codes (133 in total) and looked at ways to reduce these to a workable number, keeping in mind the philosophy of the Plass Data® DVI System International program. René Pape (Plass Data) was the "engineering" guide through this difficult exercise (De Valck 2013).

Participants were given a demonstration of the prototype system of INTERPOL's FAST and efficient international disaster victim IDentification

(FASTID) project. When fully implemented, the FASTID project will serve as the first centralized, global database of information that can be used to quickly identify and link missing persons and unidentified bodies (MPUB). Developed with experts from five European partners, the MPUB database includes search capabilities for DNA and dental records and interfaces with other INTERPOL databases such as fingerprints.

21.5.1.1 General

This DVI form set is intended for use in cases of major disaster as well as in single cases; in particular, when data concerning a known missing person or an unknown dead person are to be forwarded to another country. Provided the same form set is used, simple reference to the item number (e.g., AM-18/2 or PM-43/02/4) will ensure correct transmission of data.

21.5.1.2 Filing of Report When a Case Is Closed

Whenever an identification has been made and the Comparison Report filled in, the AM and PM forms are to be joined into one report. All AM forms should be punched with holes along the right margin, and all PM forms punched along the left margin; the pages C1 and following should be placed in such a way that corresponding page numbers face one another (yellow–pink, yellow–pink), so that corresponding data can be directly compared page by page. The Victim Identification Report is the final document to be filled in; this closes the case. The INTERPOL DVI form (version 2002) has been updated in English, French, Spanish, and Arabic.

21.6 PM Team

The PM Team collects all relevant dental medical and forensic data obtained from the bodies of deceased victims for the purpose of identifying said victims. A temporary morgue, where the PM information will be collected, needs to be constructed for body storage and examination, and should be established on the premises affording the best possible facilities in the given circumstances. In the morgue, the body will be thoroughly examined by a multidisciplinary team of specialists (fingerprint experts, policemen, pathologists, odontologists, and DNA experts) who will register their findings on the pink PM INTERPOL forms. Wherever possible, existing facilities should be used for the examination of bodies. If no such facilities are available, the site selected must meet certain minimum requirements (Fig. 21.3), i.e., availability of running water, drainage, and electricity as well compliance with safety regulations. The first autopsy room at the tsunami disaster was set up after a couple of days.

Each body to be moved into the examination room for physical description should be placed under the custody of a PM records officer, who follows the body through all of the examination stages until the body is returned for storage. The PM records officer should be in possession of all PM DVI forms for each body.

The first step is finger/palm print analysis by specialists from forensic police labs. The recovered fingerprints will be entered into the AFIS system for comparison with existing AM data.

In the second phase, bodies will be photographed, followed by an extensive external description of the body, clothing, and personal belongings. All of these items are photographed, preferably in color, after being cleaned and labeled, with the reference body number clearly visible. Personal effects such as documents, jewelry, watches, clothing, and pocket contents may constitute valuable circumstantial evidence of identity, but never proof. They must be combined with other evidence to conclude to a positive identification.

X-ray images (and, if possible, CT scans) are important for the whole body and for the teeth for finding clues to the cause of death, for screening for foreign bodies such as pacemakers, implants, osteosynthesis materials, fracture sequelae, etc. They should be taken at the beginning of the autopsy. The role of 3D imaging in the forensic field is growing quickly in the whole autopsy process. Some institutions have already implemented CT in PM forensic investigations, such as at the Armed Forces Medical Examiners autopsy room (Armed Forces Institute of Pathology, Washington, DC and Dover, DE, USA), where

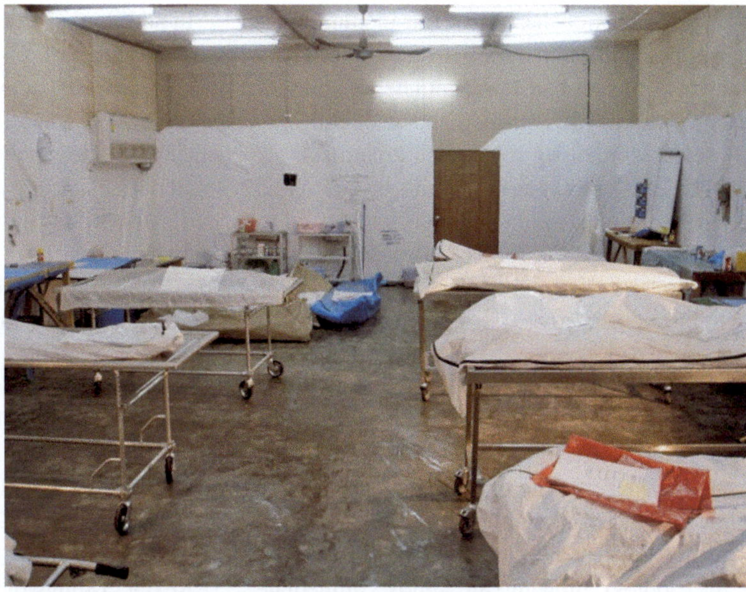

Fig. 21.3 The site selected must meet certain minimum requirements

CT scans on military personnel killed in combat are used on a routine basis. During the Victorian Bushfire in 2009, CT scanning also proved to be very useful in the victim identification process.

In Switzerland, the Virtopsy project implements a variety of imaging methods: 3D photogrammetry-based optical surface scanning, multislice CT (MSCT), and magnetic resonance imaging (MRI). Virtopsy is a noninvasive or minimally invasive approach that has several advantages over current forensic examination techniques, because it can help to provide precise, objective, and clear documentation of forensic findings for testimony in court. This technique also helps improve quality assurance through digital data archiving and transfer. Because of its minimal invasiveness to the body, it can also improve judicature in cultures with low autopsy acceptance. In most cases, physical examination should still be performed in addition to Virtopsy to provide additional physical and external information about the victims, because for some elements Virtopsy images will not produce information that is detailed enough.

During the next step, the pathologist starts the external and internal examination and description of the body. It should be standard practice to perform full autopsies on all disaster victims not only for identification and cause of death purposes, but also to assist in preventing or minimizing the effects of similar incidents in the future. The forensic pathologist takes DNA samples.

A forensic anthropologist can provide critical information for a biological profile of a given deceased person, e.g., age, gender, ethnic affiliation, stature, and other individual identifying features. The forensic pathologist decides on a case-by-case basis whether an anthropologist should be consulted.

Dental examination in this phase is carried out by forensic odontologists. As a rule, two forensic odontologists should work together to collect (dental examiner) and record (dental recorder) the dental status of the unknown body and in producing a radiographic and photographic record. All dental-related details (sound teeth, pathological teeth, restored teeth, absent AM or PM teeth, prosthetic restorations, attrition, and oral anatomical abnormalities) will be registered on the pink PM F1/F2 INTERPOL forms.

Internationally harmonized terms, the FDI two-digit tooth-numbering system, codes, abbreviations, and nomenclature must be used on the INTERPOL DVI F1/F2 forms for international DVI operations.

Many factors may compromise PM dental radiography, such as availability of X-ray equipment, electric supply, and condition of the bodies.

PM radiographs of the teeth must include bilateral molars and premolars with teeth in contact (bitewings); upper and lower molars and premolars and incisors (periapicals); and teeth with special features such as root canal treatments or crowns. These radiographs should be examined for quality so that all data can be transferred to the F1/F2 INTERPOL forms. When dealing with conventional radiography, the developed films ought to be labeled and stored in a numbered Ziplock bag. Recently developed portable and handheld digital dental X-ray units may solve some of these practical problems, as shown during the tsunami crisis, when Nomad® was introduced for the first time in mass disasters. These lightweight and autonomic working devices can be taken anywhere and can easily be brought next to the bodies, allowing an almost immediate X-ray examination of the teeth.

In addition, new technologies (Fig. 21.4) provide new accessories for X-ray viewing in the field of disasters. Some companies have launched portable X-ray machines with a viewing display attached to the machine itself. Others provide a small portable X-ray viewing gadget. When operated in a wireless environment, data and images could thus easily be transmitted in both directions. This may help to facilitate the radiographic interpretation more rapidly than previously.

Several portable dental X-ray devices are available on the market nowadays (Fig. 21.4):

1. Nomad® (Aribex, Utah, USA) was first introduced in 2005 in the identification process after the tsunami disaster
2. AnyRay® (VATECH Co., Ltd., Gyeonggi-do, Republic of Korea)
3. Rextar® (Sungwon Econet, Seoul, Republic of Korea)

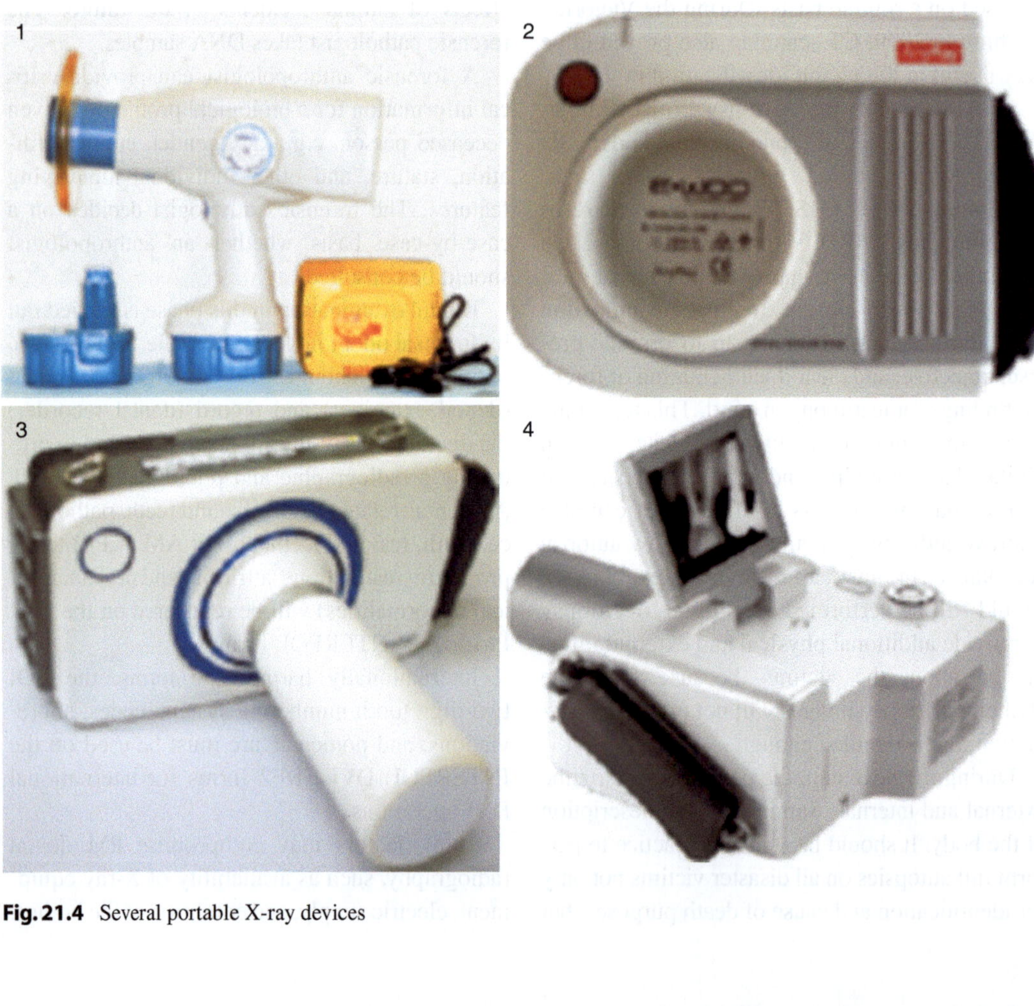

Fig. 21.4 Several portable X-ray devices

4. ADX4000 (DEXCOWIN Co., Ltd., Seoul, Republic of Korea)

As a general rule, jaws should not be removed by dental experts unless an examination that is more specific is mandatory. To create more access to the dentition, a nondestructive method of mandibular dissecting technique is recommended. This anatomical method allows easy access to both maxilla and mandible, ease for photographs and X-rays, and still enables a complete repositioning of the facial tissue after autopsy so that the body can still be shown to relatives if required.

All dental characteristics should be recorded by color photography with the body number well visible in place and by radiography. The odontologist examiner supervises the production of adequate photographic records of teeth and jaws, surrounding oral structures, and significant dental features.

Dental age estimation is a major component of the identification process. PM dental age estimation allows forensic odontologists to focus on the search for a matching AM file in a specific age range among the possible candidates for identification from the missing persons list. Dental age estimation may be performed in different ways using morphological or radiological parameters that are all age related.

In the context of identification, the most appropriately fitting age estimation method in relation to the presented evidence should be chosen out of all existing methods. This is an advantage compared with the age determination of living individuals where, for instance, the methods of age estimation performed after tooth extraction have to be excluded.

At the end of the PM examination line, the quality control officer checks all documents for completeness and legibility, and signs off on the log document.

Reconstructive identification is the first step needed to be able to achieve a comparative identification. During the reconstructive identification process, all necessary information (physical characteristics, medical, odontological, DNA, fingerprints, etc.) is gathered from the unknown body so that an objective reconstructed profile of the unknown body can be established. This reconstructed PM profile can then be matched with missing persons' AM information in a comparative identification.

21.7 Reconciliation Team

The Reconciliation Team handles and compares AM and PM documents forwarded from the AM and PM Units, respectively. Quality control and the transcription of the AM and PM documents take place in different sections of the reconciliation bureau (missing persons, AM, PM, fingerprint, odontology, and DNA). The Reconciliation Team is responsible for matching AM and PM data records, which ultimately leads to victim identification. In cases in which matches are identified, the Reconciliation Team submits the corresponding documents to the Identification Center for review and final decision.

If the use of data processing and evaluation software is possible, considerable time may be saved in comparing data. However, no computer program, no matter how effective it may be, can be more than a helpful tool. The results of the computer comparison will yield a list of probabilities of positive identification but the final judgment has to be made by professional experts and be based on a personal evaluation of the available data. Final decisions must only be made based on all relevant criteria and must have a thorough control process.

Because searches for PM findings among all AM data records is an excessively time-consuming process, the available data should be classified according to useful criteria, so that, for example, PM records for male children are compared only with AM records for male children. A simple classification by gender and age is helpful for both AM and PM records, and records should be filed accordingly (Fig. 21.5).

In the subsequent individual comparison process, the matches obtained during the initial matching are collated through individual comparison of the individual AM missing persons file with the corresponding findings in the PM file. This can result in identification, rejection, or the assumption of a possible or probable identity.

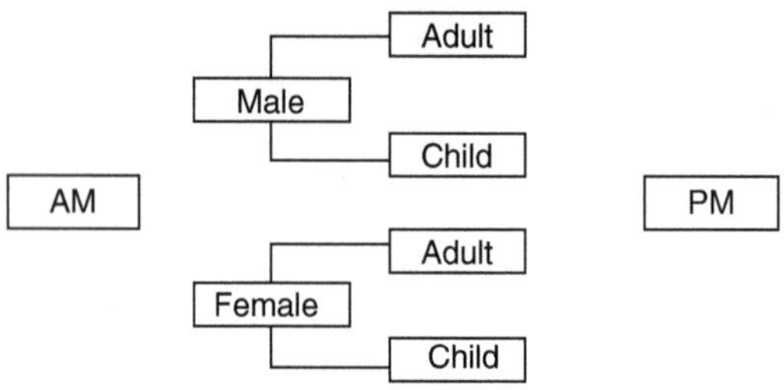

Fig. 21.5 A simple classification by gender and age

The forensic odontologists working in this section will be responsible for quality assurance of AM and PM dental data and comparison of data (Annexes 21.3 and 21.4) in the Plass Data® system. They also prepare expert opinions for matches and support the Director at the identification conference.

A large number of specific details can be compared for matching based on dental status (see Annex 21.6: Comparison Report). A further subdivision in the classification based on the presence or absence of fillings, orthodontic retainers, crowns, removable dentures, and/or implants may facilitate the matching process considerably.

21.8 Identification Board

The Identification Board is a group of senior experts with a lot of experience in identification and DVI that meets at regular intervals during the identification process to discuss and verify the different proposals submitted by the Analysis/Reconciliation Team. The responsibility of this Identification Board is to check the results of comparison made by the various specialized sections on the Reconciliation Board. The Identification Board is also responsible for scrutinizing, and for the eventual reconciliation of, possible inconsistencies and the Identification Board combines the results into a single final list of identifications.

The Identification Board produces a compilation of results in a Victim Identification Report (also part of the PM body record) and will approve this decision by signature. This record is then regarded as a formal confirmation of the identification of a deceased disaster victim.

The Identification Board is responsible for the final identification of every victim and should therefore be composed of the most experienced identification experts involved in the entire operation, i.e., the heads of the various sections/units (forensic pathology, odontology, and fingerprints) and the Director of the DVI Team (Annex 21.7: Victim Identification Report. Certificate of Identification). It may be possible to have one or two representatives (observatory) of the different countries involved in the disaster at the Identification board.

21.9 Legal Standards

Every DVI Operation is subject to the laws of the country in which the disaster in question occurs and will be handled according to the applicable national laws and under the jurisdiction of the local authorities. Considering that victims of disasters requiring DVI operations may come from different countries, approaches to cooperation with the home countries of victims should be developed in advance of such incidents in order to facilitate cooperation. A first step in this process might be to formulate agreements regarding the requirements applicable to the collection and transmission of AM data.

Agreements regarding the integration of international DVI teams in cases of need should also be worked out. The requirements imposed upon these teams are specified by the host country, and the integration of the supporting DVI teams must conform to applicable national law.

21.10 INTERPOL DVI Form

The fourth sheet (the so-called black corner) of the INTERPOL DVI AM form (yellow) (Rötzscher 1992c) contains information about the dental status of the missing person. Sheets F1 and F2 of the form are part of the dental identification about a missing person and to identify a victim of a disaster. The sheets are filled out by forensic odontologists after receiving the data from the treating dentist. The yellow INTERPOL DVI form for missing persons (Annex 21.1) contains detailed dental status, indicating the location, material and age of the fillings, crowns and extractions, etc. mentioned for comparison with the INTERPOL DVI PM form (pink) for an unidentified body (see Annexes 21.1 and 21.2).

The INTERPOL DVI form (F1/F2 for the dentist) was first presented at the meeting of the State Criminal Police Offices (State Criminal Police) in Wiesbaden, April 13–15, 1993. The computer system used in the BKA, (the so-called computer-quadrant method) Vermi/Utot, compiles the data of missing persons and unidentified dead. The information will be stored for 30 years, in some cases even longer (Hagen 1994, Hagen and Strack 1995). With the help of a computer, the AM and PM data are compared by creating a descriptor. The final identification remains reserved for the forensic odontologist (Hagen 1994; Hagen and Strack 1995). The computer only selects the data, the identification is performed by the dentist.

21.10.1 Forensic Odontostomatologic Data Exchange

The results of the comparative studies influence the final report of the legal pathologist that is sent to the police and the prosecutor.

21.10.2 Identification Programs

There are special programs for microcomputers with different interfaces for the purpose of data exchange in Australia (ODONTID), Denmark (DVI/ID DONT), Germany (four-quadrant method), Finland (IDENTIFY), Netherlands (RITSYS), Norway (VISTA), Sweden (OD), and the USA (CAPMI4, TOOTHPICS) (Clark 1990; Hagen 1983; Mäkelä 1995; Mäkelä and Tenhunen 1995; Rand 1988; Solheim et al. 1992).

It is not necessary that a DVI team change its way of working. It is important that all teams use the FDI two-digit system to detect recorded findings. Access (worldwide) to the various databases reduces the time to compare the AM data with the PM data (Bell 1995; Kullman et al. 1993; Lorton et al. 1989; Rötzscher 1992a; Soh and Keng 1990; Williams et al. 1989).

The first computer-based systems that used DVI were mainframes. Today, microcomputers are more suitable. There are two fully automated programs: CAPMI4-Windows (US Army Institute of Dental Research) and Identify 3.0 by the Finnish Air Force (Mäkelä 1995, Mäkelä and Tenhunen 1995). The other programs have no algorithm for calculations. CAPMI4 is more characteristic oriented, which is a disadvantage toward a comparison with graphic interface. Graphic interfaces avoid the dental nomenclature problem (internationally varying systems and different spelling of dentists) of the characteristic-based programs. Nowadays, the Danish computer program Plass Data® is the most common program and is part of the INTERPOL identification system.

Moving toward international cooperation in the identification of unknown living and/or dead, competent institutions will be challenged to provide communications or to expand existing ones (Nelson 1991).

Annex 21.1 and 21.2

INTERPOL Disaster Identification (DVI) AM Form (F1/F2) for missing persons (yellow)

Ante Mortem (yellow) **VICTIM IDENTIFICATION FORM** **F1**

MISSING PERSON

Family name: ____________________ No: ________

Forename(s) : ____________________

Date of birth: ☐☐ Day ☐☐ Month ☐☐ Year Male ☐ Female ☐

DENTAL INFORMATION		
76	Missing Person´s address (see 10)	
77	Reported missing	☐☐ Day ☐☐ Month ☐☐ Year
78	Circumstances of the disappearance	
79	Dental information obtained from family members and/or others (see also 45)	
DENTAL DATA PROVIDED BY		
80	Dentist / Institution...... Address............ .... Phone............ Period covered.. DOCUMENTS filed with......	From ______ To ______ ☐ Records ☐ X-rays ☐ Models ☐ Photos
81	Dentist / Institution...... Address............ .... Phone............ Period covered.. DOCUMENTS filed with......	From ______ To ______ ☐ Records ☐ X-rays ☐ Models ☐ Photos
82	Dentist / Institution...... Address............ .... Phone............ Period covered.. DOCUMENTS filed with......	From ______ To ______ ☐ Records ☐ X-rays ☐ Models ☐ Photos

Odontologist	Signature
Name..............: Address............: Phone number..:	

A~nte~ M~ortem~ *(yellow)* **VICTIM IDENTIFICATION FORM** **F2**

MISSING PERSON

Family name: ------------------ **No:** ________

Forename(s) : ------------------

Date of birth: ☐☐ *Day* ☐☐ *Month* ☐☐ *Year* *Male* ☐ *Female* ☐

86	DENTAL INFORMATION		
51-11			21-61
52-12			22-62
53-13			23-63
54-14			24-64
55-15			25-65
16			26
17			27
18			28

18 17 16 15 14 13 12 11 21 22 23 24 25 26 27 28

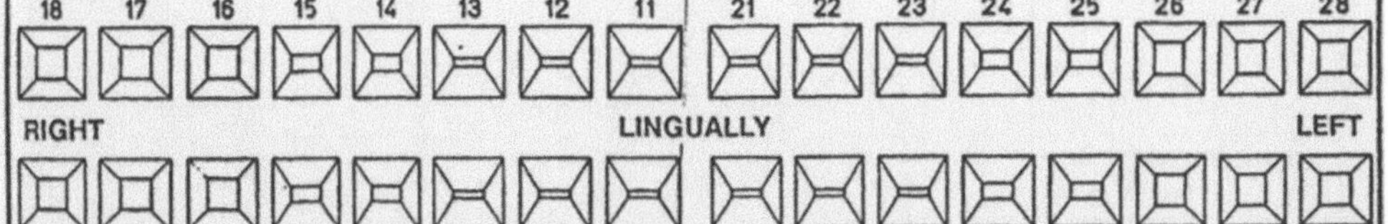

RIGHT LINGUALLY LEFT

48 47 46 45 44 43 42 41 31 32 33 34 35 36 37 38

48			38
47			37
46			36
85-45			35-75
84-44			34-74
83-43			33-73
82-42			32-72
81-41			31-71

87	**Specific data:** Crowns, bridges and dentures	
88	**Further data:** Occlusion, attrition, anomalies, smoker, periodontal status, etc.	
89	**X-rays available**	
90	**Further material**	
91	**Age at time of disapp.**	

Odontologist Name..............: Address...........: Phone number..:	Signature

Annex 21.3 and 21.4

INTERPOL Disaster Victim Identification (DVI) PM Form (F1/2) for unknown corpses found (rose pink).

P~ost~ M~ortem~ (pink) VICTIM IDENTIFICATION FORM F1

DEAD BODY

Nature of disaster: ____________________ No: ________

Place of disaster: ____________________ *Sex unknown* [ ]

Date of examination: [ ][ ] *Day* [ ][ ] *Month* [ ][ ] *Year* *Male* [ ] *Female* [ ]

DENTAL FINDINGS

83	**In single cases** Site of recovery.. Recovery No. .... Date.................... Police Agency.... Address............. .... Phone................. DENTAL EXAMINATION Requested(date) Performed at...... Date....................	
84	**Material** 01 Jaws present?..... 02 Fragmentary remains.............. 03 Single teeth......... 04 Other...................	*Upper* 1 [ ] *Lower* 2 [ ] — Specimen taken? Specimen taken? Specimen taken? Specimen taken?
85	**Supplementary details**	

Odontologist

Name.................:

Address..............:

Phone number..:

Signature

Post Mortem *(pink)* **VICTIM IDENTIFICATION FORM** **F2**

DEAD BODY

Nature of disaster: __________________ No: __________

Place of disaster: __________________ *Sex unknown* ☐

Date of examination: ☐☐ *Day* ☐☐ *Month* ☐☐ *Year* *Male* ☐ *Female* ☐

86	DENTAL FINDINGS		
51-11			21-61
52-12			22-62
53-13			23-63
54-14			24-64
55-15			25-65
16			26
17			27
18			28

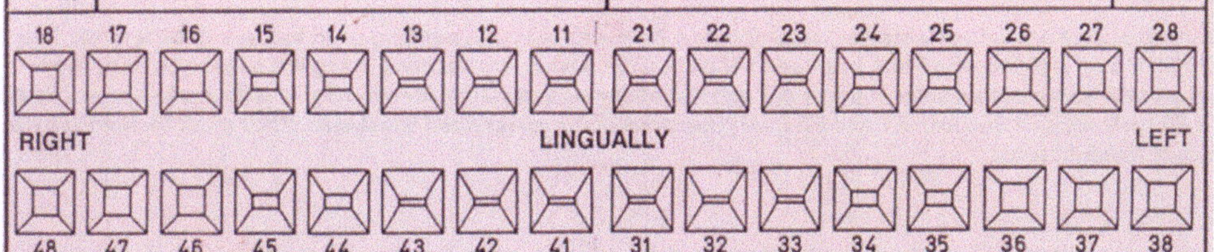

48			38
47			37
46			36
85-45			35-75
84-44			34-74
83-43			33-73
82-42			32-72
81-41			31-71

87	**Specific description of** Crowns, bridges and dentures	
88	**Further findings:** Occlusion, attrition, anomalies, smoker, periodontal status, etc.	
89	**X-rays taken of:**	
90	**Supplementary examination**	
91	**Age evaluation** (method?)	

Odontologist Name................: Address.............: Phone number..:	Signature

Annex 21.5

General Information and Instructions for Use (INTERPOL 2013)

The INTERPOL Victim Identification Form, Sections F1 and F2

GENERAL INFORMATION

The INTERPOL Victim Identification Form consists of several sections - divided into two groups:

1) YELLOW FORMS for listing latest known data concerning a mission person;
2) PINK FORMS for listing all findings concerning a dead body.

Identification of a dead body may become possible if data listed on the pink forms concerning this body can be compared with, and shown to match, data listed on the yellow forms concerning one particular missing person. If an identification is made, the experts involved will complete an Identification-Report - as a prerequisite to issuing a death certificate and releasing the body for burial.

The identification of a dead body may be accomplished in several ways, depending upon the type of data used. The INTERPOL Victim Identification Form has been set up in such a way, that sections listing the same type of data are marked with the same capital letter in the upper right-hand corner. For dental identification, the forms to use are Sections F1 and F2 (yellow), and Sections F1 and F2 (pink); because of the specialized vocabulary, they must be filled in by a forensically trained dentist.

INSTRUCTIONS FOR USE - SECTION F1 AND F2 AM (yellow)

These forms are designed for listing all dental information collected from dental practitioners' records or other sources.

In Section F1, make sure that the reference number is clearly shown - and that the sex is clearly indicated (boxes at the top). Fill in all the details requested further down. Under "Circumstances of the Disappearance", give the shortest possible extract of the police report. Under "Dental information", list any supplementary information obtained by the police from family members and/or others. Request from the police - and list - exact name, address and telephone number of the dentists/institutions from which records etc. have been obtained; also list the respective periods covered (whole years). Written records should be originals or good photostat copies. Ensure that all record X-rays, models, and photographs are clearly marked with patient's name, dentist's name, and date of exposure or production; if they are not, you must do it yourself.

In Section F2, the missing person's latest known dental status is to be listed. The status can only be established by extraction from - and re-arrangement of - the data listed in one or more dental records - or apparent from X-ray, models, photographs, or other material produced. Start with the latest entry in the written record and work your way backwards; in this way, all previous treatment now covered by later treatment can be left out. Indicate surfaces by using Capital-Letter System: M = mesial, O = occlusal, D = distal, V = vestibular, L = lingual; if other abbreviations are used, please explain them in one of the boxes further down. (NOTE: there will be a notation only for treatment/conditions actually described or seen in the material) - Next, sketch on the dental chart the location and extent of all fillings and other conditions listed as present according to your re-arrangement of data. For colour distinction, use black for amalgam, red for gold, and green for tooth-coloured material. For teeth extracted or not formed, put large cross (X) over the appropriate tooth square. If the practitioner's record includes an dental chart, compare it with your own and make sure they tally. Do not hesitate to contact practitioner for clarification of dubious points. If X-rays and/or other material are available, indicate - in the appropriate boxes - type, year of exposure or production, and teeth concerned. Finally, record age at time of disappearance.

Once Section F2 has been completed, type your name, address and telephone number (or use your professional stamp) in the box at the bottom of Section F1. Finally, enter the date of completion above your personal signature. Remember - this is a legal document, so keep a full copy for your own file. Likewise, make copies of all original record material, before returning it to the practitioner.

Annex 21.6

Comparison Report

COMPARISON REPORT

DEAD BODY — **No:** ________ Barcode

Nature of disaster : ____________________

Place of disaster : ____________________

Date of disaster : ☐☐ Day ☐☐ Month ☐☐☐☐ Year — Male ☐ Female ☐ Sex unknown ☐

MISSING PERSON — **No:** ________ Barcode

Family name : ____________________

Forename(s) : ____________________

Date of birth : ☐☐ Day ☐☐ Month ☐☐☐☐ Year — Male ☐ Female ☐

Findings in the unknown DEAD BODY have been compared with information of MISSING PERSON

Conclusions mainly based on evidence by:

☐ Police investigation	Possible identity ☐	Probable identity ☐	Established identity ☐
Reasons:	*Place and date* / *Signature*		*Stamp/institution*
☐ Fingerprint	Possible identity ☐	Probable identity ☐	Established identity ☐
Reasons:	*Place and date* / *Signature*		*Stamp/institution*
☐ Pathologist	Possible identity ☐	Probable identity ☐	Established identity ☐
Reasons:	*Place and date* / *Signature*		*Stamp/institution*
☐ Odontologist	Possible identity ☐	Probable identity ☐	Established identity ☐
Reasons:	*Place and date* / *Signature*		*Stamp/institution*
☐ DNA scientist	Possible identity ☐	Probable identity ☐	Established identity ☐
Reasons:	*Place and date* / *Signature*		*Stamp/institution*
☐ Anthropologist	Possible identity ☐	Probable identity ☐	Established identity ☐
Reasons:	*Place and date* / *Signature*		*Stamp/institution*
☐ Other: ________	Possible identity ☐	Probable identity ☐	Established identity ☐
Reasons:	*Place and date* / *Signature*		*Stamp/institution*

[IOB] Version 2008]

Annex 21.7

Victim Identification Report. Certificate of Identification

VICTIM IDENTIFICATION REPORT

DEAD BODY		(pink forms enclosed)
Site of body examination Police Agency Address Phone		PM File: Date

MISSING PERSON		(yellow forms enclosed)
Family name Forename(s) Street/No. Postcode/Town Country		AM File: Nationality
Date of birth	Day Month Year	Reported missing

CERTIFICATE OF IDENTIFICATION

According to the data here enclosed the above dead body has been IDENTIFIED as the above missing person.

Identification was mainly based on (see comparison report)		
Authorized signature Type the name	Reviewed by:	Place and date Signature
Stamp / Director: Victim Identification		Place and date Signature
Stamp / Local authority		Place and date Signature

[(GB) Version 2008]

Annex 21.8 and 21.9

The new INTERPOL DVI Forms (dental part). AM (yellow), 600´s

Ante Mortem (yellow) **INTERPOL DVI Form - Missing Person** Odontology **600's**

Family name: AM No:

First name(s):

Date of birth: Day Month Year | Age | Male | Female | Unknown

a = Data not available b = Attachment c = Further info on page Sup. Info. (700's)

ODONTOLOGY			a	b	c
600	**Dentist/clinic** Name Street / No. Postcode / Town State / Country Phone / Email				
	01 Period covered	Records 1☐ From: To:			
	02 Enclosed	Radiographs 1☐ Casts 2☐ Photos 3☐ Other (specify): 4☐			
605	**Dentist/clinic** Name Street / No. Postcode / Town State / Country Phone / Email				
	01 Period covered	Records 1☐ From: To:			
	02 Enclosed	Radiographs 1☐ Casts 2☐ Photos 3☐ Other (specify): 4☐			
615	**Dental images available**	1 Digital : 2 State number of : 3 Non digital : 4 State number of			
	01 PA	☐ : ☐ :			
	02 BW	☐ : ☐ :			
	03 OPG	☐ : ☐ :			
	04 CT	☐ : ☐ :			
	05 Other radiographs	☐ : ☐ :			
	06 Photographs	☐ : ☐ :			
620	**Further material**				

Collected by		Signature / Date
	Duty Title :	
	Name :	
	Address :	
	Phone / Email :	

[(EN) Version 2013] 10 of 12

Ante **M**ortem (yellow) **INTERPOL DVI Form - Missing Person** Odontology **600's**

Family name: .... **AM No:** ________

First name(s): ....

Date of birth: ☐☐ Day ☐☐ Month ☐☐☐☐ Year Age ☐ Male ☐ Female ☐ Unknown ☐

a = Data not available b = Attachment c = Further info on page Sup. Info. (700's)

ODONTOLOGY

630	Dental findings (for primary teeth change specific FDI code)		
11			21
12			22
13			23
14			24
15			25
16			26
17			27
18			28

18 17 16 15 14 13 12 11 21 22 23 24 25 26 27 28

RIGHT LEFT

48 47 46 45 44 43 42 41 31 32 33 34 35 36 37 38

48			38
47			37
46			36
45			35
44			34
43			33
42			32
41			31

			a	b	c
635	**Specific data** 01 Specify	1☐ Crowns 2☐ Pontics 3☐ Implants 4☐ Dentures 5☐ Other			
640	**Other findings** 01 Specify	1☐ Occlusion 2☐ Tooth wear 3☐ Periodontal status 4☐ Supernumeraries 5☐ Stains 6☐ Other			
645	**Type of dentition** 01 Specify	1☐ Primary dentition 2☐ Mixed dentition 3☐ Permanent dentition			
650	**Quality check** FOd 1 FOd 2 (If available)	Date: Signature: FOd 1 Name: Date: Signature: FOd 2 Name:			

Collected by Duty Title : Name : Address : Phone / Email :	Signature / Date

[(EN) Version 2013] 11 of 12

Annex 21.10 and 21.11

The new INTERPOL DVI Forms (dental part). PM (pink), 600´s

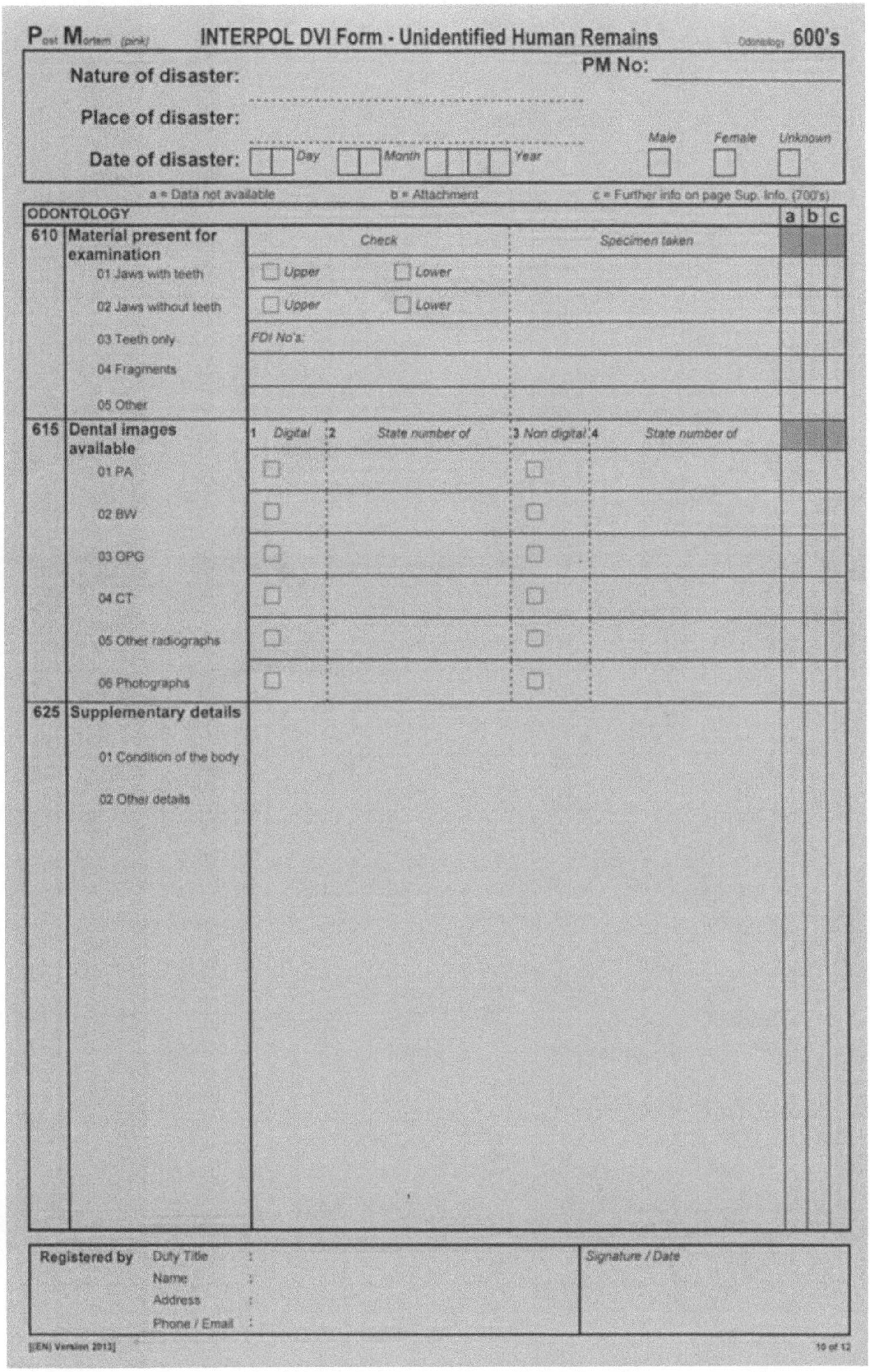

P~ost~ M~ortem~ (pink) INTERPOL DVI Form - Unidentified Human Remains Odontology 600's

Nature of disaster: PM No:

Place of disaster:

Date of disaster: Day Month Year Male Female Unknown

a = Data not available b = Attachment c = Further info on page Sup. Info. (700's)

ODONTOLOGY						a	b	c
610	Material present for examination	Check		Specimen taken				
	01 Jaws with teeth	Upper	Lower					
	02 Jaws without teeth	Upper	Lower					
	03 Teeth only	FDI No's:						
	04 Fragments							
	05 Other							
615	Dental images available	1 Digital	2 State number of	3 Non digital	4 State number of			
	01 PA							
	02 BW							
	03 OPG							
	04 CT							
	05 Other radiographs							
	06 Photographs							
625	Supplementary details							
	01 Condition of the body							
	02 Other details							

Registered by Duty Title :
Name :
Address :
Phone / Email :

Signature / Date

(EN) Version 2013 10 of 12

Post **M**ortem (pink) **INTERPOL DVI Form - Unidentified Human Remains** Odontology **600's**

Nature of disaster: PM No: ____________

Place of disaster:

Date of disaster: ☐☐ Day ☐☐ Month ☐☐☐☐ Year

Male ☐ Female ☐ Unknown ☐

a = Data not available b = Attachment c = Further info on page Sup. Info. (700's)

ODONTOLOGY

630 Dental findings (for primary teeth change specific FDI code)

11			21
12			22
13			23
14			24
15			25
16			26
17			27
18			28

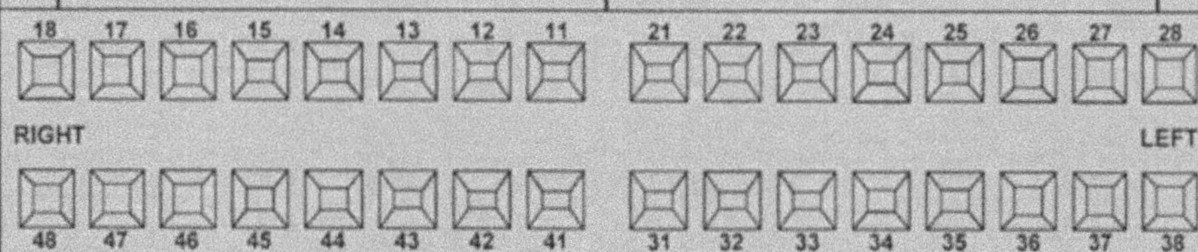

48			38
47			37
46			36
45			35
44			34
43			33
42			32
41			31

					a	b	c
635	Specific data 01 Specify	1☐ Crowns 4☐ Dentures	2☐ Pontics 5☐ Other	3☐ Implants			
640	Other findings 01 Specify	1☐ Occlusion 4☐ Supernumeraries	2☐ Tooth wear 5☐ Stains	3☐ Periodontal status 6☐ Other			
645	Type of dentition & estimated age 01 Dentition	1☐ Primary dentition	2☐ Mixed dentition	3☐ Permanent dentition			
	02 Age (Fill either year or month)	Min ______ year /	Max ______ year	Min ______ month / Max ______ month			
650	Quality check FOd 1	Date FOd 1 Name		Signature			
	FOd 2 (If available)	Date FOd 2 Name		Signature			

Registered by Duty Title : Name : Address : Phone / Email :	Signature / Date

[EN] Version 2013] 11 of 12

Annex 21.12

The new INTERPOL DVI Forms Unidentified Human Remains PM (pink), 700´s

Post Mortem *(pink)* **INTERPOL DVI Form - Unidentified Human Remains** Supporting information **700's**

Nature of disaster: **PM No:**

Place of disaster:

Date of disaster: Day Month Year *Male* *Female* *Unknown*

Supporting information (if referring to data given on a previous page, please indicate field number)

700 1 *Field No.* 2 *Description*

705 *Additional Supporting Information page (700's)* 1 No 2 Yes

[(EN) Version 2013] 12 of 12

Annex 21.13

The new INTERPOL Comparison Report (AM Form)

COMPARISON REPORT

	MISSING PERSON	AM No:
Family name:		
First name(s):		Male ☐ Female ☐ Unknown ☐
Date of birth:	☐☐ Day ☐☐ Month ☐☐☐☐ Year	

	HUMAN REMAINS	PM No:
Nature of disaster:		
Place of disaster:		Male ☐ Female ☐ Unknown ☐
Date of disaster:	☐☐ Day ☐☐ Month ☐☐☐☐ Year	

HUMAN REMAINS have been compared with information of MISSING PERSON

Identification Evidence Evaluation

Primary Identifiers

Fingerprint expert	☐ Not applicable	☐ Data not available/insufficient data	Possible ID ☐	Probable ID ☐	Established ID ☐
Reasons:			*Place and date* / *Signature*		*Stamp/institution*
DNA scientist	☐ Not applicable	☐ Data not available/insufficient data	Possible ID ☐	Probable ID ☐	Established ID ☐
Reasons:			*Place and date* / *Signature*		*Stamp/institution*
Odontologist	☐ Not applicable	☐ Data not available/insufficient data	Possible ID ☐	Probable ID ☐	Established ID ☐
Reasons:			*Place and date* / *Signature*		*Stamp/institution*

Secondary Identifiers

Police investigator	☐ Not applicable	☐ Data not available/insufficient data	Possible ID ☐	Probable ID ☐	Established ID ☐
Reasons:			*Place and date* / *Signature*		*Stamp/institution*
Pathologist	☐ Not applicable	☐ Data not available/insufficient data	Possible ID ☐	Probable ID ☐	Established ID ☐
Reasons:			*Place and date* / *Signature*		*Stamp/institution*
Anthropologist	☐ Not applicable	☐ Data not available/insufficient data	Possible ID ☐	Probable ID ☐	Established ID ☐
Reasons:			*Place and date* / *Signature*		*Stamp/institution*
Other: ______			Possible ID ☐	Probable ID ☐	Established ID ☐
Reasons:			*Place and date* / *Signature*		*Stamp/institution*

Annex 21.14

The new INTERPOL Certificate of Identification

CERTIFICATE OF IDENTIFICATION

MISSING PERSON		AM forms enclosed
Family name **First name(s)** Street / No. Postcode / Town State / Country		*AM No:*
		Nationality
Date of birth	Day Month Year	*Date reported missing*

HUMAN REMAINS		PM forms enclosed
Site of body examination		*PM No:*
Police agency Name Street / No. Postcode / Town State / Country Phone / Email		*Date*

According to the data here enclosed the above human remains have been IDENTIFIED as the above missing person.		
Identification was based on (see comparison report)		
Authorised signature Type the name	*Reviewed by:*	*Place and date* *Signature*
Stamp or logo / Director: Victim Identification		*Place and date* *Signature*

Stamp or logo / Local authority	*Place and date* *Signature*

References

Bell GL (1995) CAPMI 4 (computer aided post mortem identification version 4.0), chapter 7. In: Bowers CM, Bell GL (eds) Manual of forensic odontology. ASFO, AAFS, Colorado Springs, pp 200–226

Beyer G, Materne H, Schröder R (1966) Katastrophenkommission im Einsatz. Kriminalistik 20:241–248

Clark DH (1990) Forensic odontology in six mass disasters. In: Presented at the 12th IAFS meeting, Adelaide, 1990

De Valck E (2013) 24th meeting of the INTERPOL Standing Committee on DVI. IOFOS Newsl 35(1):24

Endris R (1982) Forensische Katastrophenmedizin, 7.6.1 Identifizierungskommissionen. Kriminalistik, Heidelberg, S 214ff

FBI (1961) FBI disaster squad stand ever ready to give assistance. FBI Law Enforc Bull 30:17–19

Hagen M (1983) Forensisch-odontologische computerunterstützte Identifizierung unbekannter Leichen. Zahnmed.Diss. Mainz

Hagen M (1994) Die Computer-Quadranten-Methode. Pers. Mitt

Hagen M, Strack SJ (1995) The Computer-Quadrant-Method running on a PC. In: Jacob B, Bonte W (eds) Advances in forensic sciences, vol 7, Forensic odontology & anthropology, in coop. with Alt KW, Pieper P. Köster, Berlin, S 247–249

Heidemann D (1988) Identifizierungsarbeiten in Ramstein. Zahnarztl Mitt 78(19):2116–2123

Hugret B (1973) The identification teams. Chir dent France 43:46

INTERPOL (2013) Forms. Instruction for use of the Interpol DVI Form Set. http://www.interpol.int. 31 May 2013 – Media release

Johnson LTH (1995) Forming a disaster team. In: Bowers CM, Bell GL (eds) Manual of forensic odontology. ASFO, AAFS, Colorado Springs, pp 249–250

Keiser-Nielsen S (1980) Person identification by means of the teeth, preface. V. J Wright Sons Ltd, Bristol, pp 1–114

Kullman L, Solheim T, Grundin R, Teivens A (1993) Computer registration of missing persons. A case of Scandinavian cooperation in identification of an unkown male skeleton. Forensic Sci Int 60:15–22

Lorton L, Rethman M, Friedman R (1989) The Computer-Assisted Postmortem Identification (CAPMI) system: sorting algorithm improvements. J Forensic Sci 34(4):996–1002

Mäkelä H (1995) Computer assisted identification of disaster victims. Med. Dissertation. Med Fak, Universität Helsinki

Mäkelä H, Tenhunen M (1995) Identify, ID-pro and DVI-logistics, 2000, computer usage in mass disaster. AKFOS Newsl Jg 2(3):97–100

Nelson GD (1991) Kanadischer Polizei-Informations-Dienst (CPIC) der Königlichen Kanadischen Berittenen Polizei (RCMP), Ottawa. Report

Rand M (1988) A computer system to help police cope with major disasters. Int Crim Police Rev 43(413): 18–24

Rotondo G (1967) Contributo allo studio dei problemi medico-legali relativi alla lesivita da disastri aerei. Riv Med Aeronaut 30:251

Rötzscher K (1992a) Computer Assisted Disaster Victim Identification Systems. Vortrag, Joint meeting of A.S.F.O. and B.A.F.O., New Orleans, Feb 1992

Rötzscher K (1992b) The origins and development of FDI, INTERPOL and IOFOS: international co-operation in identification. J Forens Odontostomatol 10(2):58–63

Rötzscher K (1992c) Heutige Erkenntnisse der Identifizierung aus Forensisch – Odonto-Stomatologischer Sicht: Das INTERPOL-DVI-Formblatt. Das Two-Digit-System. Die Internationale Zusammenarbeit bei Identifikationen, Vortrag 110, 71.Jahrestagung Dtsch Ges Rechtsmed, Berlin, 17 Sept 1992

Rötzscher K (1995) Techniques for evaluation of forensic odontological findings. In: Jacob B, Bonte W (eds) Advances in forensic sciences, vol 7, Forensic odontology & anthropology in coop. with Alt KW, Pieper P. Köster, Berlin, S 250–253

Rötzscher K, Benthaus S, Höhmann B (1998) Schutz oder Management? Katastrophenschutz in der Bundesrepublik Deutschland. Rechtsmedizin 8: 201–206

Soh G, Keng SB (1990) Applications of computer technology in dentistry. Ann Acad Med Singapore 19(5):720–730

Solheim T, Lorentsen M, Sundnes PK, Bang G, Bremnes L (1992) The "Scandinavian Star" ferry disaster 1990 – a challenge to forensic odontology. Int J Legal Med 104:339–345

Sperber ND (1979) Disaster Victim Identification – An example of Professional Cooperation. In: FBI Law Enforcement Bulletin, May 1979

Warnick A (1995) Mass disaster dental identification, chapter 8, mass disaster management. In: Bowers CM, Bell GL (eds) Manual of forensic odontology. ASFO, AAFS, Colorado Springs, pp 236–249

Williams AB, Friedman RB, Lorton L (1989) A new algorithm for use in computer identification. J Forensic Sci 34(3):682–686

Clinical Postmortem Findings

22

Klaus Rötzscher, Tore Solheim, and Claus Grundmann

22.1 INTERPOL Postmortem (PM) Form (Pink)

INTERPOL form F1 (see Annex 21.3) contains information about the location and time the body was found and information on when the forensic examination was performed, followed by a description of the test material.

22.2 Examination Technique

The postmortem (PM) examination is to be performed like an ordinary dental examination. The teeth and oral cavity are inspected. This is not complicated, even on a putrid corpse. Rigor mortis significantly impedes the examination, especially in fire victims and bodies that have been in water. In such cases, an oral autopsy must be conducted to allow the examination. The best results can be achieved, especially in mass disasters, if the upper and lower jaw can be removed. This can lead to difficulties if family members have objections or want to see the body. In all cases, the legal coroner or the investigating authority must approve before the jaws are removed.

Depending on the individual case, the examiner may decide to cut only the cheek structures to enter the oral cavity (Fig. 22.1a, b) or may decide to remove the jaw *en bloc* (Heidemann 1988). The latter allows recording of an exact diagnosis and is preferable for photographic or radiographic purposes (Hühn and Gärtner 1974; Sopher 1986).

In cases of mass disasters, removal of the jaw allows subsequent investigations (without exhumation of a corpse). The jaws can be reunited with the rest of the corpse at a later time for burial. Problems may arise if family members have objections or want to see the body. The time for the odontological investigation, whether immediately or only after the forensic findings, will be decided in consultation with legal pathologists and criminologists.

A dentist may work alone, but the examination is more effective with the cooperation of two dentists. In this case, one dentist conducts the examination and the other records and controls the findings (Solheim et al. 1992; Stene-Johansen et al. 1992). Then the results can be compared and, if they do not correspond, they can be reexamined. Finally, the data must be entered in the INTERPOL F2 disaster victim identification (DVI) form with a signature and date (Solheim et al. 1992).

K. Rötzscher, Dr. med. Dr. med. dent. (✉)
German Academy of Forensic Odontostomatology (AKFOS),
Wimphelingstraße 7, 67346 Speyer, Germany
e-mail: roetzscher.klaus.dr@t-online.de

T. Solheim, Prof. (em) Dr. odont.
Institute of Oral Biology,
Pathology and Forensic Odontology,
University Oslo, Oslo, Norway
e-mail: tore.solheim@odont.uio.no

C. Grundmann, Dr. med. Dr. med. dent.
Municipal Medical-Superviser,
Duisburg (North-Rhine-Westphalia),
Arnikaweg 15, 47445 Moers, Germany

K. Rötzscher (ed.), *Forensic and Legal Dentistry*,
DOI 10.1007/978-3-319-01330-5_22, © Springer International Publishing Switzerland 2014

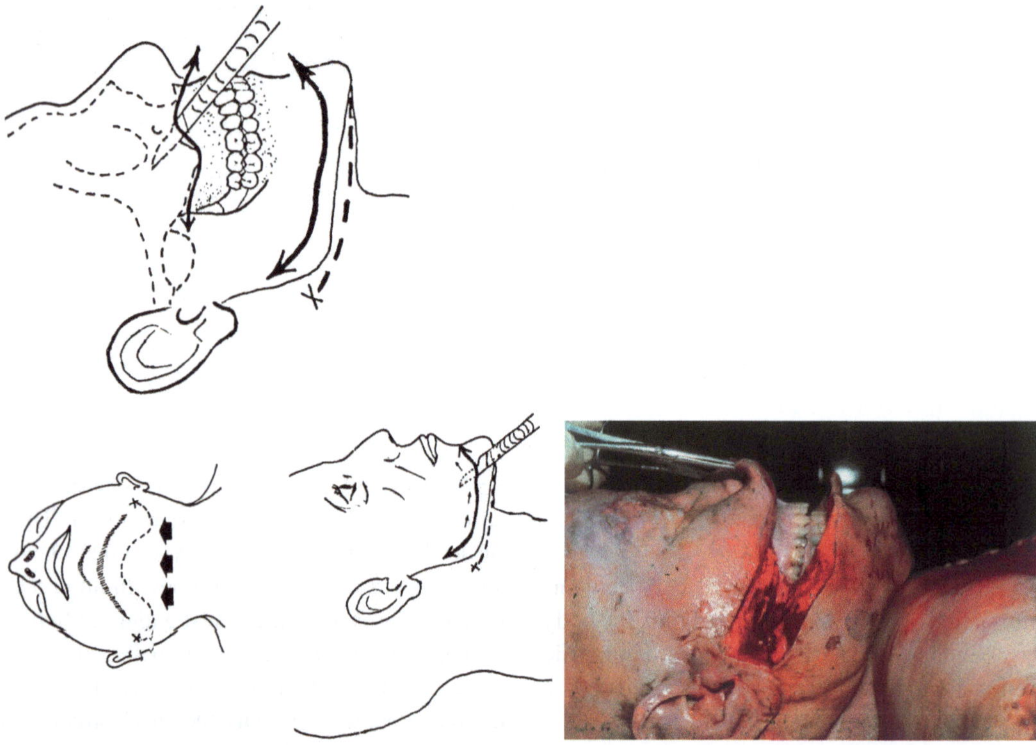

Fig. 22.1 (**a**, **b**) Orofacial autopsy technique. Incision (Courtesy of Prof. Dr. Dr. R. Endris, Mainz)

22.2.1 Technology of Oral Autopsy

Requirements for an oral autopsy are anatomic and surgical tweezers, suture holders, sutures, scissors, scalpel handle and blades, tongue clamp, curved and straight clamps, gauze swabs to clean the teeth, robust autopsy gloves, plastic bags, and photographic equipment and tapes. The basic equipment for a dental emergency examination should include an air blower, magnifier, mirrors, probes, cheek hooks, mouth gag, wedge (for the mouth), bow divider, toothbrushes, and extraction forceps for the various groups of teeth (for the upper and lower jaw).

The mouth must be opened if the investigation of the jaw is performed in situ. A special mouth pliers (mouth gag) or a mouth wedge is useful. The best results are achieved (especially in mass disasters) if the upper and lower jaw can be removed. First the jaw muscles are cut and the mandible is disarticulated in the mandibular joint. Note that removal of the jaw by a horizontal saw cut through the upper jaw parallel to the occlusion of the teeth can lead to damage to the root tips of the maxillary teeth. The removal of the upper jaw is easier if the nasal septum and the lateral sinus wall are separated with a chisel. This is known as a Le Fort I osteotomy. Afterward, the jaw parts are fixed in formalin (Grundmann and Rötzscher 1999a, b).

22.2.2 Maceration

Previous methods (potassium hydroxide, antiformin) have many deficiencies (toxicity, odor, calcification, disposal problems, etc.) (Table 22.1). After possible maceration, the obtained specimens are to be placed for several hours in a 5 % sodium hypochlorite solution (bleach).

The preparations, which can be seen in the search display, were macerated with ENZYRIM®, which has been proven for 6 years in the medical and biological field.

Table 22.1 Comparison of conventional maceration method and ENZYRIM OSA OSS

Previously (conventional maceration method)	New (ENZYRIM OSA OSS)
Rot maceration	"Fluid" or granulated
Toxic	Not toxic
Strong odors	No odor
Potassium soap developing/ chalking	Bone material is not affected
Disposal problems critical in the application	Fully biodegradable
Important bone parts under some circumstances will also be macerated under certain circumstances	Simple handling
Time needed for preparation	The bones will remain; minor mechanical work

After "*arte copia*", R. and W. Nusser/Zurich

22.2.2.1 Maceration by Enzymes

Enzymes are able to enormously accelerate the catalyzed reactions. The reaction rates often are millionfold or even billionfold times the rate of a noncatalyzed reaction. The enzymes themselves remain unchanged during these reactions (Nusser 1996). The most important factors of enzymatically controlled reactions are:

1. Solution temperature 55–60 °C (enzymes only work at temperatures between 20 and 60 °C)
2. pH 8.5 (most enzymes optimally work within a narrow pH range). In extreme cases, the enzyme is altered in its structure (denatured) and loses all catalytic features.

   As a buffer for the pH value, sodium carbonate (soda) is most suitable. The pH value is measured by an indicator stick or paper (Merck).

22.2.2.2 Standard Protocol

Solution: 2 % ENZYRIM® (granular or fluid), 1 % detergent concentrate THH (to support the enzymes, 1 l of warm water, not demineralized). The solution can be repeatedly used, but must be kept at 60 °C, otherwise it decomposes (Fig. 22.2a–d). If the solution is poured into a bath of an ultrasound unit, the 35-kHz frequency allows an accelerated maceration within 2 h. Cooled or frozen material should be kept in warm water.

If the aesthetic aspect is not crucial, the facial soft tissues can be severed starting from the mouth basis or by an oval autopsy with removal of parts of the lip and cheek. The tissue can be put back after the investigation (Grundmann and Rötzscher 1999a, b). In cases of mass disasters, transparent plastic bags with labels ensure a safe transport of body parts to the location of the examination (Grundmann and Rötzscher 1999a, b). A tooth that was dropped during maceration should be fixed into the correct position by cementum.

22.3 Documentation

In order to submit a final report, all findings must be recorded in written form and signed by the forensic odontologist (indicating the date and place of study). The use of a scheme with columns reminds the investigator to do a systematic and complete recording.

22.3.1 Written Form

The report should be typed on computer, not written by hand, in order to provide an overview. Non-odontologic information should also be included. Dentists are familiar with the odontogram and recognize the nature of the dentition in the dental chart with the aid of the fillings. Further information that otherwise is not easy to describe can be inserted into the odontogram.

22.4 Comparison by X-Ray Images

Whether X ray images are significant for the identification depends on whether X-ray images or references to endodontic and/or previous surgical procedures are recorded the patient file. The technical effort is justified by the information yield and may justify the cost. The X-ray finding is an additional forensic odontological method for the assessment. Morphological objectivity is the basis for the assessment (Stene-Johansen et al. 1992).

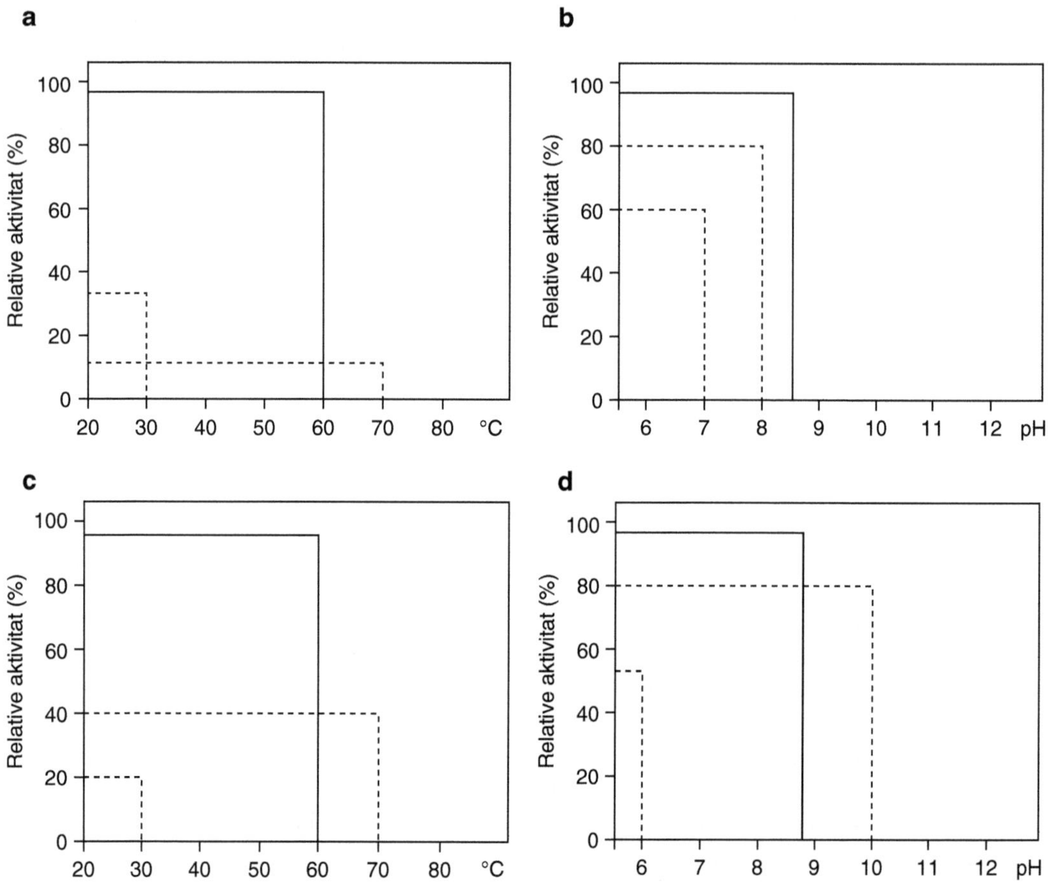

Fig. 22.2 (**a–d**) Relative activities of ENZYRIM OSS (**a**) at different temperatures; (**b**) at various pH values. Activities of ENZYRIM-OSA (**c**) at different temperatures; (**d**) at various pH values

Intravital X-ray images can be compared with PM X-ray images (secondary X-ray identification) (Rötzscher et al. 1974) (Fig. 22.3a–d).

For the radiographic documentation of findings, the following shots are recommended (Happonen et al. 1991):

- Shots of single tooth and tooth groups
- Bitewings
- Panoramic shots
- Lateral skull cephalometric (FRS)
- Anterior–posterior images of the skull, which allow an assessment of the jaw structures and the adjacent areas

Intraoral digital X-ray technology offers an opportunity for global data exchange without the use of conventional X-ray film and development (Endris 1979; Rötzscher 1991a). For head shots, Clement (1998) recommends the fixing of the skull for lateral and anterior–posterior recordings in a cephalostat (Fig. 22.4a, b). See Annex 22.1 for the input facilities for PM X-ray technology according to Clement (1998).

Because a positioning aid for the setting of the X-ray tube is not yet available, Benthaus (1997) uses the method of PM X-ray production of Du Saucey and Brown added to a film holder by Updegrave, as used in dental practice (Fig. 22.5). The film holder is equipped with a balloon catheter that is fixed in the inflated state syringe. Subsequently, a large-caliber bronchial tube is introduced intraorally and also blocked between the teeth. This balloon simulates the bite on the film holder. The catheter is attached to the plastic block connected to the holder. After positioning in the mouth, the balloon is inflated by a syringe. The film is fixed in the mouth by a second balloon at the inside of the lower jaw. If the soft tissue completely remains, the exposure times are

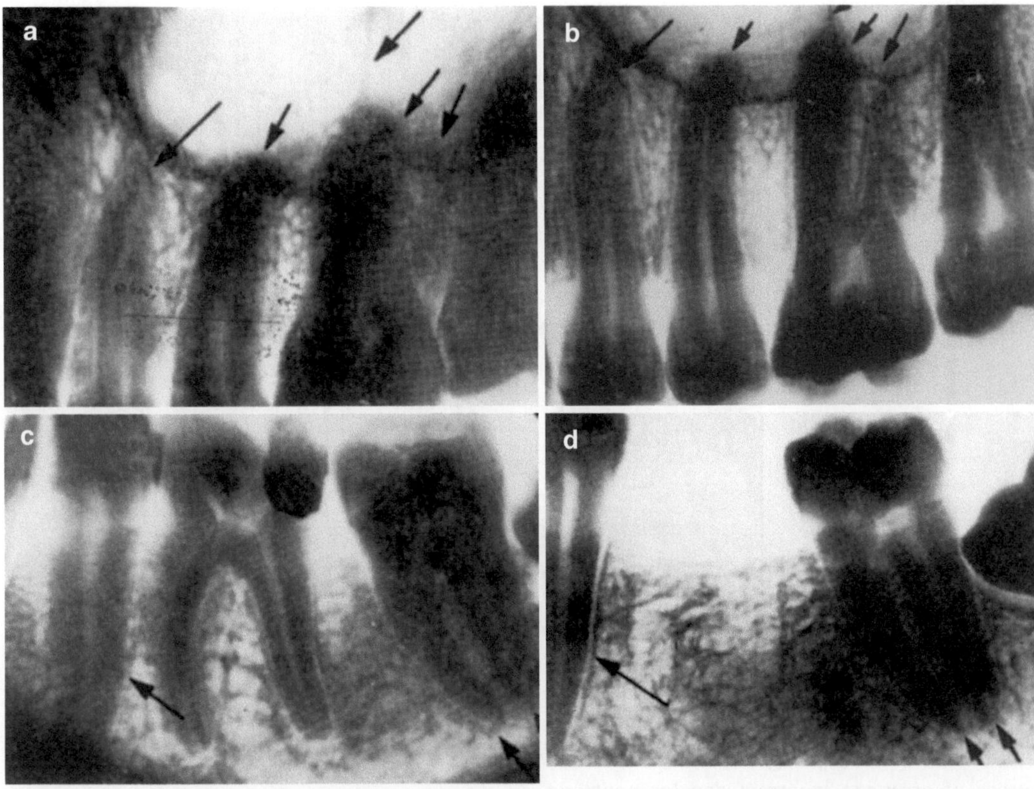

Fig. 22.3 (**a–d**) Dental identification. (**a**) Radiography of the left upper jaw; (**b**) comparison exposure of the skull of a body that was in water; (**c**) radiography of the left mandible of the missing person; (**d**) comparison exposure of the body that was in water (**b** and **d**, courtesy of Prof. Dr. R. Kluge, University Hospital Charité, Berlin)

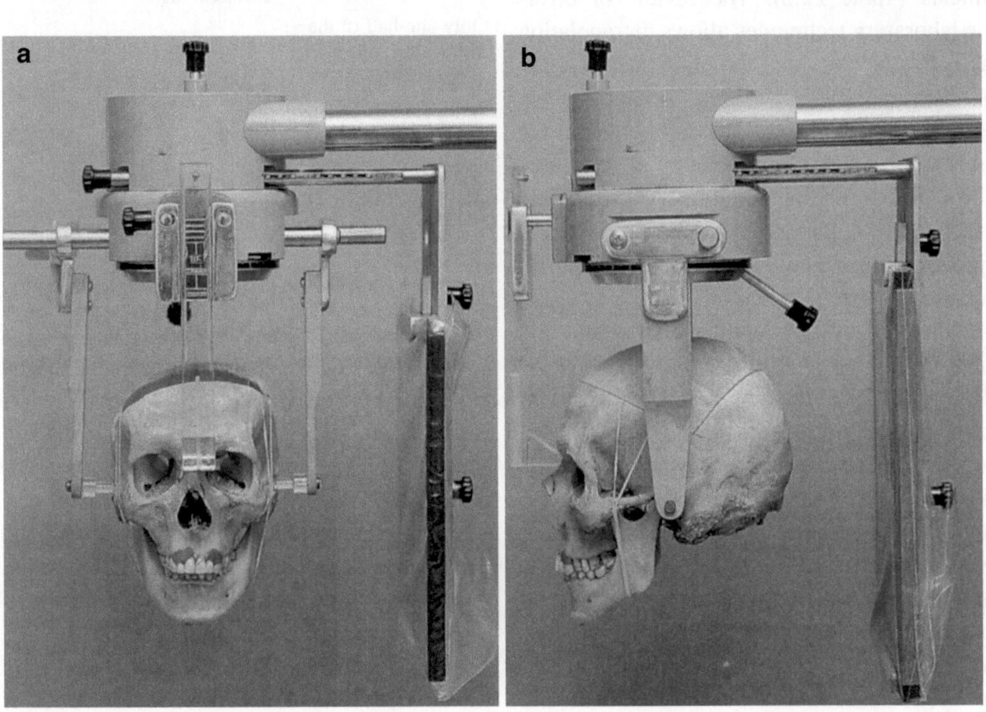

Fig. 22.4 (**a, b**) Skull in cephalostat (From craniofacial identification in forensic medicine, courtesy of Dr. J. Clement, Melbourne and A. Publishers, London)

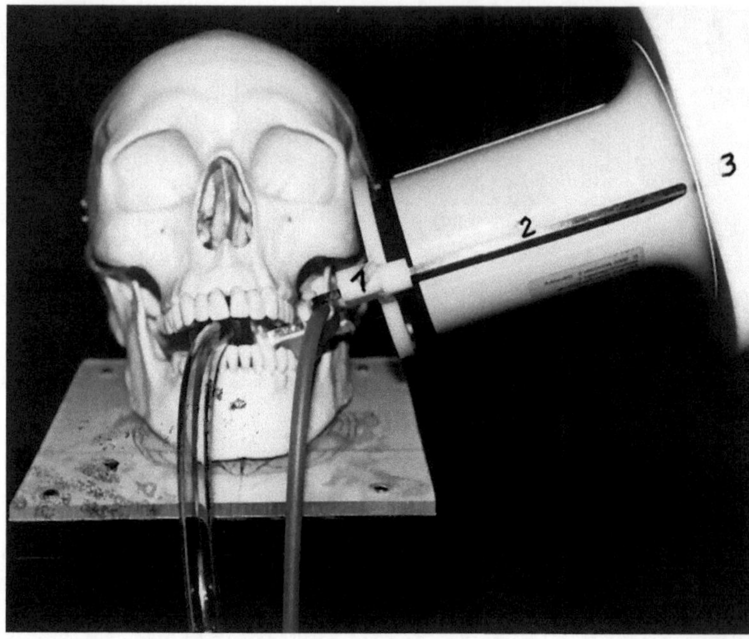

Fig. 22.5 The film holder is locked by the bite. A plastic ring (*1*) with a metal rod (*2*) is used for the X-ray tube (*3*) (Courtesy of Dr. S. Benthaus, Munster-Westfalia)

similar to those of living persons. In cases of loss of soft tissue, the exposure time is reduced, with the tube voltage remaining the same. The main sources of error are incorrect development and washing times through using incorrectly tempered solutions and contamination of the films by chemicals (Table 22.2). The review of error-prone laboratory techniques allows extrapolation from the visible failure of the film material to the cause (Benthaus 1997).

Post-mortem X-ray images can be useful for identity determination in that they can:

1. Provide information about internal structures such as root fillings or apical pathological processes (especially in fire victims with charred teeth)
2. Be directly compared with antemortem (AM) radiographs.

To prevent the destruction of evidence by mechanical stress during the course of the investigation, the objects are first fixed with an aqueous sodium silicate solution, which is easily absorbed by hydrophilic fragments. After evaporation of the water, the crystal structure of sodium silicates causes a stabilization of the fragments, which can withstand mechanical pressure. In this way, jaw bone and tooth fragments are repositioned and fixed by translucent dental wax (Benthaus and Teige 1998).

Table 22.2 Juxtaposition of causes and false processing

Errors on the film	Errors during developing
Dark spots on the film	Splashes of developer
Bright transparent strip	Uneven immersion into liquid developer
Strip	Inadequate fluid volume in the chemical trays
Only one-half of the film is developed	
Melting of the film surface	Too hot drying Too long rinsing
Yellow haze	Developer or fixer exhausted
Low-contrast film	Too short or too cold developer
Dense dark X-ray image	Too warm or over-concentrated developers

If only a few teeth or only few or no fillings are present, the X-ray comparison will be the only way to determine the identity. Therefore, AM X-ray images need to be available. In many countries, including England, dentists only rarely take X-rays of public health patients. Usually there are no requirements for X-ray examinations for the purpose of identification. The PM images should have the same projection as the AM images.

Recommendations:

1. For single identifications, X-ray images are not necessary. This will only make sense if a patient file with previous images is available.

2. If a body is unidentified and the police urge proceeding to the burial, then either the jaw should be removed or X-ray images should be taken.
3. In cases of mass disasters, images of the molars or bitewings should be taken. If the jaw is not removed during autopsy, it may be difficult to produce the images at a later time. Bitewing images are often included in the patient's file.

Computer-based comparisons of AM and PM bitewing images digitized by reducing image histograms with standard deviations (SD) of the gray tones show existing fillings that are statistically significant (especially plastic fillings), more clearly than the typical X-ray technique (Aagaard et al. 1991; Borrman and Grondahl 1990; Depenau et al. 1987; Prevost et al. 1990; Sainio et al. 1990; Wenzel and Andersen 1994).

22.5 Photographic Comparison

Because of the variety of details, a single photo can provide high-quality information. In general, black/white photos (Endris 1979) are sufficient, but color photos are preferable. All photographs must be numbered in order to avoid errors. A photograph status should consist of five shots.

In autopsies of unknown dead bodies, the following images are recommended:

1. Before removing the jaw, radiographs of the head:
   - 1.1. Image of the head *en face*
   - 1.2. Image of the head in profile
   - 1.3. Upper and lower jaw in occlusion
   - 1.4. Upper and lower jaw separated
2. After the autopsy, photographic documentation of the jaws:
   - 2.1. Frontal images of the upper and lower jaw asservates in occlusion
   - 2.2. A top shot of the upper and lower jaw

     For example, the supervision of the mandible from the left side is shown in Fig. 22.6.
3. In cases of removable prosthetic dentures:
   - 3.1. Image without a prosthesis
   - 3.2. Image with prosthesis

     This type of evidence is convincing. After maceration, the jaws (evidence objects) are photographed for demonstration in any necessary investigation (Fig. 22.7a, b). If the picture of the upper and macerated mandibular is taken from only the frontal viewpoint, important findings may be overlooked. The existing partial denture (model cast) is clearly recognizable only in the lateral view of the upper and lower jaw in occlusion and in additional supervision images of the lower jaw from the right and from the back (dorsal) (Fig. 22.8a, b). Unusual dental work has enough characteristics; even a few images are sufficient. *Example*: Cover denture = telescopic full denture prosthesis = tooth supported restoration with telescoping primary crowns on the abutment teeth 33, 43 (Fig. 22.9a, b).

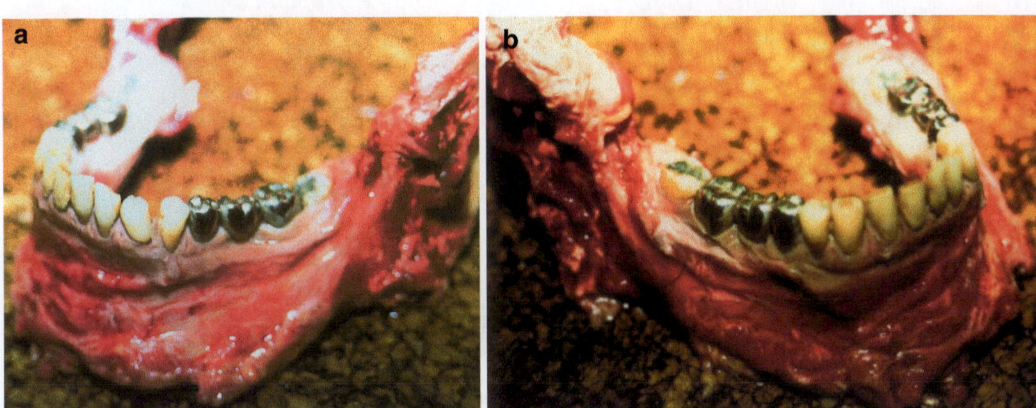

Fig. 22.6 (**a**, **b**) Supervision of the mandible from the left side and laterally from the right

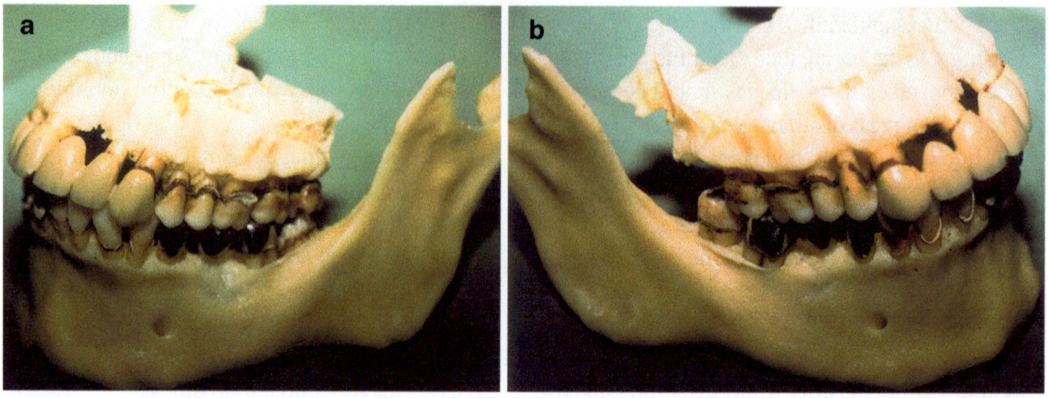

Fig. 22.7 (**a**, **b**) View of a macerated upper and lower jaw in occlusion of (**a**) left side; (**b**) right side

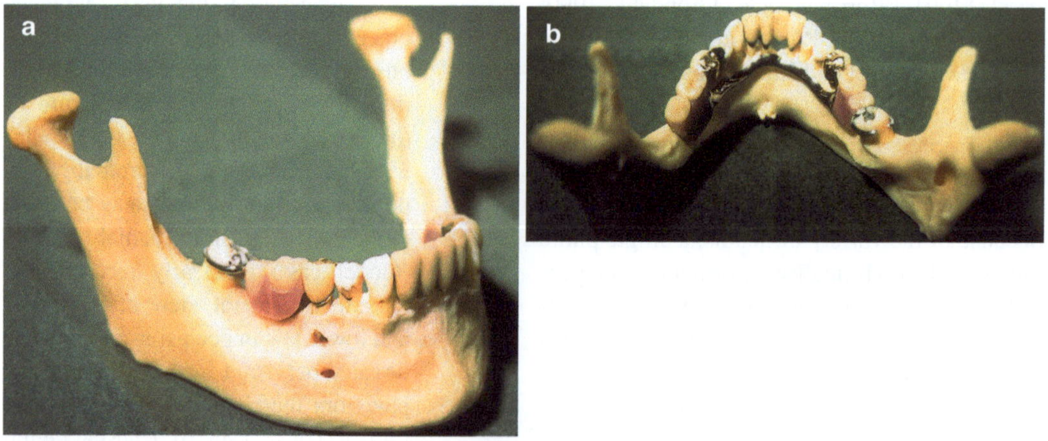

Fig. 22.8 (**a**, **b**) Lower jaw from the right side and from the back (dorsal); the partial denture (model cast) is visible

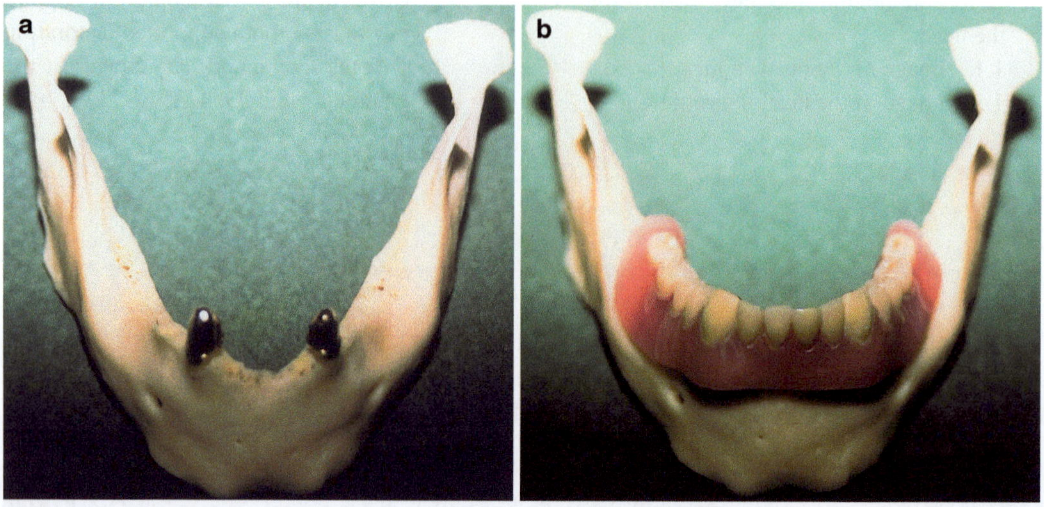

Fig. 22.9 (**a**) Telescopic primary crowns on the abutment teeth 33, 43; (**b**) cover denture (Courtesy of Dr. Dr. C. Grundmann, Moers)

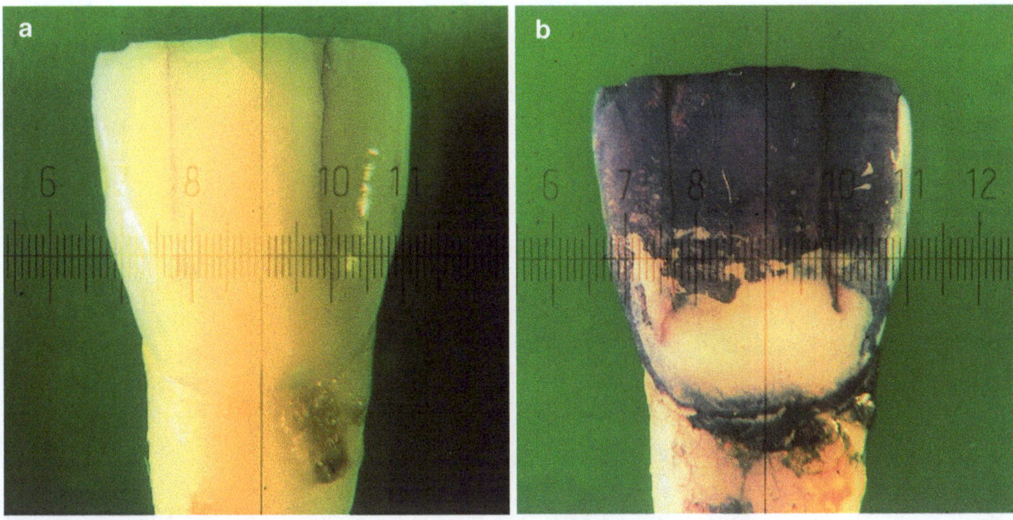

Fig. 22.10 (**a**) Vestibular view of a front tooth, incisor. (**b**) The same after staining. The vestibular filling has become clearly visible

4. Detailed pictures and clips are recommended for:
   - 4.1. Tooth position anomalies
   - 4.2. Dental anomalies
   - 4.3. Tooth diseases (e.g., caries)
   - 4.4. Special fillings
   - 4.5. Fixed restorations (e.g., crowns, bridges, combined dentures)
   - 4.6. Traumatic injuries (e.g., fractures, fracture lines in teeth and jaw bones)

     The localization of tooth-colored filling materials is difficult. Fillings may be overlooked or not visible in photographs (Fig. 22.10a, b). The translucency and color characteristics do not allow a reliable diagnosis of fillings. With the help of the melt-dyeing method (Fig. 22.11a, b), a simple localization of very small plastic waste is possible. Confusion with enamel cracks is avoided (Benthaus 1998; Benthaus and Teige 1998).
5. The enamel-dyeing method:
   - 5.1. The teeth are cleaned with water and toothbrush. Subsequently, the clinical crown (after photographic securing of the native preparation) is etched with 35 % phosphoric acid for 2 min.
   - 5.2. Next, the tooth is dyed with blue ink as an indicator.

     The color pigments are absorbed by the roughened enamel surface, but they drip off from smooth plastic surfaces and bonding residues. The extension of the fillings now can be evaluated and documented.

22.6 Comparison of AM and PM: INTERPOL Form

If the INTERPOL AM and PM forms are filled out as accurately as possible, the comparison begins. Both sheets have the same shape but different colors, which is of great advantage and makes a comparison easier (the AM form is yellow and the PM form is pink). See Annexes 21.1, 21.2, 21.3, and 21.4. The sheets are placed side by side and compared tooth by tooth. Another possibility is the direct comparison of AM and PM radiographs. Comparison and assessment are the basis for the expertise of forensic odontologists.

The validity of the forensic odontologic comparison is to evaluate the congruent odontological information. The dentists are not responsible for the identification, the police and the Identification Commission (IdCo) who evaluate all details are responsible. Incorrect conclusions by self-appointed experts are significant risks.

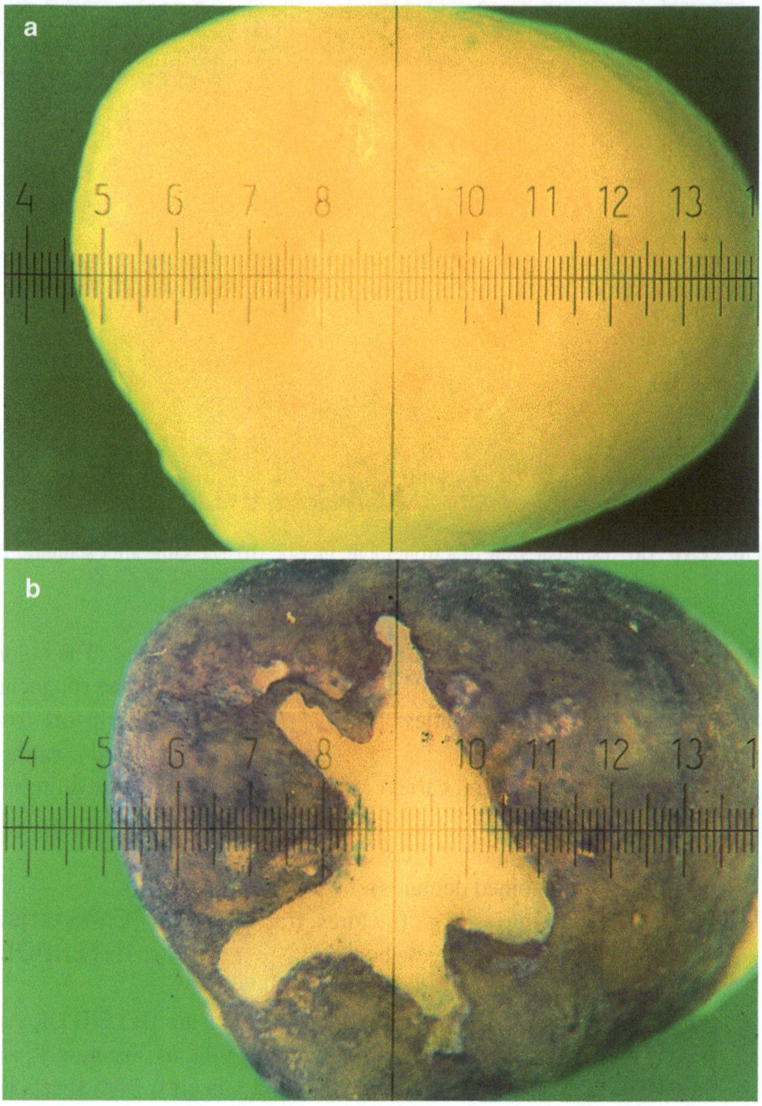

Fig. 22.11 (**a**) Molar (occlusal view). A filling is not recognizable. (**b**) The same molar after staining. The occlusal filling is now visible (Courtesy of Dr. S. Benthaus, Munster-Westfalia)

22.7 Identity Exclusion

Tore Solheim

In certain cases, an identity cannot be excluded, even though the AM and PM information do not match, e.g., if a tooth was extracted at an earlier time but this tooth is present in the unidentified body (or a filling was made and the tooth of the body does not have any fillings). If the identity is excluded in that way, the authorities must be informed. But it is also possible that there is no scientific explanation for nonmatching features (Fig. 22.12).

The following is an authentic case of a flight accident in Norway. Most fillings match; however, the vestibular (buccal) filling on tooth 16 (see arrow), which was indicated by the treating dentist, was not found on the body. Inaccurate file management may be the cause. In contrast, the vestibular filling on tooth 46 (see arrow) found on the corpse was not in the patient's file.

1. If the data was correctly transferred from the patient file to the AM form, but errors cannot be excluded, the question is whether the data from the patient file is correct. If the treating dentist did enter a wrong tooth, this is not

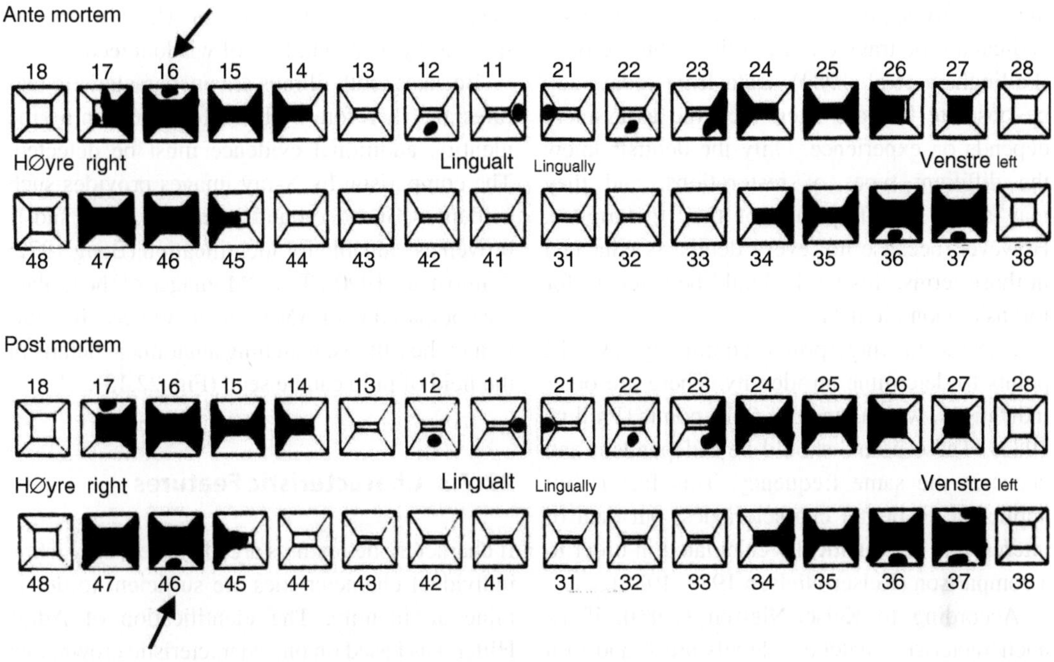

Fig. 22.12 AM to PM comparison of a Norwegian odontogram

significant for the billing, but these errors do inhibit an identification by computer. The expert must always evaluate the matching and the nonmatching results. In such cases, the forensic odontologist is advised to contact the treating dentist.

2. Often, treatments entered in the patient file are exclusively those that were performed by the treating dentist. In that case, the descriptions of previous treatments are missing. Therefore, it is important to know how old the described treatments are.
3. If the PM findings are correctly recorded, the AM findings may be faulty. The transfer from the patient file and X-rays to the AM INTERPOL form, if available, are easy to control. For this reason, all radiographs and the original card files are given to the forensic odontologists in order to transfer them to the INTERPOL AM form. This procedure is common, e.g., in Norway.
4. The next question that must be asked is whether the documentation of evidence on the body is faulty. If X-ray images are available or the jaws could be secured, a check is simple. Therefore, jaw removal is recommended.
5. What remains are the cases in which the nonmatching findings cannot be explained and the identity can be declared as excluded.

If two forensic odontologists have examined a corpse and compared their results, it is probably a safe conclusion that the recording of the findings is correct and a reinspection is not required.

22.7.1 Matching Features

All matching odontological information in the AM and PM form must be recorded. At this time, it must be considered that tactical (nonodontologic) information is not included. The forensic odontologist is supposed to evaluate only the odontological information. The investigators and forensic scientists are responsible for all other information and must evaluate all information for a definitive identification.

How must congruent odontological data be assessed? The difficulty with statistics is that they usually apply only to a specific population and cannot be transferred to other ethnic groups (Fellingham et al. 1984). Data from today may be obsolete 5 years later, then the assessment depends on experience. Only the dentists know the different types of restorations, and they may assess the frequency of their occurrence. However, because not every dentist is educated in those terms, this work should be reserved for forensic odontologists.

Experts in fingerprints commonly use 12 points to determine an identity. There are other indications, with a range of 6–16 points (Phillips 1983). These points should be independent and occur in the same frequency. This fact is not applicable to dental characteristics, but data of interest can be statistically calculated in order to a comparison (Keiser-Nielsen 1977, 1980).

According to Keiser-Nielsen (1980), if 12 uncharacteristic matching details are found in a dentition, the possibility of repetition with 1:225 million is small and an identity can be concluded. Phillips and Scheepers (1990) asserted that, if seven odontological congruent features are matching, the probability of erroneous conclusions is negligible. According to another study, six coincident features are sufficient to reduce the probability of erroneous conclusions to 1:100,000 (Eastwood et al. 1984).

22.7.2 Uncharacteristic Features

It is difficult to determine the exact frequency of a feature. An attempt was made to quantify the frequency of features, but it is not relevant whether the features are found in 30 % or 60 % of cases if no reliable information is given. It is more important whether features occur in 1 % or 50 %, of cases, which constitutes a significant difference to the assessment. Many features on the teeth are so common that they are found in 50 % of a population. Such features are considered as uncharacteristic (Keiser-Nielsen 1977).

In young people, there are often unspecific fillings (Gustafson and Johanson 1963); fillings on the mesial, occlusal, and/or distal tooth surface are uncharacteristic features that are not meaningful for a determination. This also applies for healthy teeth and lack of wisdom teeth.

Because tooth fillings are uncharacteristic features and therefore no basis for determining the identity, additional evidence must be detected. The comparison by X-ray images provides such evidence (Gustafson and Johanson 1963) and is proven as valuable for identification (Bang 1972; Sainio et al. 1990). Two PM images of the molars are compared with AM bitewing images. In addition to the fillings, matching anatomical details in the field of pulp can be seen (Fig. 22.13).

22.7.3 Characteristic Features

If characteristic features are identified, only a few individual characteristics are sufficient to determine an identity. The identification of Adolf Hitler was based on one characteristic crown, one bridge, and information regarding periodontal reductions (Sognnaes and Strøm 1973).

How characteristic fillings or combinations of fillings are may be calculated as a "measure of uniqueness" according to an epidemiological population study (Phillips and Scheepers 1990). Some fillings (composites, ceramics, etc.) and filling materials, such as gold, can be seen as characteristic; additionally, prosthetic work such as crowns and bridges can be characteristic because of the materials and techniques used. Often, special details in this work are evident to make the work more characteristic.

22.8 Assessment

The assessment is the most difficult part of identification and requires all of the knowledge and experience of a forensic odontologist. Some experts claim to determine the identity solely on the basis of their experience. This is not sufficient. The conclusions must be justified not only for themselves but also to convince others (Dahlberg 1957). In order to draw correct inferences, the error probability must be calculated, i.e., for the case that another person has the same tooth features. If the characteristics are independent

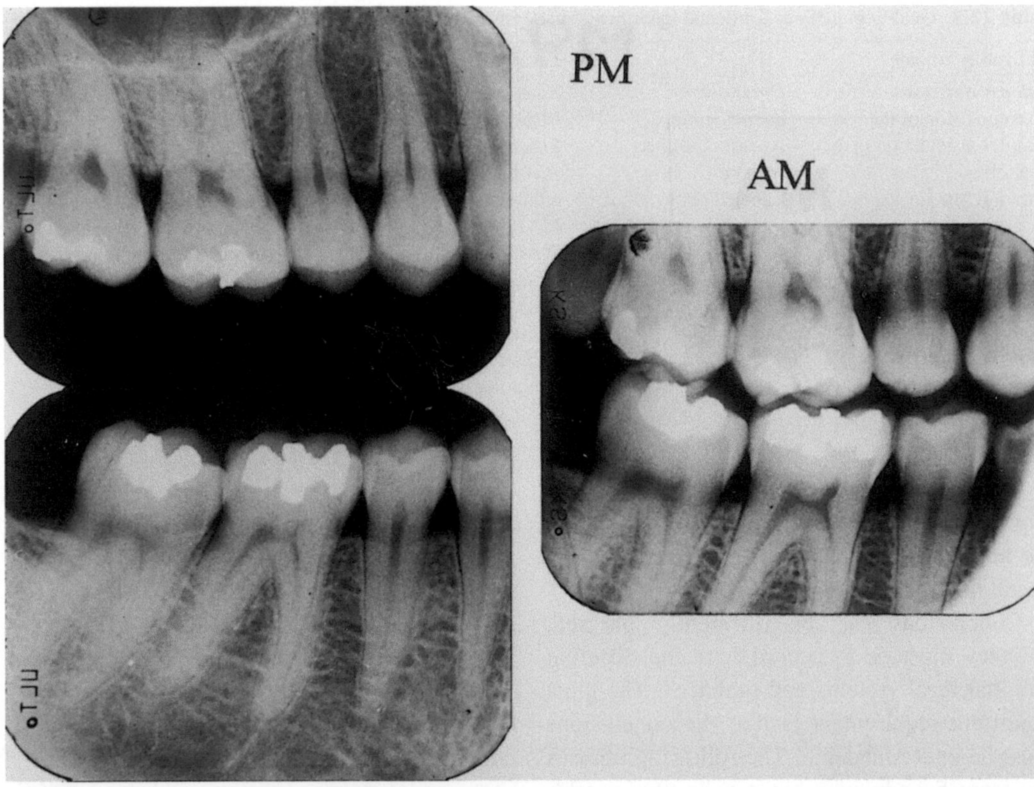

Fig. 22.13 Comparison of a Norwegian odontogram (bitewing)

from each other, this corresponds to a probability = probability 1× of a probability 2×, 3× probability probability *n* (Eastwood et al. 1984).

Difficulties may arise if the probabilities are not known. They can be estimated, but this is not reliable and cannot be a basis for an assessment. A combination with a probability of, e.g., less than 1:10,000, can be regarded as a definitive statement. An experienced dentist knows the frequency of various restorations, and, therefore, is able to propose that a certain restoration was made in a maximum of one or two people, for instance. The correct frequency of course is unknown but could be 1:7. The probability that this specific combination of characteristics also exists in another person is less than 1:1,000. The specified frequency can be used to estimate (better than the really vague statement) and should always be the basis for conclusions.

The probability of identity should always be estimated. It depends on the number of applicable characteristics and their frequency in the population. Rules about the minimum number of necessary characteristics do not exist, because it is linked with the frequency; congruence in a few rare characteristics is more useful than congruence in many common characteristics. Most features can be difficult to quantify (Rösing 1999). Benthaus et al. (1999) developed and listed quality guidelines for dental identification (Table 22.3).

22.8.1 Conclusions from the Comparison

After odontological comparison and evaluation, the dentist must outline the results to the police and IdCo in order to let them know the matching odontological features. The phrasing must be precise and obvious and contain exclusively ondontological findings. The odontological conclusion can only be a statement about the scientific probability of an identity. The final identification

Table 22.3 Quality guidelines for dental identification (Benthaus et al. 1999)

Obligatory findings		Facultative findings	
Autopsy diagnosis	*Diagnosis documentation*	*Assessment in written form*	*National findings form*
Size/condition of the samples articulation in the final bite	Anatomical chart with key	Medical history	Impression
Intraoral bite image	Labeled photo status	Size and condition of samples	Palatography
Disarticulation	INTERPOL form	AM findings with source citation/source	Maceration
Numerical results		PM findings	X-ray microanalysis
Location and size of fillings		PM radiographic findings (comparative)	Macroscopic examination
Prosthetics		Result	Special radiographic examination
Materials		"Certainty factor"	"Slice interposition"
Photo status		Signature of two forensic odontologists	DNA examinations
X-ray survey/single image			Contrast-medium radiology

happens later. The dentist is not responsible for the final identification, the dentist only provides dental findings.

Conclusions can be differently phrased, but they must be in accord with the different national legal systems and practices. The most important requirement is that the conclusions must be understandable. The following phrases are from Scandinavia, but can be used worldwide and are recommended by INTERPOL (Keiser-Nielsen 1977):

1. Odontologically excluded identity: "identity excluded"

   One or more nonmatching features
2. Odontologically possible identity: "identity possible"

   Identical characteristics occur in several persons with the ratio <1:100, there are only few comparable details, and several persons have the same characteristics; usually between one and six individual characteristics.
3. Odontologically probable identity: "identity probable"

   There is a chance that another person has the same characteristics, there are many comparable details with the ratio <1:1,000; 7–12 individual features.
4. Odontologically established identity: "identity established"

   There are several comparable details with the ratio <1:10,000, it is hardly possible that someone else has similar characteristics to be considered as a sole identification; more than 12 congruent features.

The task of the forensic odontologist is to phrase and to document conclusions that are understood by the other members of the IdCo. All relevant features of the result, not only matching details, must be described (Keiser-Nielsen 1980; Solheim et al. 1992). The assessment of the comparative data is the most difficult part of the odontological identification (Solheim 1998).

22.9 Final Identification

After the analysis of all congruent and non-congruent characteristics, a decision must be made regarding whether it is the very same person. This question must be answered without any doubt. Both the authorities and the relatives have to get a clear yes or no with regard to the identity. If doubts exist, how to eliminate them must be discussed. If this is not possible, further investigations must be performed. In cases where doubt cannot be eliminated, a decision that the body cannot be identified must be reached.

If the list of the missing persons (e.g., in a flight accident) is 100 % correct, a body can also be identified by exclusion, that means that this body without doubt is none of the other missing persons on the list. Although the congruent characteristics are not sufficient, the identity can be established. For the final identification, the identification chart should be used. The identification chart allows a summary. In the final stage, the chart can also be used as an elimination graph. If not enough congruent information is available, the identity can be excluded because the characteristics are not matching those of the other people on the list. This requires that the list be correct.

22.10 Mass Disasters

An incident with more than five victims is defined as a great accident (Fig. 22.14a, b). If there are more than 100 victims, it is a large disaster or a mass disaster. The dead cannot be laid into a mass grave before the bodies are identified (Keiser-Nielsen 1963).

In case of a flight or ship accident with 100 or more deaths and little time and few experienced personnel for the identification, a team of forensic experts as part of the DVI teams should be assigned at the site of the accident (Mason 1986; Sopher 1986).

22.10.1 General Considerations

The PM forensic odontological investigation should start at the place where the body was found. It cannot be assumed that the police recognize all dental remains in the surrounds of a burnt and maimed body (Gilliland et al. 1986).

Furthermore, rescue forces are not always aware of the significance of a single dropped

a

Missing person	Body-Nr. 1	2	3	4	5	Conclusion
A	IP					IP identity probable
B				IA		IA identity ascertained
C						
D		IA				IA identity ascertained
E						

b

Missing person	Body-Nr. 1	2	3	4	5	Conclusion
A	IP					IP identity probable
B				IA		IA identity ascertained
C						
D		IA				IA identity ascertained
E						

Fig. 22.14 (**a**) Identification chart (Norway). Five missing persons and five bodies. For No. 1, identity can be regarded as probable (assigned to A). Bodies Nos. 2 and 4 were identified (IA). Only where the identity has been established may the other categories not be filled. (**b**) After the final identification of the bodies (such as Person A), the identification chart can be used for elimination (exclusion); thus, body No. 5 must be missing person E and body No. 3 is missing person C

tooth, jaw fragment, or dental prosthesis (Mason 1986). If the forensic odontologist is consulted after the body is removed to the morgue, this often leads to the loss of remains of the dentition, because they were lost at the place the body was found or during transport (Sopher 1986). The removal of remains of a body should be performed by an IdCo (Beyer et al. 1966; Hooft et al. 1989; Keiser-Nielsen 1963; Solheim et al. 1992; Stene-Johansen et al. 1992), as is routine, e.g., in Scandinavia (Solheim et al. 1992).

Usually, all victims of a disaster are autopsied to determine not only the identity but also the cause of death. The necessity of this is still under discussion (Hooft et al. 1989).

22.10.2 Operational Readiness of the Identification Commission (IdCo)

The members of the IdCo must always be accessible and available because they might be deployed all over the world in cases of disaster. The team members must be prepared for missions in foreign countries and have valid passports, global insurance coverage and all required vaccinations. They also must be aware that the operation may last for an unknown number of days and might be under adverse conditions and temperatures (Clark 1992, 1994).

22.10.2.1 Operation at Home

IdCos are divided into two groups. The first group, the "home team," provides file cards and all other required documents for the AM DVI form. The home team is responsible for the transfer of these data to the second group, the so-called "go team" (Warnick 1995) or "away team" (Clark 1994; Solheim et al. 1992).

Possible problems for the home team (Clark 1992) are:

The relatives of the alleged victim do not know the name of the treating dentist or give a false name.

The treating dentist has no treatment records.

The team cannot reach the treating dentist.

Different time zones complicate making contact.

Because of long distances, treatment records cannot be brought to the place of the incident within 10–12 h.

The victim is a foreigner and no or poor dental records exist.

22.10.2.2 Operations at the Place of the Accident

The away team (go team) of the IdCo is in place at the location of the incident and the forensic odontologists provide dental examinations of each victim. They prepare the PM DVI Form (pink) for comparison with the AM DVI Form of the missing persons (Clark 1992). In order to accelerate the comparison of PM and AM findings, computer programs were developed that sort the findings (Solheim et al. 1992; Stene-Johansen et al. 1992). Nowadays the Danish Plass-Data program is in use.

Clark (1994) reviewed 54 disaster reports (1951–1988) where, in 43 % of the cases, the odontological characteristics lead to an identification. The range of 6.25–91.6 % point to the difficulties in practice: 6.25 % (112 victims) were Asians without dental recordings, in 91.6 %, dental recordings were available (70 victims, 2 exceptions) (McCarty et al. 1987).

22.11 Final Remarks

Only a precise documentation of dental findings and treatments with consideration of retention periods allows a dental identification of living and dead persons. In case of a disaster, it is important to establish a collection point for dental evidence at the earliest possible time. The AM forms should always list the treating dentist (the use of INTERPOL forms is optimal).

In victims of different nationalities, it is recommended that an experienced forensic odontologist of the concerned nationality be consulted, who communicates with the dentists in the home country of the victims. Dental treatment records often are incomplete, with a deficient status praesens, and sometimes right or left side are confused (mostly within the groups of front teeth, premolars, and molars).

In our experience as forensic ondontologists, good identification aids such as prostheses or plaster models of the jaws were only rarely available, more frequently available were dental X-ray images. For an effective stomalologic identification, jaw removal is always advised (Heidemann 1988; Hunger et al. 1992). Note that the ethnic, cultural, or religious origin of victims must always be considered and respected.

Annex 22.1

Input Equipment for X-Ray Equipment for Application of Postmortem (PM) X-Ray Technology

(From cranio-facial identification in forensic medicine, with permission from Dr. J. Clement, Melbourne, Arnold Publishers, London)

Radiographic exposure factors/section/bone intact body region

		mAs	kVp	mAs	kVp
Calvarium	Anteroposterior/posteroanterior	20	70	8	70
	P-A ↓ 25°	16	70	6	70
	Townes (A-P ↓ 3.5°)	16	70	6	70
	Lateral	16	70	6	70
	Anterosuperior	16	70	6	70
Facial bones	Posteroanterior	20	70	8	70
	P-A ↓ 25′ (orbits etc.)	16	70	6	70
	Waters (P-A; 35″ ↑ head tilt)	20	70	8	70
	Reverse Townes	16	70	6	70
	Inferosuperior	12	70	4	70
	Lateral	8	70	3	70
Maxillae (with teeth)	Posteroanterior	20	70	8 (4)[b]	70
	Lateral	8	70	3 (1.5)	70
	Waters	20	70	N/A	N/A
	Inferosuperior	12	70	3 (1.5)	70
Mandible (with teeth)	Posteroanterior	16	70	3 (1.5)	70
	Lateral	8	70	1.5 (0.75)	70
	Lateral oblique[a]	8	65	1.5 (0.75)	65
Teeth (individually)	Dental X-ray unit, 40-cm focus–film distance, D-speed dental film	N/A	N/A	1–2	70

[a]All exposure factors, except lateral oblique mandible, dissected maxillae/mandible, and teeth, assume modern radiographic equipment, 100-cm focus–film distance, buckly/stationary grid, and regular green-emitting intensifying screens. Factors are for *guidance only* and will vary according to variations of equipment, film types, and intensifying screen speed/sensitivity (if used)
[b]Bracketed values are for use with a dental radiographic unit and dental/occlusal film, D speed

References

Aagaard E, Donslund C, Wenzel A, Sewerin I (1991) Performance for obtaining maximal gain from a program for digital subtraction radiography. Scand J Dent Res 99:166–172

Bang G (1972) Factors of importance in dental identification: five case reports. Forensic Sci 1:91–102

Benthaus S (1997) Systematik der Röntgenidentifikation – Praktisches Vorgehen und neue Hilfsmittel. Arch Kriminol Bd 200(3/4):95–106

Benthaus S (1998) Forensische Odontologie in Deutschland – Eine Fachdisziplin für den Spezialisten ? Quintessenz 49:411–416

Benthaus S, Teige K (1998) Ist die Identifikation stark verbrannter Leichen aussichtslos? Arch Kriminol Bd 201,1 u.2:31–38

Benthaus S, DuChesne A, Brinkmann B (1998) A new technique for the post mortem detection of tooth coloured dental restorations. Int J Legal Med 111: 157–159

Benthaus S, Rötzscher K, Brinkmann B, Knell B, Waes van H, Bonnetain JC, Hutt JM (1999) Qualitätsrichtlinien

bei der zahnärztlichen Identifikation unbekannter Leichen. Definition eines international verbindlichen Standards. Newsl AKFOS 6,3:56–65
Beyer G, Materne H, Schröder R (1966) Katastrophenkommission im Einsatz. Kriminalistik 20: 241–248
Borrman H, Grondahl HG (1990) Accuracy in establishing identity by means of intraoral radiographs. J Forensic Odontostomatol 8:31–36
Clark DH (1986) Dental identification problems in the Abu Dhabi air accident. Am J Forensic Med Pathol 7:317–321
Clark DH (1989) Postmortem dental identification in mass disasters. PhD thesis, University of London, London
Clark DH (1992) Practical forensic odontology. Wright, Butterworth-Heinemann Ltd. Oxford, pp 111–127
Clark DH (1994) An analysis of the value of forensic odontology in ten mass disasters. Int Dent J 44:241–250
Clement JG (1998) Guides for post mortem cranial radiography. Appendix VI. In: Clement JG, Ranson DL (eds) Craniofacial identification in forensic medicine. Arnold, London/Sydney/Auckland, pp 287–289
Dahlberg AA (1957) Criteria of individuality in the teeth. J Forensic Sci 2:388–399
Depenau J, Hansen A, Kirkegaard BB, Knudsen FB, Lassen AS, Nielsen PS, Specht M (1987) Substraktion af intraorale röntgenbilleder. Aalborg Universitetscenter, Aalborg
Eastwood BA, Fletscher J, Laird W (1984) The value of dental restorations in post-mortem identification. J Forensic Sci Soc 24:569–576
Endris R (1979) Praktische Forensische Odonto-Stomatologie, Kriminalistik, Wissenschaft & Praxis. Kriminalistik, Heidelberg, S 203ff, 242ff, 233ff
Engel H (1995) Organisation der Personenidentifikation in der IDKO des BKA. AKFOS Newsl 2,3: 81,82
Fellingham SA, von Kotze TJ, Nash JM (1984) Probabilities of dental characteristics. J Forensic Odontostomatol 2:45–52
Gilliland MGF, McDonough ET, Fossum RM, Dowling GP, Besant-Matthews PE, Petty CS (1986) Disaster planning for air crashes. A retrospective analysis of Delta Airlines flight 191. Am J Forensic Med Pathol 7(4):308–316
Grundmann C, Rötzscher K (1999a) Zur Sektionstechnik im orofazialen Bereich. Die Mazeration mit Enzyrim. Rechtsmedizin 9:115–117
Grundmann C, Rötzscher K (1999b) Autopsy techniques in the orofacial area (part 1). Maceration using Enzyrim (part 2). News For Odont ASFO 18(2):4–5
Gustafson G, Johanson G (1963) The value of certain characteristics in dental identification. Acta Odont Scand 21:367–389
Happonen RP, Laaksoonen H, Wallis A, Tammisalo T, Stimson PG (1991) Use of the orthopantomographs in forensic identification. Am J Forensic Med Pathol 12(1):59–63
Heidemann D (1988) Identifizierungsarbeiten in Ramstein. Zahnarztl Mitt 78(19):2116–2123
Hooft PJ, Noji EK, van de Voorde HP (1989) Fatality management in mass casualty incidents. Forensic Sci Int 40:3–14
Hühn H, Gärtner F (1974) Identifizierung unkenntlicher Leichen mit Hilfe der forensischen Odontologie. ZWR 83:197–201
Hunger H, Scholz D, Lessig R (1992) Untersuchungen bei Massenunfällen in der ehemaligen DDR. Erfahrungen und Probleme der Leipziger Arbeitsgruppe "Identifikation". Beitr Ger Med Bd L: 261–266
Keiser-Nielsen S (1963) Dental investigation in mass disasters. J Dent Res 42:303–311
Keiser-Nielsen S (1977) Dental identification: certainty and probability. Forensic Sci 9:87–97
Keiser-Nielsen S (1980) Person identification by means of the teeth, preface. V. J Wright Sons Ltd, Bristol, pp 1–114
Mason JK (1986) Death and disaster (editorial). Forensic Sci Int 14:49–57
McCarty VO, Sohn AP, Ritzlin RS, Gauthier JH (1987) Scene investigation, identification, and victim examination following the accident of Galaxy 203: disaster preplanning does work. J Forensic Sci 32:983–987
Midda M (1975) The role of dental identification in mass disasters. J Ir Dent Assoc 20:51–62
Morlang WM (1986) Mass disaster management update. J Calif Dent Assoc 14:49–57
Nusser W (1996) ENZYRIM, arte copia, R. + W.Nusser, Muschellenstraße 41, Zürich
Phillips VM (1983) The uniqueness of amalgam restorations for identification. J Forensic Odontostomatol 1:33–38
Phillips VM, Scheepers CF (1990) A comparison between fingerprint and dental concordant characteristics. J Forensic Odontostomatol 8:17–20
Prevost AP, Forest P, Tanguay R, Degrandmont P (1990) Radiopacity of glasionomer dental materials. Oral Surg Oral Med Oral Pathol 70:231–235
Rösing FW (1999) Standards für die anthropologische Identifikation lebender Personen auf Grund von Bilddokumenten. Grundlagen, Kriterien und Verfahrensregeln für Gutachten. Rechtsmedizin 9: 152–154
Rötzscher K (1991a) Die Radio-Visio-Graphie im Einsatz mit Computer-Systemen. Identifikation durch Datenspeicherung und Datenübertragung. Internationales Symposium über Massenkatastrophen, Poster S48, 70.Jahrestagung Dtsch Ges Rechtsmed, Lausanne, 10–14 Sept 1991
Rötzscher K (1991b) Die Internationale und Interdisziplinäre Zusammenarbeit auf dem Gebiet der Forensischen Odonto-Stomatologie,Vortrag S16,70. Jahrestagung Dtsch Ges Rechtsmed. Internationales Symposium über Massenkatastrophen, Lausanne, 10–14 Sept 1991
Rötzscher K, Mende S, Kötzschke R (1974) Zur Personenidentifizierung an Hand stomatologischer Merkmale. Stomat DDR 24:162–167
Sainio P, Syrjänen SM, Kolmakow S (1990) Positive identification of victims by comparison of ante-mortem and post-mortem dental radiographs. J Forensic Odontostomatol 8:11–16

Sognnaes RF, Strøm F (1973) The odontological identification of Adolf Hitler. Definitive documentation by X-rays, interrogations and autopsy findings. Acta Odont Scand 31:43–69

Solheim T (1992) The Alexander L. Kielland disaster. Politiavdelingssef Knut Berglia Kriminalpolitisentralen, Oslo. In: Clark DH (ed) Practical forensic odontology. p 126

Solheim T (1998) 10.10. Vergleich AM-PM-INTERPOL-Formblatt. 10.11 Beurteilung. In: Leopold D Identifikation unbekannter Toter. Schmidt-Römhild, Lübeck, S 419–427

Solheim T, Lorentsen M, Sundnes PK, Bang G, Bremnes L (1992) The "Scandinavian Star" ferry disaster 1990 – a challenge to forensic odontology. Int J Legal Med 104:339–345

Sopher IM (1986) Kap.6: Gesichtspunkte für das Vorgehen bei der postmortalen zahnärztlichen Untersuchung: Allgemeine Erwägungen. Forensische Zahnmedizin. Quintessenz, Berlin, S 81–85

Stene-Johansen W, Solheim T, Sakshaug O (1992) Dental identification after the Dash 7 aircraft accident at Torghatten, Northern Norway, May 6th, 1988. J Forensic Odontostomatol 10:15–24

Wagner GN (1997) Scientific methods of identification. In: Stimson PG, Mertz CA (eds) Forensic dentistry. CRC Press, Boca Raton/New York, p 1

Warnick A (1995) Mass disaster dental identification, chapter 8, mass disaster management. In: Bowers CM, Bell GL (eds) Manual of forensic odontology. ASFO, AAFS, Colorado Springs, pp 236–249

Weedn VW (1997) DNA identification. In: Stimson PG, Mertz CA (eds) Forensic dentistry. CRC Press, Boca Raton/New York, p 37

Wenzel A, Andersen L (1994) A quantitative analysis of subtraction images based on bite-wing radiographs for a simulated victim identification in forensic dentistry. J Forensic Odontostomatol 12:1–5

23 Bite Marks and Tooth Marks

Klaus Rötzscher, Wolfgang Pilz, and Tore Solheim

23.1 Preliminary Comments

Human teeth leave more or less characteristic marks on bodies and objects (Pilz et al. 1980; Sweet 1995). These marks appear on the human skin as bite marks (without cutting through the epidermis) or bite wounds. Although bite or tooth marks caused by humans are rather common, they are of only little forensic importance; however, it often happens that people use their teeth as a weapon for attack or defense (self-defense, fighting). The motivation for biting ranges from disturbed partner relations (conflict, jealousy, revenge) or abnormal sexual drive or self-mutilation (Ulrich 1963; Haak 1970; Trube-Becker 1973; Rotzscher and Reimann 1975; Pilz et al. 1980; Sobel and Perper 1985; Ligthelm and van Niekerk 1995).

The literature talks of bite marks, and indeed most tooth marks are caused by bites. If impressions of the upper and lower teeth (mostly the front and canine teeth) are visible, a bite mark is suggested. However, not all tooth marks are also bite marks, and the cause must be investigated. Tooth marks can be caused by a punch/strike or if the teeth are used as a tool. Therefore, the neutral term *tooth mark* should be used until the investigation about the cause is completed (Humble 1933). Human tooth marks are caused by ingestion, work activities, and by sexual activities. If tooth marks are related to a crime (e.g., physical violence), an investigation should be started to determine the time, scope, and cause of the crime and, of course, the identity of the perpetrator.

23.2 Tooth Marks

Tooth marks can be found in foods but also in other objects such as wood, plastic, or metal (Mills 1976). In burglaries, strangely, the burglar often has an appetite for food, fruit, or candy. Indentations in the teeth can leave marks, in most cases by impressions of the incisors of the upper and lower jaw. Such traces are often well visible and can serve as evidence (Euler 1937; Pilz and Zerndt 1963); for example, a tooth mark left in cheese is uncontradicted evidence (Kerr 1977).

The first question is whether the marks are caused by teeth or by an item. Items can leave rounded, curved, and arched tracks (Rotzscher 1972). Note that tooth marks must at least have individual details to serve as evidence. However, it also happens that items are unevenly designed and thus a mark could look like an individual

K. Rötzscher, Dr. med. Dr. med. dent. (✉)
German Academy of Forensic Odontostomatology (AKFOS), Wimphelingstraße 7, 67346 Speyer, Germany
e-mail: roetzscher.klaus.dr@t-online.de

W. Pilz, Univ.-Prof. (em) Dr. med. dent.
Department of Preservative and Pediatric Stomatology, Academy Carl Gustav Carus, Dresden, Germany

T. Solheim, Prof. (em) Dr. odont.
Institute of Oral Biology, Pathology and Forensic Odontology, University Oslo, Oslo, Norway
e-mail: tore.solheim@odont.uio.no

K. Rötzscher (ed.), *Forensic and Legal Dentistry*,
DOI 10.1007/978-3-319-01330-5_23, © Springer International Publishing Switzerland 2014

tooth mark. Solheim (1980) reported a case with tooth marks on the crown caps of beer bottles (Figs. 23.1, 23.2, and 23.3). After a burglary, the police found two beer bottles at the scene, obviously opened by teeth (two teeth marks were clearly visible). Two suspects were arrested and, on the way to the police station, they got thirsty. The officers got them bottles of mineral water that also had crown caps. One of the suspects opened the bottle with his teeth and proudly claimed that he always opens bottles like this. Thus, the police were in possession of three crown caps that could serve as evidence (reference material) (Solheim 1980). It was concluded that both bottles were opened by the same person.

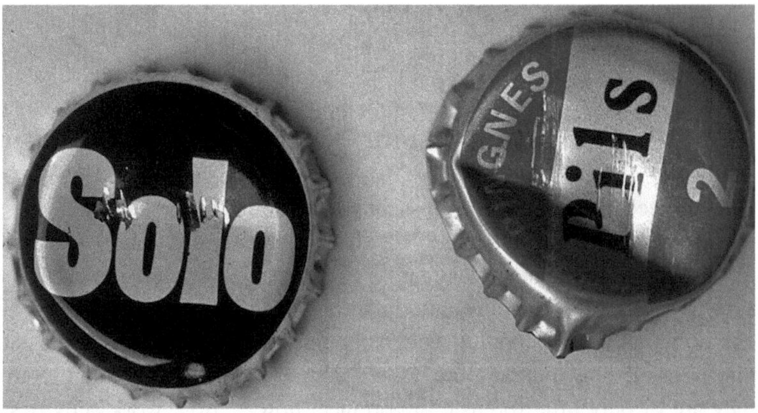

Fig. 23.1 Traces of tooth marks on crown caps of beer bottles (Solheim 1980)

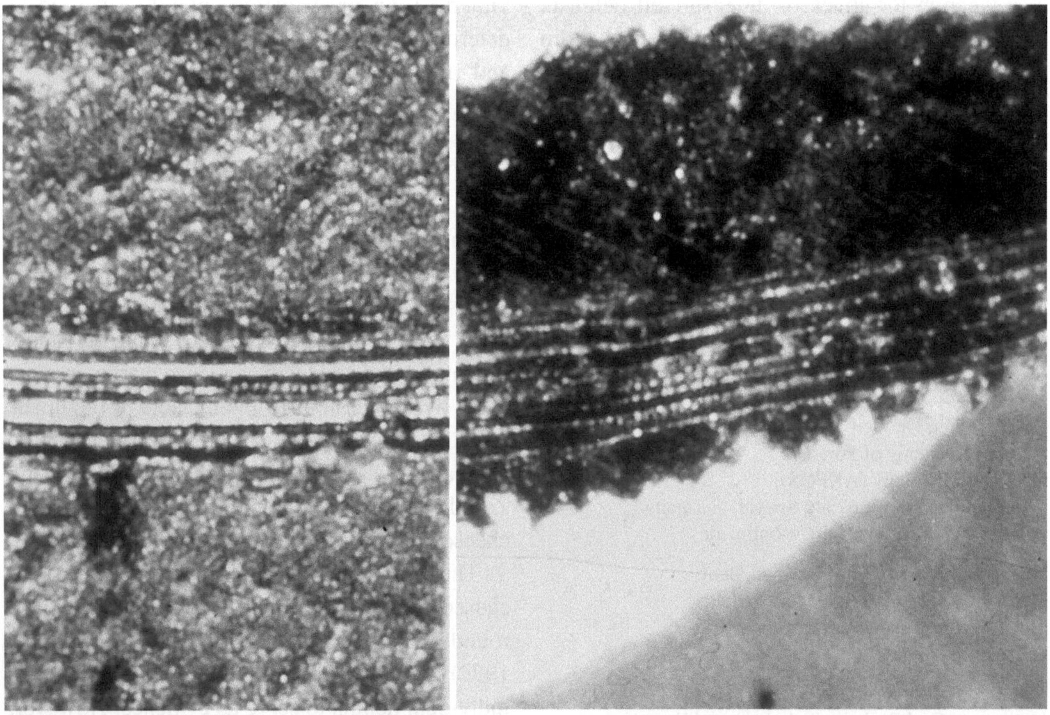

Fig. 23.2 Trace comparison (comparative microscopy: crown cap of a beer bottle (*left* - *right*)). Many indentations show conformity

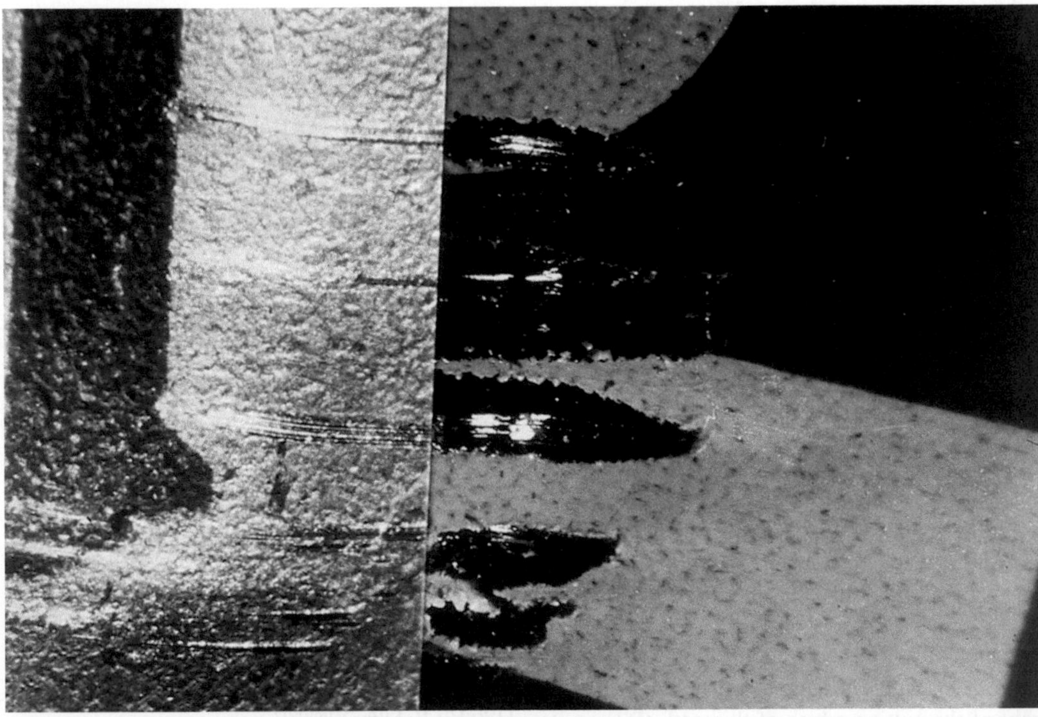

Fig. 23.3 Trace comparison (at higher magnification): the microfurrow on the crown cap of the mineral water bottle (*left*) and the beer bottle (*right*) match exactly

However, teeth may also leave marks during a fall or because of a punch against the teeth. In such cases, the teeth often are damaged or fractured. Then, the scene must be searched for the dropped or fractured teeth. Most often, tooth marks occur in the skin (Ligthelm and van Niekerk 1995). The skin can be cut and/or a piece of skin could be bitten out (Graw et al. 1998). In a conflict, both parties, perpetrator and victim, may have tooth marks on the skin.

Particularly in the investigation of sexual crimes, bodily injuries, and other violent crimes, bite marks can be found on the body of the injured person and, as a result of defensive actions, also on the body of the perpetrator (Prokop 1966; Free 1995; Graw et al. 1998). In all cases where bite marks are found, attention must also be paid to traces of blood and/or saliva. This is useful for the reconstruction of the course of the crime and to determine any possible intoxication of the perpetrator (Zerndt and Simon 1962).

In cases of rape, tooth marks (only with impressions and subepithelial hemorrhage) often resemble a love bite. If the victim survives the attack, these marks disappear after few hours. Therefore, the tooth marks must be examined as quickly as possible. Subepithelial bleeding is still visible after several days and may become even more obvious. Therefore, the victim should be examined on several consecutive days. In addition, an investigation under infrared or ultraviolet light makes the marks more obvious (Ruddick 1974). However, subepithelial bleeding only shows little detail and is of limited importance. Frequently found are bites with ring-shaped subepithelial bleeding as a result of a suction process. The dimensions of the bite may change (Thompson and Phillips 1994).

Unlike animals, humans suck more often than they bite. Animals do not leave central subepithelial hematomas between the dental arches. In case of a suspected animal bite, the investigation and bite comparison should be done in cooperation with a veterinarian (Ligthelm and Niekerk 1995).

The mechanics of bite injuries with cuts of the epidermis, "pull bite" (Fig. 23.4), is

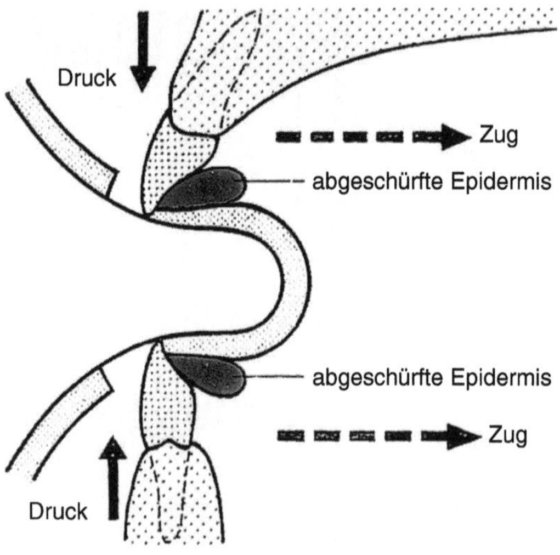

Fig. 23.4 Mechanics of the bite injury with cut of the epidermis by the "distortion-pull bite"

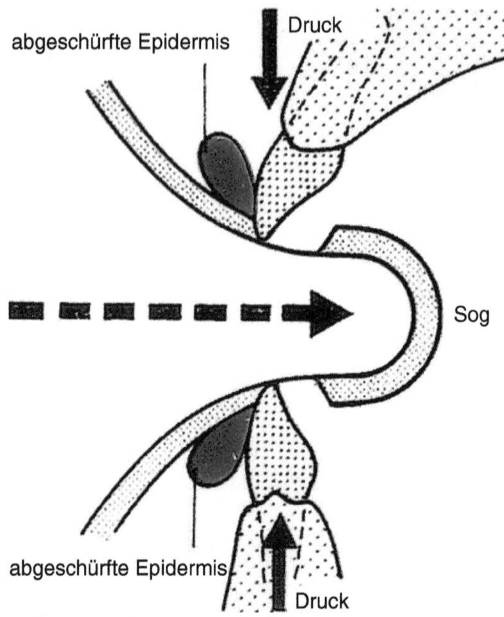

Fig. 23.5 Mechanics of "suck bite" with "enrichment" of the epidermis (Modified after Zerndt, with courtesy of Prof. Dr. W. Pilz, Arnstadt)

fundamentally different from the "suck bite" (Fig. 23.5), with enrichment of the epidermis in front of the cutting edges of the teeth (Pilz et al. 1980). Experimenting with suction cups on the skin (Fig. 23.6) produces a circular mark that develops into an oval shape after removal of the suction cup (Pilz et al. 1980). This behavior corresponds to the cleavage lines, as described by Langer (1861).

The nature of the force acting on the skin, i.e., whether the bite was made with "burrowing" movements or if the skin was in a stretched or warped condition, is also important. In this case, moving into a relaxed state also shifts the bite mark. This is particularly true for arms and legs (surveys on human volunteers), and is another uncontrollable unknown in the analysis of bite marks (Pilz et al. 1980).

In order to test the validity of evaluations of bite marks, Pilz et al. (1980) conducted bite mark comparisons (native trace setting in the human skin) on different models in a blind test. The accuracy of the evaluation by photographs was very dependent on the time when the photos were taken. The evaluation of the 24-h model showed a precision value of only 9 %! A high percentage of accuracy is achieved when the bite mark provides clear imprints and is photographed as soon as possible.

Nehrkorn and Sturm (1974) studied the problem of whether:

1. Typelike normal teeth have recognizably different impressions at all
2. Active bites into vital, responsive, and movable substrate are comparable to bite mark copies.

In typical normal teeth, comparisons are worthless because pseudo-identities bear the risk of false positive statements. In case of congruence only, the reference "not to be excluded" is allowed, with reference to the high rate of nonspecific similarity in typical teeth.

Abused children often have tooth marks in the skin (Fulton 1984). These traces only show impressions and subepithelial bleeding, especially if the perpetrator had no intention to kill. If the examination of the child takes place after several days, the marks usually are no longer visible and thus are hardly suitable as evidence.

Bite marks on the same object can be single or multiple, and may be spread over various regions of the body, so the entire body must be examined. Furthermore, the traces can be caused by one or several perpetrators (Pilz et al. 1980).

The localization of bites (frequency) shows that the fingers are most commonly involved (due to defensive reactions), followed by the female mammary gland (sexual crimes), and the

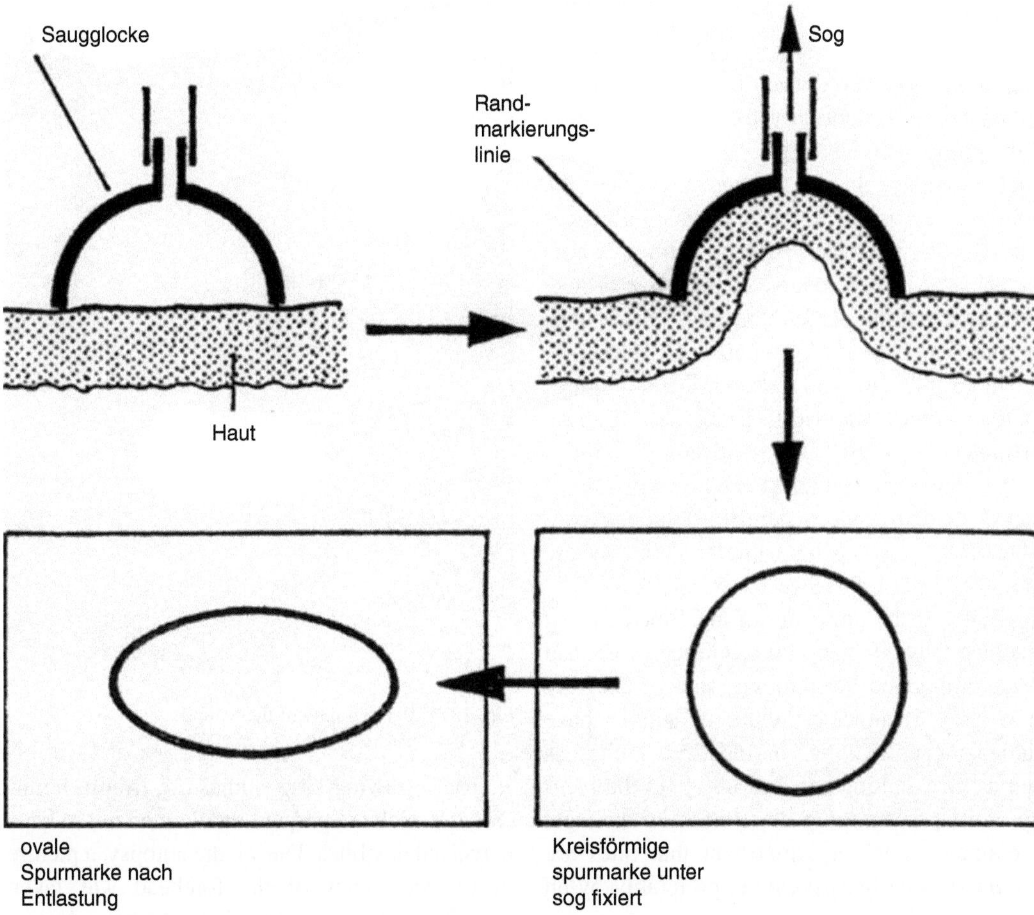

Fig. 23.6 Experimental suction marks on the skin (Courtesy of Prof. Dr. W. Pilz, Arnstadt)

extremities. The neck and torso are relatively rarely involved (Ulrich 1963). The locations of bites with respect to their frequencies, from most to least frequent, are (Ulrich 1963): fingers, breasts, legs, nose, hands, ears, cheeks, lips, neck, chin, shoulders, abdomen, genitals, and armpit.

A further study on the frequency of bite marks in homicides regarding the sex of the perpetrator (trace causer) and the sex of the victim (trace carrier) clearly shows that the male sex is in the majority, while the female gender predominates as a trace carrier (victim) (Ulrich 1963).

23.3 Examination Methods

Pathologically altered or dentally treated dentures are more useful for an assessment of bite marks than "normal teeth." Note that the mechanics of the bite must be considered (Pilz et al. 1980; Sweet 1995; Zerndt 1964):

- Simple hack bite
- Tear or pull bite
- Raising of soft tissues that are grasped with the teeth
- Intensity and location of the bite
- The vital reactions
- The nature of the affected tissue
- The respective base

Nevertheless, many details must be minded to avoid faulty assessments. In this regard, it is advantageous that "normal teeth" appear less than pathologically altered dentures.

The examination of bite marks in violent crimes requires great expertise. The dental expert must be included in the investigation as early as possible. The dental assessment must be stated in an opinion that is justified by proper scientific methods. Even the securing of evidence bears the risk of incorrect assessments. All traces at the scene must be secured, even the smallest details can be of great importance for the identification of the perpetrator. Under the principle of "do not touch anything, do not change anything," the crime scene must be protected against influences that may alter the traces. False or fictitious traces can be caused by the course of the crime or may be targeted by the perpetrator. Such traces must be immediately secured (Hennis et al. 1981a).

The examination of bite/tooth marks requires interdisciplinary teamwork. Detectives, forensic scientists, serologists, and dentists are involved in the detection, securing, and evaluation of traces. An experienced dentist should be consulted in all cases where bite/tooth marks are present (Endris 1985; Sweet 1995).

Searching the literature on legal medicine, it becomes obvious that bite injuries have had greater importance in court only since a relatively short time. Meanwhile, numerous authors have studied the possibilities of identifying bites as well as the resulting conclusions about the identity of the perpetrator (Selle 1966). For the legal assessment, it is very important that bites are examined as early as possible, preferably by an experienced forensic odontologist.

Graw et al. (1998) reported a morphological finding survey on a piece of skin and its DNA typing, which led to the identification of the perpetrator. A 35-year-old woman who suffered from psychosis was found dead with multiple stab wounds. A piece of horny skin (~1 cm) was found in her oral cavity (sublingual). It could not be assigned to one of the numerous skin defects. Several men of her connections were potentially suspected and had to undergo a physical examination. One of them had a healing injury at the bending side of his left ring finger. The piece of horny skin had the contours and size and papillary lines of this wound. The DNA testing showed that the piece of skin could only be assigned to the suspect, who thereupon made a confession. The specific molecular biological study of the washed piece of skin showed a statistically computable frequency of 1:700,000 (matching feature pattern).

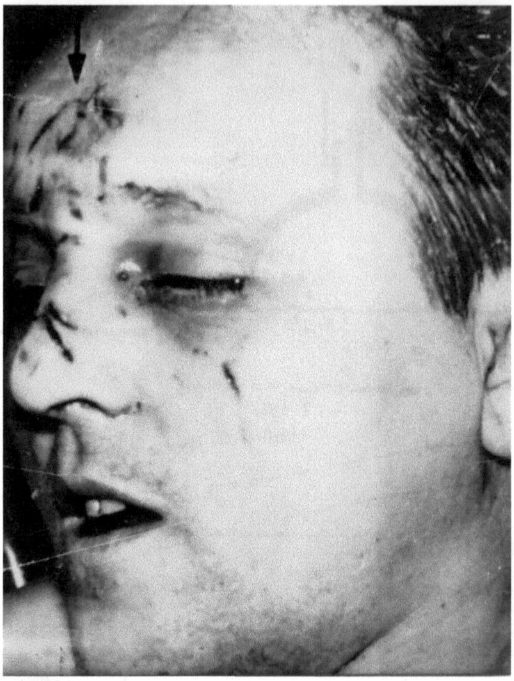

Fig. 23.7 Photography of the wound

The following case studies are from a homicide in which the perpetrator claimed not to have perceived any bites. During the autopsy, a picture of the side view of the forehead was taken (Fig. 23.7, see arrow) and showed a bow-shaped, scratch-like cut of the epidermis between the eyebrows (the other injuries of the skin, caused by a knife, were irrelevant). Initially it was assumed that the wound was caused by a broken milk bottle. The forensic odontologist supposed that the bow-shaped forehead injury was caused by a bite of the perpetrator.

The comparison with the plaster of the upper jaw of the perpetrator showed that the injury was caused by the right canine, all incisors, the left canine, and the anterior premolar. The width of the wound and also the width of the incisor was 7 mm. Remarkable is that the impression of the first right incisor is slightly inward (Figs. 23.8 and 23.9, arrow A). Those studies confirmed that the bow-shaped skin lesion was caused by a bite of the suspect (Rötzscher 1972). The tooth mark is more likely an impression than an active bite that emerged through the impact of the teeth of the perpetrator on the forehead of his victim,

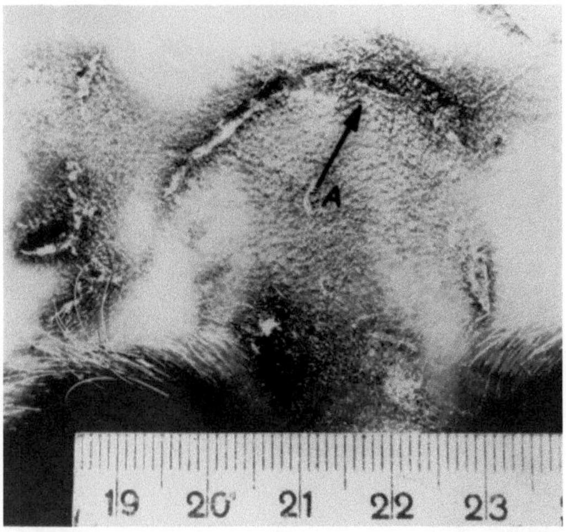

Fig. 23.8 Image of the forehead with a bow-shaped injury

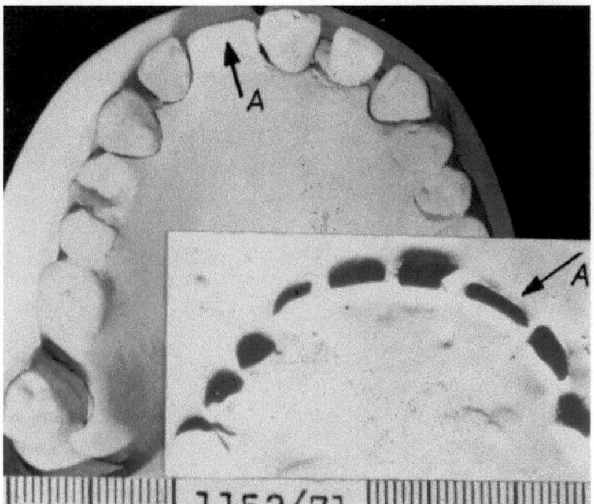

Fig. 23.9 Upper jaw plaster model of the suspect with the cutout plasticine impression

without the intent to bite. This could be explained by a violent impact (head butt) of the upper dental arch (with open mouth) during the fight with the defending victim.

An important reference criterion is an acceptable thickness of the soft tissue in the forehead area. In the area of the scalp and the soft tissues of the forehead, there is little deviation of the thickness, as the scalp, on average, is about 5- to 7-mm thick. The measurement of the soft tissue thickness according to Helmer (1998) is determined by sex, age, and type of constitution:

1. Measuring point 17: stm — middle of the forehead, point in the center of the upper orbital margin on the line of frontotemporal to metopion
2. Measuring point 30: mt — M. temporalis above zygion, at the height of the ectoconchion
3. Measuring point 31: zy — zygion (the most protruding point on the cheek bone)

In the presence of an anomaly, its characteristics are valuable in identifying the bite/tooth mark. The morphological assessment has priority over the measurements of distance and angle, which only have complementary functions (Hennis et al. 1981b, c).

Prerequisite for a judicial assessment of bites is accurate anatomical knowledge of the shape and appearance of the wounds as well as profound knowledge of the dentition and the bite behavior of animals in order to determine whether the bite injury was caused by an animal or by a human (Endris 1979).

23.4 Traces Caused by Animals

Animals bite (at least during the attack) indiscriminately into covered and uncovered parts of the body. Humans usually bite into bare or bared body parts: fingers, breasts, arms, legs, nose, hands, ears, cheeks, lips, neck, jaw, shoulders, abdomen, genitals, and armpits. In particular, the fingers, ears or the nose may completely or partially be bitten off. Animals that may become a danger because of their bites are primarily pets such as dogs, cats, and horses. The owner is liable for the legal consequences of animal bites. Because many bite injuries by animals are serious and even lethal, these cases are subject to criminal law. In the USA, an estimated two to three million dog bites occur each year (60 % of the victims are children). Approximately 20 children in the USA die each year from dog bites (Berk et al. 1997).

Injuries caused by bites of nondomestic animals, such as rats, mice, wild cats, and other predators, are important during an investigation because the time of the bite (intravital or postmortem) may help to solve a crime. Postmortem injuries caused by wild animals, even smaller animals, may be confusing because they massively alter the condition of the body and must be carefully examined in order to detect whether the injuries were caused intravital or postmortem.

Tsokos and Schulz (1999) reported two cases with postmortal injuries by domestic animals that mangled their owners who had died natural deaths. The owner of two pitbull terriers laid dead and dressed in his house. The two dogs mangled his head and neck region; the larynx, the thyroid gland, parts of the carotid artery of both sides and the upper part of the esophagus and the trachea could not be found at the scene.

A 41-year-old woman had died from an acute pneumonia and laid dressed in her house. Rats gnawed her neck and upper thorax. The larynx, the thyroid gland, parts of the carotid artery of both sides and the upper part of the esophagus and the trachea could not be found at the scene. Rat bites are also found on living persons. This etiological difficulty increases the significance of the cases.

Strauch (1927) studied cases of bite injuries by cats: "Felids are markedly predators which put the main emphasis on the hunt of living, warm prey." Nevertheless, there are cases where cats ate dead bodies. Commencing or advanced decay does not keep them from the corpse.

In identification of animal bites it is difficult to recognize a bite because most of the tissue is destroyed by tearing bites and, thus, it is difficult to detect individual features. Houtrow (1963) reported a case of a 14-year-old boy who was found dead in a park in Vienna, maimed by injuries that seemed to be stab wounds. Investigations and the forensic autopsy revealed that the injuries were from several German Shepherd dogs who had largely mangled the body.

Comparative studies of skulls of dogs (German shepherd, Boxer) and a polar bear (Du Chesne and Rötzscher 1968) provided both surprising similarities and differences between the species and the sets of their bites. The dentition of the Boxer shows physiological prognathism (reverse front bite) with expected bite ratios strains and bruises in the tissue. In the German shepherd, the front teeth rows slide like scissor branches close to each other. In dog bites, the relatively long canines (carnassials) leave impressions that are similar to injuries (Figs. 23.10 and 23.11) by conical objects (Pilz et al. 1980).

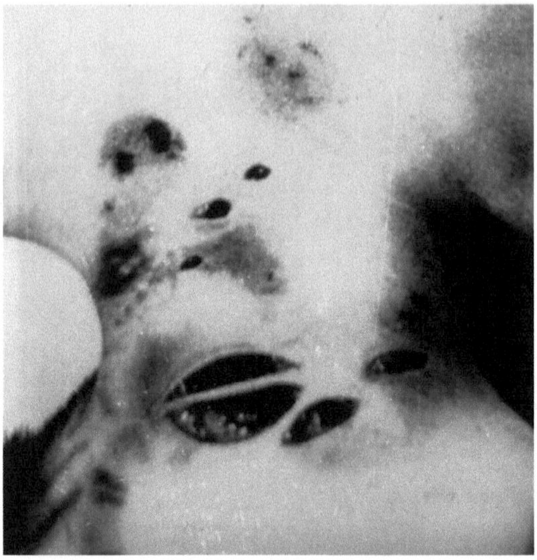

Fig. 23.10 Animal bite (shepherd dog), similar to stab wounds

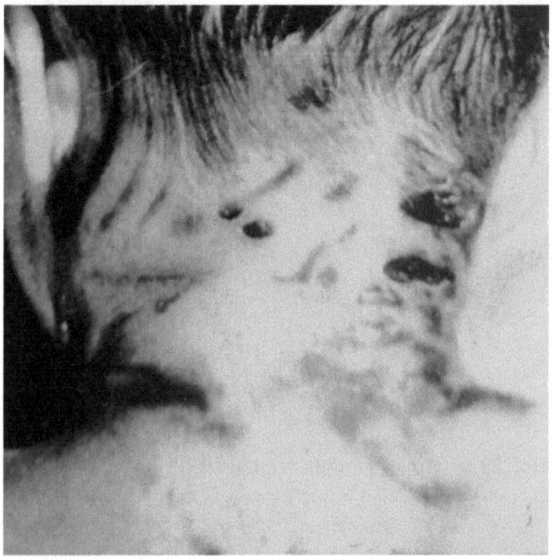

Fig. 23.11 Bite wounds; tooth marks, slide traces, and subdermal bleedings

Conclusions about the nature and course of the injury can only be drawn by comparative analysis of teeth and bite injuries. For example, the Forensic Institute in Leipzig had to examine the body of a 2.5-year-old boy who had fallen over the railing into the pool of a polar bear compound. First the child was submerged and brought up into the paws of the polar bear. He brought the child back to land where he was rescued by the guards after 10–20 min. The child died on the way to the hospital. The autopsy showed numerous bites, abrasion injuries, and scratches on head and body. The pericranium was scalped. The right lower leg had a characteristic ring-shaped discoloration of the skin with abrasion injuries. It was assumed that the polar bear pressed his slightly opened mouth against the skin and sucked. This type of bite was interpreted for the playful behavior of the polar bear during the accident. It would have been easy for the polar bear to mangle the child's leg (Du Chesne 1968). Note that the main danger of animal bites is less the injury itself as its infectivity.

Minor injuries are underestimated by the patient and can be starting points of infections, such as pasteurellosis (*Pasteurella multocida* and *septica*), septicopyemia (*Streptobacillus moniliformis*), Sodoku ("rat bite fever"), and Weil's disease (*Leptospira icterohaemorrhagiae*) (Mollaret 1969).

Tsokos and Schulz (1999) compiled literature about bites by domestic animals and their localization; this information is presented in Chart 23.1.

Chart 23.1

Domestic animal bites and their locations in a literature collection

Authors	Age/gender	Cause of death	Animal	Time between death and postmortem injuries	Location	Traces of blood
Böhmer (1925)	Newborn/(u)	(u)	Mouse	(u)	Extremities	(u)
Böhmer (1925)	3 days/m	Cerebral hemorrhage	Rats	3 days	Face	No
Mttmeyer et al. (1976)	49 years/m	Cerebral hemorrhage	Dog	(u)	Penis	On carpet
Mätzler (1977)	66 years/m	Natural death	Dog (poodle)	(u)	Abdomen, penis, anus	No
Weiler (1978)	77 years/m	Pneumonia	Dog	8 days	Abdomen, pelvis, penis	No
Pötsch-Schneider and Endris (1984)	53 years/m	Cerebral hemorrhage	Dog	(u)	Decapitation	Large amounts on head and neck
Haglund (1992)	27 years/m	Suicide by propane gas inhalation	Rats	3 days	Skeletonization of the head and (u)	(u)
Hayase et al. (1994)	59 years/m	Ischemic heart disease	Dog	3 days	Front chest wall was missing, internal organs intact	no
Rossi et al. (1994)	53 years/m	Pneumonia, diabetes, heart disease	Dog (German shepherd)	(u)	Skeletonization of head and neck, internal organs missing	Tracks
Rossi et al. (1994)	82 years/m	Myocardial ischemia	Dog (German shepherd)	(u)	Skeletonization of head and neck, internal organs partially missing	Tracks

Rossi et al. (1994)	42 years/f	Pulmonary edema, alcohol intoxication	Dog (Setter)	16 h	Face	(u)
Rossi et al. (1994)	32 years/m	Suicide by intoxication	Cats	3 days	Skeletonization of head and neck, internal organs partially missing	(u)
Patel (1994)	(u)/m	Ischemic heart disease	Rats	48 h	Face	No
Ropohl et al. (1995)	43 years/f	Pneumonia	Golden hamster	(u)	Face, neck	Little amounts
Schumann et al. (1996)	65 years/m	Myocardial ischemia	Dog	12 h	Face, neck	No
Rothschild and Schneider (1997)	31 years/m	Suicide by shooting	Dog (German shepherd)	45 min	Lower part of the face, neck	Large amounts near the body

After Tsokos and Schulz (1999)
Unknown (u)

23.5 Traces in Food and Objects

Tooth marks (or mucosal impingement bite) in food (chilled butter, cheese, cakes, fruit, chocolate, sausage, etc.) can also lead to the identification of the offender (Marshall et al. 1974). Indentations are subject to progressive abrasion of the teeth and, thus, unpredictable changes are possible. The incisors leave obvious indentations on food, e.g., chocolate (Fig. 23.12). These results were gained in systematic studies of teeth (even with deciduous teeth) and dental prostheses (Pilz and Zerndt 1963). Longer intervals (>2 months) between the crime and the comparison limit the reliability of the results because of possibly progressive wear of the teeth. Comparison of indentations from a single individual showed that, after approximately 2 months, individual features may be lost or replaced by a new feature (Pilz et al. 1980). The shape and the number of teeth allow conclusions regarding possible abnormalities, such as changes in tooth number, size, site, position, abrasion, or caries, or tooth replacement.

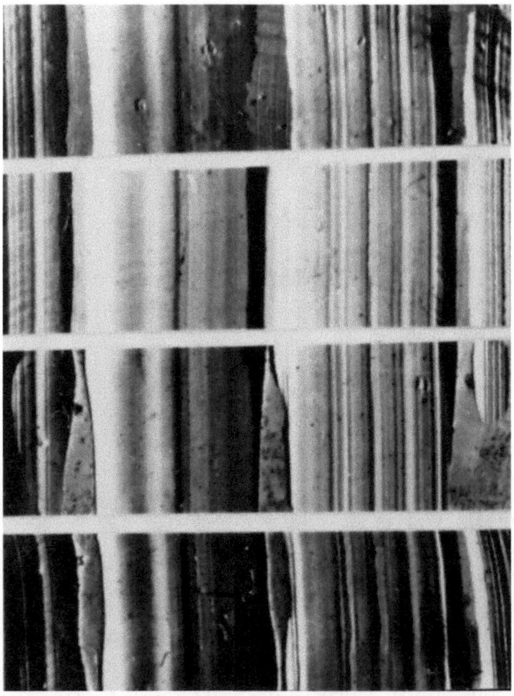

Fig. 23.12 Indentations in chocolate

If traces of saliva exist, the blood type must be determined; controlled absorptions with the food are necessary, and individualizing studies at the DNA level may be indicated in special cases (Sweet 1995).

23.6 Methodology of Preservation of Evidence

It is very important that bite marks are secured as soon as possible because they may become nonspecific in a short time, especially marks that are in the skin or on food. Ideally, the forensic odontologists should secure the evidence because they know best which steps are necessary to maintain the chain of evidence.

23.7 Securing of Evidence

23.7.1 In Food and Objects

The following principles should be considered:

1. The evidence must be immediately secured to avoid any contact (contamination) with other objects and bodies.
2. Several different and precise investigations must be conducted for each piece of evidence; the results must be reproducible and verifiable.

   The evidence material (the object with the original traces) must be preserved and treated such that a subsequent second opinion can be obtained. This might be problematic with easily perishable foods. Preservation in fixatives is possible; however, shrinkage is expected and destruction of the marks cannot be excluded.
3. The original material is in possession of the police and only may remain with the expert by special agreement with the police. The technique of securing of evidence in food is equal to that of securing of evidence in skin.

The uncertainty factor is the incorrect use of the methods or often the careless interpretation of the results. Knowledge of these weaknesses and the uncritical use of forensic methods can reduce this source of danger to a barely effective minimum.

23.7.2 In the Skin

The investigation depends on whether the person is alive or dead. In the latter case, the first examinations should be performed at the scene before the body is brought to the institute in order to avoid possible destruction of evidence. Finally, the dental status (as a precautionary measure) of the victim must be documented, because the victim might have caused bite injuries to the perpetrator. All present persons (witnesses of the autopsy; pathologist) must be documented by name.

Depending on the case, the circumstances of the crime that have become known so far, the time elapsed since the crime, and also the time elapsed until the examination of the suspect (as causer of the marks) must be documented; this procedure should be standard practice in any crime investigation (Clark 1992).

23.7.2.1 Saliva Sample

Saliva from the suspect is mostly found in the vicinity of the bite/tooth mark. Blood-type antigens or the characteristic DNA profile should be examined for a comparison with the suspect. If the skin of the victim has already been washed, useful material for DNA analysis may have been destroyed. The sample should be removed from the body with filter paper (cigarette paper placed on the body and then documented by photos is very practical) or by dry cotton (Stimson and Mertz 1997). Furthermore, the timing of when the tracks arose must be investigated (Mittleman et al. 1980). This work must be performed with gloves to avoid distortion of the results by contamination. A control sample should be taken from body parts that were not in contact with the evidence. If the saliva trace is older, the saliva sample can be resolved with some water.

23.7.2.2 Photography

All bite/tooth marks must be numbered. Then the bite marks must be drawn and photographically secured (color photos, b/w photos, plus slides). It is important that the scale does not cover any parts of the trace itself. The images should be taken with artificial light from various directions in order to obtain better shading and markings. A picture of the whole body is recommended in order to document the location of the track. The same applies if traces are found on the body of the suspect. If possible, the photographs should be repeated after 24 h for 3–5 days. Pieces of skin that are cut from the "context" are worthless because of the inevitable warping and should be histologically/histochemically investigated.

In 1937, Manczarski recommended use of infrared light to detect bleeding in the subcutaneous fatty tissue, e.g., bite marks in human skin. Pictures with UV light provide a more obvious display of traces (Ruddick 1974).

The detection and examination of human bites that did not cut through the epidermis depend on the location on the body and also the gender. According to Saar (1952), bites on the male arm are traceable up to 3 h after occurring and up to 48 h on the female face. If possible, the skin or the organ should be in the same position as when the injury was caused.

Serial photographs of the dentition of the suspect should be taken (with scale ABFO No. 2 or other millimeter scale):

1. *En face* and in profile
2. Two right and left lateral images of the closed teeth rows (cheek retractor)
3. Right and left canines
4. Upper arch, if possible, parallel to the tooth longitudinal axis
5. Lower dental arch, if possible, parallel to the tooth longitudinal axis
6. Additional use of a spatula (mirror) (Sweet 1995)

Photographs of plaster models of the upper and lower jaw of the suspect should be taken in surveillance and occlusion, left and right side, and also with a scale and parallel to the arch, so that a comparison with the trace is possible. The sides should always be labeled to avoid side confusions (R = right; L = left).

23.7.2.3 Drawings

Although photographs are taken, a drawn sketch of the marks and the surrounding area is advantageous for further orientation (Annexes 23.1, 23.2, 23.3, 23.4, and 23.5: FO Form SMD (Rev.1/91© 1989 by JB & MN Sobel). In addition to a normal sketch, placing a transparent film over the marks and tracing the marks with ink is highly recommended.

23.7.2.4 Description

A verbal description of the marks is necessary for better orientation. The description should include the storage conditions (such as how the marks were set) and the time and temperature, along with an estimate of possible dimension changes. The extent of subcutaneous bleeding, especially in corpses, must be documented. Slight or no subcutaneous bleeding may mean that the marks were made temporally close to the time of death, which may be of utmost importance (Luntz and Luntz 1973).

23.7.2.5 Impression

A silicone impression is recommended, but, with a good technique, a cast (at least as a template for the silicone) can also be used (Bang 1976). Strøm (1963) recommended making a second silicone model of the marks for comparison if not all details were displayed. It may also be advantageous to have an unused impression as evidence. The impression must be taken as soon as possible, before shrinkage or drying of the marks. However, the impression can only be made at the last moment of the investigation.

Impressions of the marks should be made in every case, even if only subcutaneous bleeding is obvious. In cases where no impressions in the skin are visible, they could become obvious in the casting under good lighting (Luntz and Luntz 1973).

23.7.2.6 Conservation

In cases with tooth marks on a corpse, it must be considered whether it is advantageous to cut a piece of skin and preserve it as evidence. This must be decided in consultation with the forensic pathologist and the police (Bang 1976; Endris 1979).

The human skin as *integumentum commune* is a complex organ with a highly developed nerve plexus, blood vessels, sweat glands, and sebum. The skin consists of three layers of tissue (Fig. 23.13):

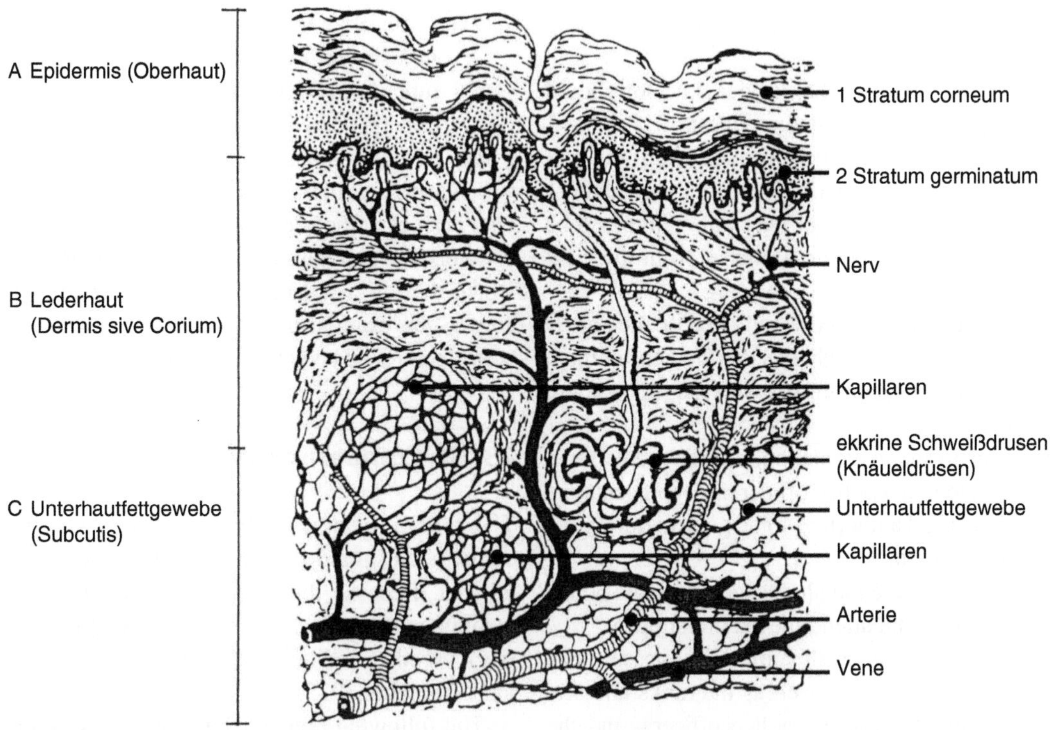

Fig. 23.13 The human skin of the hand (After Lundevall (1989); courtesy of Universitetsforlaget, Oslo)

- A: The very thin skin (epidermis: *stratum corneum* and *stratum germinativum*)
- B: The leathery skin connective tissue (dermis: *corium*)
- C: The subcutaneous fatty tissue (subcutaneous tissue: *tela subcutanea*)
- A and B comprise the cutis (skin) and C corresponds to the subcutis (subcutaneous tissue).

After the mark is photographically secured, it should be excised 3–5 cm around the marking. The body temperature should be around 21 °C and the skin must be dry (Dorion 1995). Excising only the piece of skin with the tooth marks is not recommended because the shrinking of the skin may destroy the trace. Shrinkage can be avoided by fixation with pins on a cork tile (Endris 1979).

23.8 Questioning

If the injured person is alive, they must be interviewed about where, when, and how the tooth marks were caused. Some forensic odontologists think that they may not talk to the suspect. However, the suspect has the same rights to express themself as the victim does. All facts of a case should be known to the expert in order to conduct a qualified assessment.

23.9 Investigation of a Suspect

The fact that tooth marks can be used as evidence is justified in the individuality of teeth. Studies have shown that teeth may even identify twins (Sognnaes 1977). Some details may change during chewing, by accident, or because of multiple lesions, or they may even disappear. Therefore, the teeth must be examined as soon as possible (Luntz and Luntz 1973). Often the suspect is in a different city. In that case, a dentist in the other city can perform the examination of the teeth (after consultation with the forensic odontologist). This saves time and effort.

The examination should include the following steps:

1. The examination of a suspected person should only be conducted upon request.
2. The suspect must be informed about the reason of the examination in order to obtain consent that the results of the examination will be given to the police (release from medical confidentiality).
3. The suspect is asked whether he or she knows the tooth marks: whether she/he caused them or whether she/he knows who caused the tooth marks.
4. Prior to the examination, arrangements must be made for a police officer or a representative of the legal authorities to be present during the examination.
5. In the case of a female suspect, a female police officer should attend the examination.
6. The names and occupations of witnesses must be documented; as well as the ranks and service numbers of the police officers, and the date, time, and place of the examination.
7. Photos (slides and prints) must be taken *en face* and in profile to identify and document the physiognomy (Endris and Hilgert 1975).
8. The teeth should be photographed in black and white and in color, if possible, with a scale.
9. The examination of the teeth and jaws should include the following details:
   (a) Description of dental status, caries, and restorations.
   (b) Description of dental characteristics.
   (c) Description of tooth positions, occlusion, and articulation. The plaster models should be articulated (not only in an occludator, but also in an articulator).
   (d) Description of damage to the teeth and jaws.
   (e) Impressions of upper and lower jaw (for removable dentures: cast with and without dentures). Most suitable are silicone or alginate impressions. The impressions (models) should be photographed with a scale that is equal to the cutting edges of the front teeth to allow comparisons with the bite marks. To avoid confusion, the photos must be labeled (R = right; L = left).
   (f) If possible, impressions (for comparison) in a similar material, e.g., in a cardboard tube that is covered with red dental wax (Endris and Hilgert 1975).
   (g) Saliva samples.

DNA profiles of these samples can be compared with profiles of the bite in order to identify the perpetrator. The prerequisite is that the material from which the bite is taken be suitable. In case of a corpse, the examination should start right at the scene, before the body is transported for autopsy.

23.10 Comparison of Traces

The further treatment of the material and the comparison should be done by a forensic odontologist. Because this analysis is difficult, it is recommended that two forensic odontologists work together and achieve a consensus of opinion (Rötzscher 1972).

The following prerequisites are necessary for a viable identification:

1. Realistic drawing and photograph (scale 1:1) in color and black and white.
2. Consideration of the natural warp of the skin during the bite, especially if the bite marks are in an area with a soft base (subcutaneous fat, e.g., female breast) (Rotzscher and Reimann 1975; Sweet 1995).
3. Development of a method that vividly shows the relation between the dentition of the suspect and the bite.
4. If several persons are suspected, they must each be examined in the same way. Thus, a later expert will be able to draw their own conclusions about the identity of the perpetrator.
5. All bite marks must be examined for shreds of epidermis (Zerndt and Simon 1962; Zerndt 1964), which may be relevant for the reconstruction of the crime and the assessment of the activity of the perpetrator(Zerndt and Simon 1962; Graw et al. 1998).

The marks (on the body of the victim) and the teeth (of all suspected persons) must be analyzed and compared (Keiser-Nielsen 1947). Many techniques are available. Sörup (1926) was one of the first to describe a special technique.

23.10.1 Odontoscopy

The cutting edges and cusps of the plaster models are dyed and the prints are made on copper printing paper and afterwards transferred on a transparent film. The impressions on this transparent paper can be compared 1:1 with the original photographs.

Melchior (1929) described securing the bite marks by using finely pulverized cast material distributed by a fine sieve all over the bite wound. After accumulation in sufficient quantity, the wound is covered with a wet cloth, until clear water appears on the cloth. Because the impression of the bite is a negative, the cast impression is a relief (*positive*) of the teeth that caused the bite.

According to Buhtz and Erhard (1938), this method is not very reliable because of:

(a) Shrinkage of the dissected tissue
(b) Neglect of the shape of the bitten body part
(c) Neglect of the bite mechanic (distortion of the tissue at the bite)
(d) Inappropriate recording technology
(e) Comparison of the jaw model with the distorted impressions of the suspects or their bites photograms

It is important to ascertain whether the marks are caused by the front and/or side teeth. Transparent films with simple sketches of the images or models of teeth can also be very helpful in demonstrating the matching details in court (Rötzscher 1972). Transparent wax is soft and molds easily to the cutting edge or occlusal surface. The photos must be labeled to avoid side confusions (R=right; L=left).

Paraffin wax impressions can be laid over the track. This method might be more objective than the application of a transparent film. Comparative microscopy is used less often, except in cases where grinding marks at the cutting edges are obvious and must be compared with test marks (Solheim 1980).

23.10.1.1 The Stereometric Drawing

Teeth and tooth marks can reproduced into different levels with the help of lines in a stereometric plan drawing (stereometric graphic plotting), a technique similar to the drawing of maps.

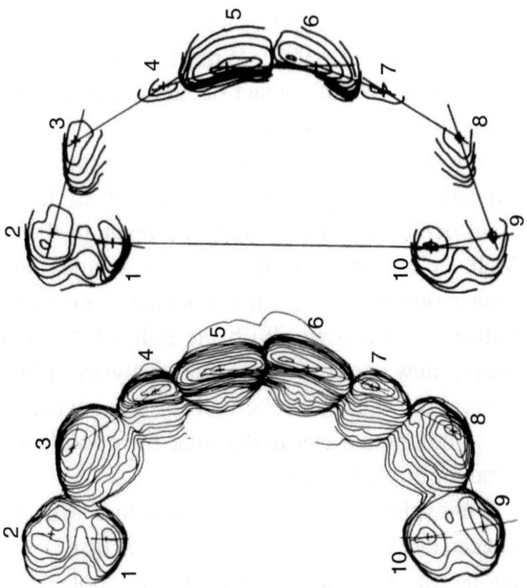

Figs. 23.14 and 23.15 Principle of the stereometric reconstruction of a bite mark in two levels. First level (*less teeth are visible*), Second level (*all teeth are visible*) (Frykholm et al. 1970)

Frykholm et al. (1970) included the canines and premolars in their analysis (Bang 1976). The distance between the teeth and the angle to each other are used as an identity criteria (Figs. 23.14 and 23.15). The method requires complicated equipment, which is available for PCs.

23.10.1.2 Scanning Electron Microscopy (SEM)

Scanning electron microscopy (SEM) produces a detailed picture of surfaces and is suitable for the analysis and comparison of tooth marks on the skin (Bang 1976) and in food (Solheim and Leidal 1976).

23.10.1.3 Computer-Assisted Image Analysis

Image analysis with the computer is available and images can be easily compared (Wood et al. 1994); manipulations are also possible (Aboshi et al. 1994).

Superimposition three-dimensional laser scanners can digitize individual chewing surfaces and also plaster models, and the results can be measured on the computer (Mehl et al. 1996, 1997). Changes in the occlusal surfaces (such as sanding and abrasions) can be statistically analyzed (Mehl et al. 1997). With this method, it is also obvious which contact occurs in each phase of the movement of the position.

Any type of sectional plane can be constructed, thus, the cusp–fissure relief in functional occlusion can be analyzed layer by layer (Mehl et al. 1997). Both sectional images and contact points can be simultaneously generated in different windows. With the help of "virtual reality," new perspectives for the analyses of bite marks are available. Nevertheless, the uncritical use of computers can undermine the confidence in the tooth mark analysis.

If unexplained incongruities are found, the suspect can be excluded. This is a safe conclusion and can be of great importance for the police. If matches are found, how likely it is that a particular suspect caused these marks must be judged. This is a very difficult task, and 100 % confidence in the results is not possible. Only rarely are the marks so obvious that all details can be deciphered.

Only few studies provide useful details for the frequencies of the comparison of tooth marks (MacFarlane et al. 1974; Hennis et al. 1981c). For most details, however, no such data exist. The experience of the forensic odontologist is requested. For an evaluation of the marks, the mutual covariates for all of the details should be taken into account. For instance, if a tooth is in an unusual position, it is likely that the contralateral tooth has a similar position. Unfortunately, there is very little scientific data for these covariates.

23.11 Conclusions

Berg and Schaidt (1954) conducted interesting experiments that showed the difficulty of the question of whether and what evidence should be attached to a line of human bite marks with tooth impressions of suspects. Technically accurate marks are not always available to the experts, but usually there are more or less good contour images of the outer profile of the incisors and of the canines.

The simultaneous contour coverage of at least four or five teeth next to each other is required before the evidence of identity in "normal dentition" can be called "provided" (Hammer 1956; Simon et al. 1971). However, the nature of the bite marks may allow conclusions about the age of the perpetrator. Above all, whether the bite marks are caused by permanent or deciduous teeth can be proven.

Martin (1959) notes that the results obtained should be interpreted very carefully. The conclusion should be a synthesis of the scientific data and the evaluation by the expert. The result is the opinion of the expert, which must be expressed clearly and unambiguously (Kerr 1977).

Tooth marks have a high significance in relation to a crime; it is important that the expert uses the power of the proof so that a guilty person is not acquitted in court. On the other hand, the conviction of an innocent person should not be risked.

Often the results of the examinations of bite marks is taken absolutely, i.e., whether the suspect has caused the track or not. From the scientific view, this is doubtful because there is no 100 % guarantee. Only in rare special cases is the comparison of tooth marks sufficient as the sole evidence (Rötzscher 1972).

If the suspicion that a certain person has caused the tracks cannot be excluded, the following conclusions are usually used (Solheim 1980):

1. It is *more likely* that the suspect has set the marks.

   With "almost absolute certainty" (reasonable medical/dental certainty). In these cases, the expert should be confident that the suspect has caused the track. This means that another expert with the same education, experience, and background knowledge would obtain the same result.
2. It is *likely* ("identity probable") that the suspect has set the marks. This phrase is used if an absolute certainty is not given, but many details do match. The conclusion is a strong

indication. Nevertheless, there is still a chance that another person has the same characteristics.

3. It is *possible* ("identity possible") that the suspect has set the bite marks.

   There are not many positive details, but the possibility that the suspect has set the traces cannot be excluded. This conclusion is dangerous because the judge may misinterpret the content of this terminology. The expert must be aware that the suspect cannot be excluded, even though only few positive evidences have been found. That means there is still a substantial probability that another person has caused the marks.

The use of the terms "actually, without a doubt ..." or "... I believe the suspect has caused the track" or "... no one else in the world could have caused the track" is not provable and negligent. The dentist must remember that lawyers have a different use of words (which is part of their job) from dentists, who use the words to convey ideas and thoughts. The dentist must be aware that in court words and terms are subject to strict scrutiny and sometimes are taken out of context (Stimson and Mertz 1997). Note that if tooth marks are linked to a crime, it is possible that the causer of the traces is not the perpetrator of the crime. It is very unlikely but not excluded that two individuals with otherwise unusual characteristics are involved in the same trial (Stimson and Mertz 1997).

23.12 Demands on the Expert

The investigation of tooth marks and the comparison with teeth of people who could have set the marks are similar to the analysis of all other evidence. However, a profound knowledge of the teeth and their variations, particularly in the frontal area, is necessary to understand the details of the marks. Also, in comparison, this knowledge is absolutely necessary to correctly determine the details.

Studies of bite marks/tooth marks are always difficult and require experience and interest (Endris 1979). The marks are not set in impression material, but in a medium that compounds the detection of details. Therefore, it is essential that the investigating authorities have a forensic odontologic consultant. Bite/tooth marks in criminal cases should always be investigated by forensic odontologists and carefully and adequately compared with all suspected persons.

The investigation of a tooth mark requires the following parameters (Stimson 1980):

1. Date, time, and approval of the investigation
2. Detailed description of the victim/suspect
3. Detailed analysis and finding (documentation)
4. Type of camera and film batch used
5. Detection of anomalies
6. Absence of dentures, etc.

If the investigator is not experienced, there is an enhanced risk that the significance of characteristic details will be overestimated or uncharacteristic details will be underestimated or completely overlooked. This bears the risk that a guilty person is not convicted (Martin 1959), or, even worse, that an innocent person is convicted.

23.13 Final Remark

The analysis and the conclusions drawn from the analysis must be documented in written form because it is a forensic report. The expert should be appointed by the court in order to give a verbal presentation of the investigation. The rules are from the Code of Criminal Procedure (CCD). In countries with the Napoleonic Criminal Procedure, e.g., Germany, the expert is a neutral advisor to the court. The expert must convince the court of their knowledge in bite/tooth mark analysis. It is of greatest importance that the expert is neutral and does not exceed their authority.

Appendix A Annex 23.1

Drawing chart of the skin, hands (for drawings form SMD) (Rev. 1/91 © 1989 by JB & Sobel MN)

Anhang H-1: Hautzeichnungsdiagramm, Hände

Case Number: ______________________ Exam. Date: ______________________

Marks Found On:

❑ Victim's Name: ______ LAST ______ FIRST ______ MIDDLE

❑ Victim's Name: ______ LAST ______ FIRST ______ MIDDLE

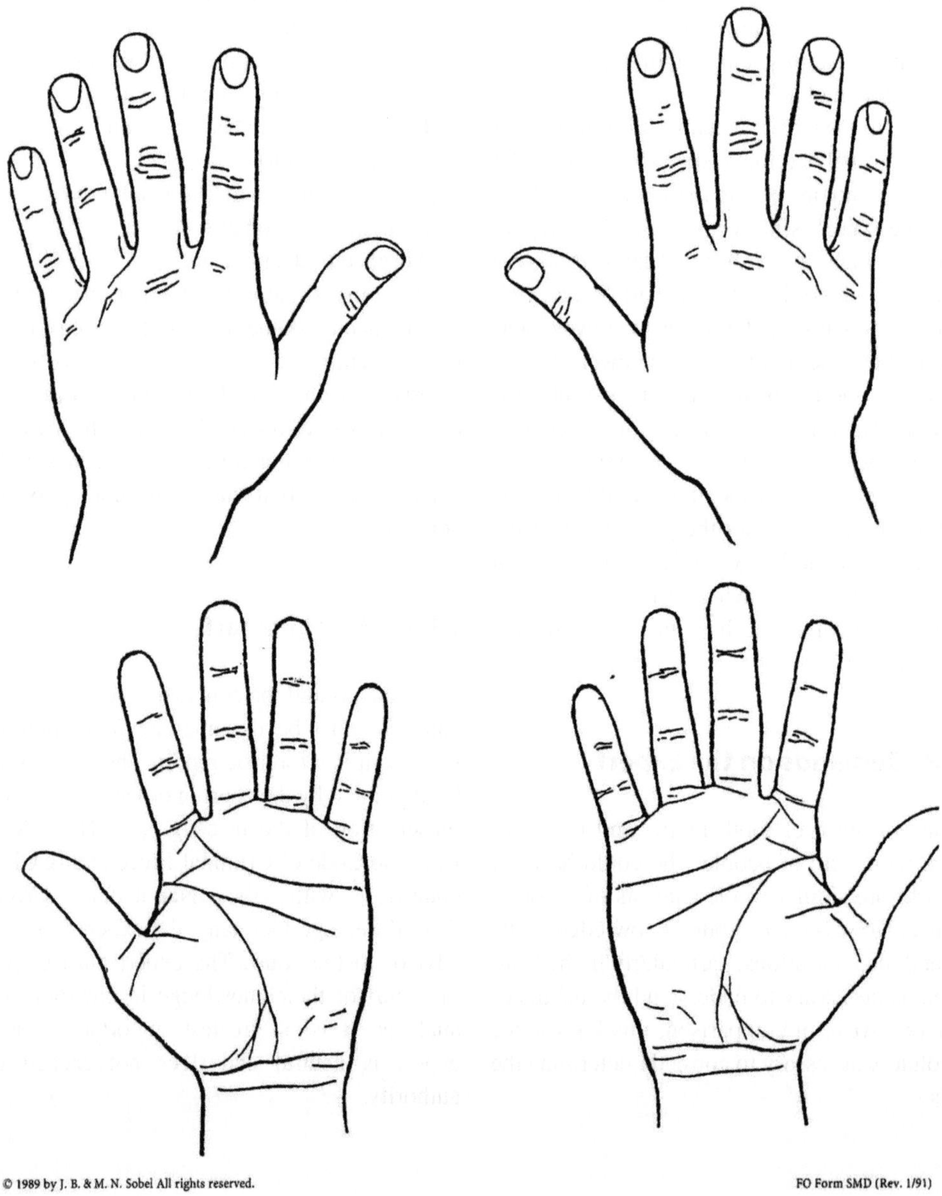

FO Form SMD (Rev. 1/91)

Appendix B Annex 23.2

Drawing chart of the skin, head (for drawings form SMD) (Rev. 1/91 © 1989 by JB & Sobel MN)

Init.: ________ **Skin Marking Diagram** ____ of ____

Case Number: ______________________ Exam. Date: ______________________

Marks Found On:

❑ Victim's Name: ______ LAST ______ FIRST ______ MIDDLE

❑ Victim's Name: ______ LAST ______ FIRST ______ MIDDLE

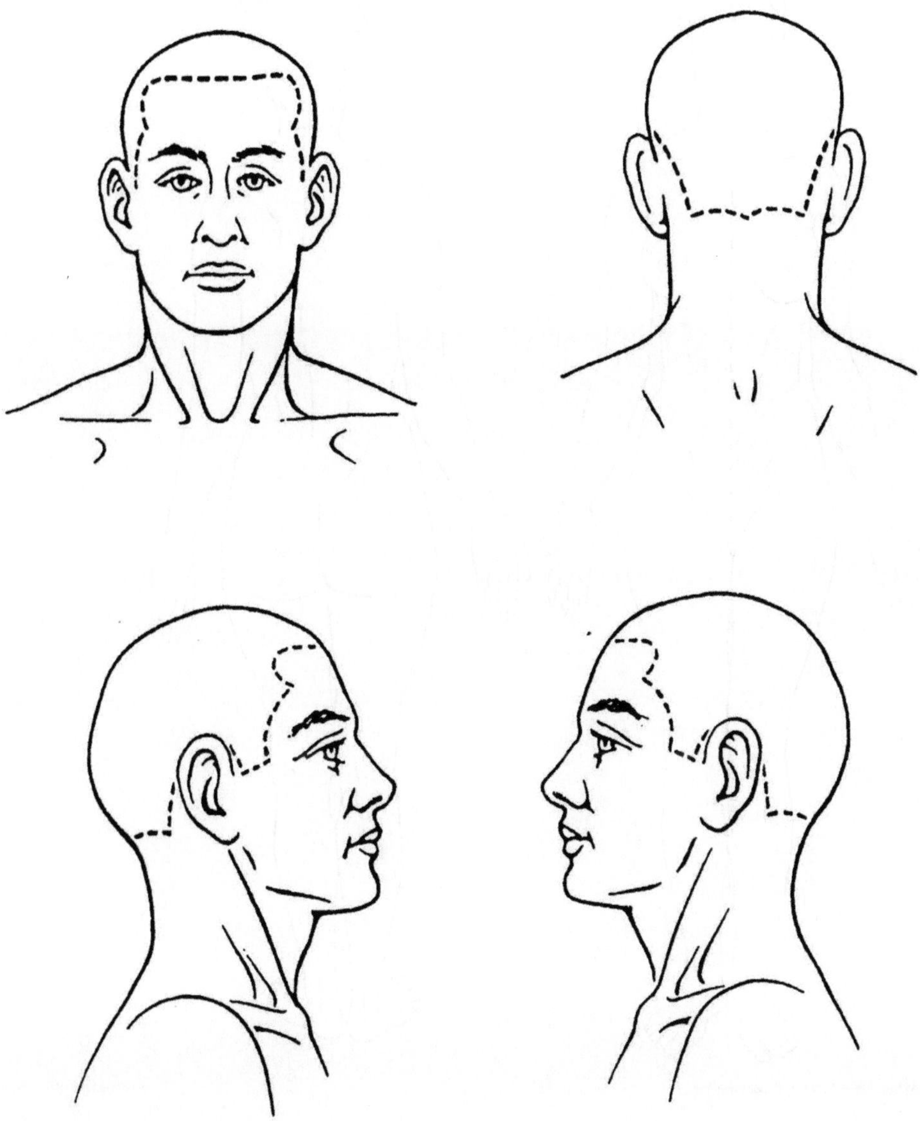

FO Form SMD (Rev. 1/91)

Appendix C Annex 23.3

Drawing chart of the skin, body, female diagram

Init.: ______ **Skin Marking Diagram** ____ of ____

Case Number: ______________________ Exam. Date: ______________________

Marks Found On:

- ❑ Victim's Name: ______________________
  LAST FIRST MIDDLE
- ❑ Victim's Name: ______________________
  LAST FIRST MIDDLE

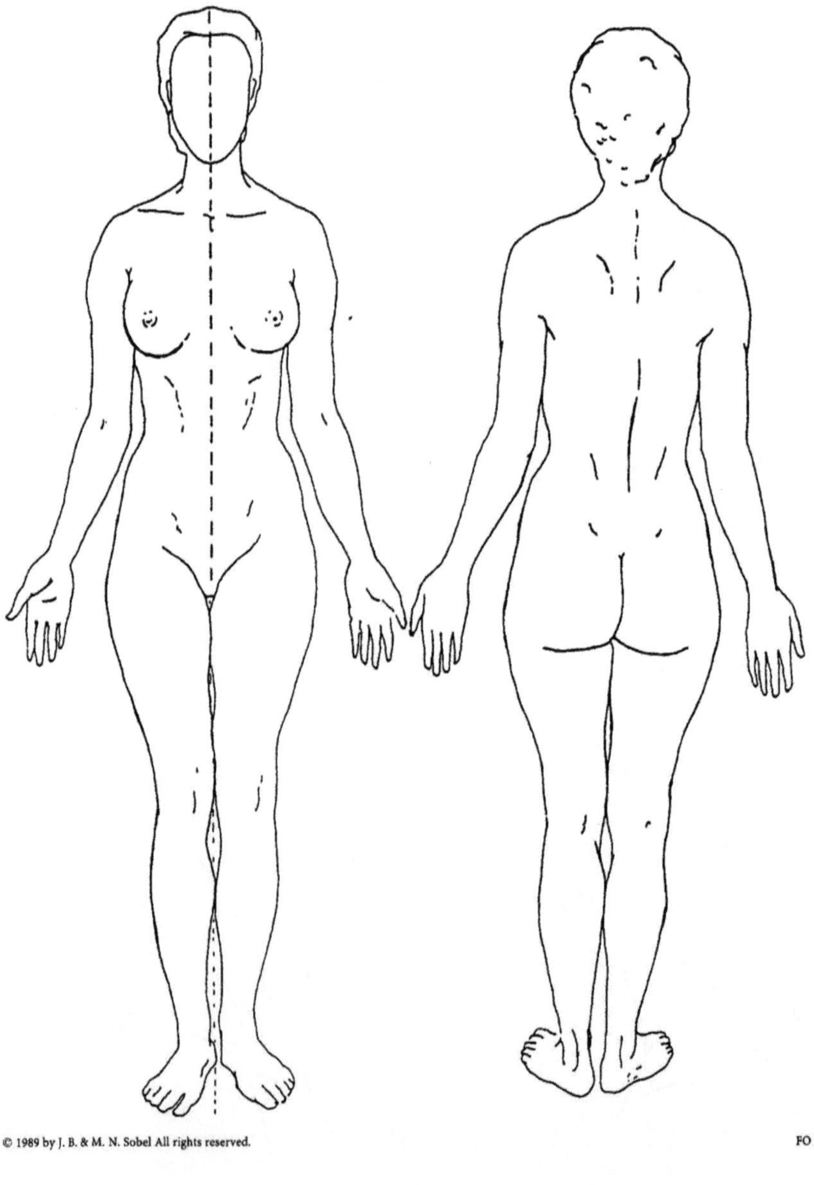

FO Form SMD (Rev. 1/91)

Appendix D Annex 23.4

Drawing chart of the skin, body, male diagram

Init.: ____ **Skin Marking Diagram** ____ of ____

Case Number: ____________ Exam. Date: ____________

Marks Found On:

❑ Victim's Name: ____________ LAST ____________ FIRST ____________ MIDDLE

❑ Victim's Name: ____________ LAST ____________ FIRST ____________ MIDDLE

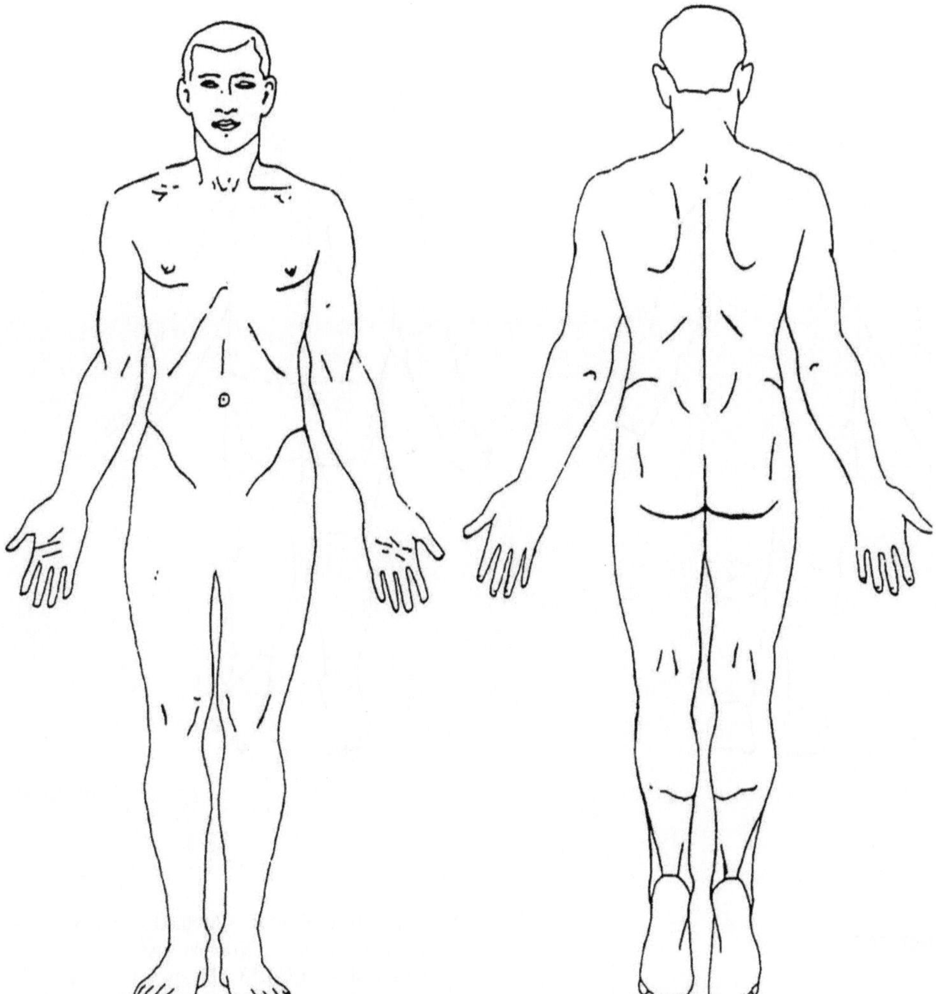

FO Form SMD (Rev. 1/91)

Appendix E Annex 23.5

Drawing chart of the skin, body, child

Init.: ______ **Skin Marking Diagram** ____ of ____

Case Number: ______________ Exam. Date: ______________

Marks Found On:

❑ Victim's Name: ______________ LAST FIRST MIDDLE

❑ Victim's Name: ______________ LAST FIRST MIDDLE

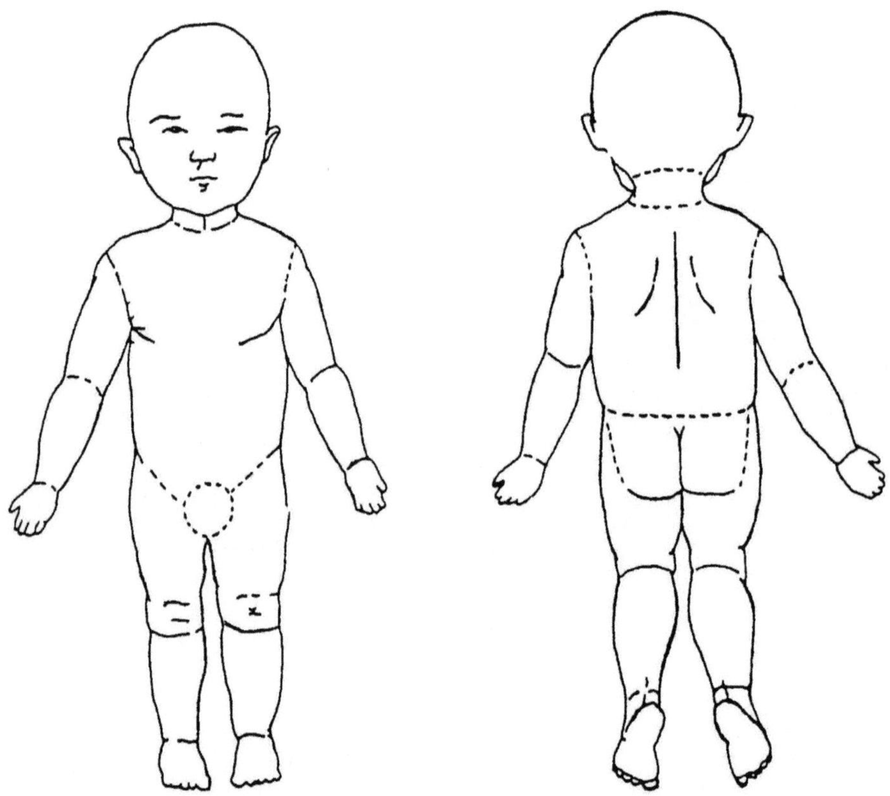

FO Form SMD (Rev. 1/91

References

Aboshi H, Taylor JA, Takei T, Brown KA (1994) Comparison of bitemarks in foodstuffs by computer imaging: a case report. J Forensic Odontostomatol 12(2):41–44

Bang G (1976) Analysis of tooth marks in a homicide case. Observation by means of visual description, stereophotography, scanning electron microscopy and stereometric graphic plotting. Acta Odontol Scand 34:1–11

Berg S, Schaidt G (1954) Methodik und Beweiswert des Bisspurvergleichs. Kriminalwiss 1:128–130, Beil z Kriminalistik 1954:53. Mitt auf dem Kongress der Dtsch Ges gerichtl und soziale Medizin, Kiel, 1.-3.Okt.1954. In: Dtsch Zschr gerichtl Med 44: 443 (1955/56)

Berk JK, Spencer DE, Mar GL (1997) Dog Bites and a "Dog Bite". F43. In: Proceedings AAFS annual meeting, New York, 17–22 Feb 1997, p 117

Bohmer K (1925) Postmortale Zerstorung durch Tiere und Rattenbis am Lebenden. Zschr Med Beamte 38(47):215–218

Buhtz, Ehrhardt (1938) Die Identitatsfragen von Biswunden (Experimentelle Untersuchungen). Dtsch Z Gesamte Gerichtl Med 29:453–468
Clark DH (1992) Chapter 10. Bite mark examination procedures: victims and suspects. In: Clark DH (ed) Practical forensic odontology. Wright Linacre House, Jordan Hill, pp 128–137
Dorion R (1995) Translumination of bitemarks. In: Bowers CM, Bell GL (eds) Manual of forensic odontology, 3rd edn. ASFO, AAFS, P.O. Box 669, Colorado Springs, p 173
Du Chesne A (1968) Bisverletzungen bei todlichen Unfallen mit Tieren. Vortrag, 1. Gemeinschaftstagung Ges Exp Med, Leipzig, 2 Oct 1968
Du Chesne A, Rötzscher K (1968) Zur Moglichkeit der Identifizierung von Tierbissen. Vortrag, 1. Gemeinschaftstagung Ges Exp Med, Leipzig, 2 Oct 1968
Endris R (1979) Bissmarken. In: Praktische forensische Stomatologie. Kriminalistik, Heidelberg, S 279–299
Endris R (1985) Biß und Bißspur, Kriminalistik - Wissenschaft & Praxis, Bd.18. Kriminalistik, Heidelberg
Endris R, Hilgert W (1975) Bissmarken bei Sexualdelikten. Spurensicherung, Abformung und Beweisfuhrung. Kriminalistik 29(9):406–409
Euler H (1937) Zahnarztliche Mitarbeit in der Kriminalistik. Nor Tannlaegeforen Tid 47:303–318
Free EW (1995) A bitemark and a fracture? Case report. J Forensic Odontostomatol 13(2):33–35
Frykholm KO, Wictorin L, Torlegard K (1970) Analysis of teeth-marks with stereometric reproduction. Sven Tandlak Tidskr 63(3):205–218
Fulton PR (1984) Child abuse and a bite mark. A case report. J Forensic Odontostomatol 2(2):53–55
Graw M, Pflug W, Benz D, Kugler M (1998) Morphologische Befunderhebung und DNATypisierung an Hornhaut als Beitrag zur Tateridentifikation. Rechtsmedizin 8:112–114
Haak HH (1970) Die Selbstverletzung aus phylogenetischer und psychiatrischer Sicht. Psychiat Neurol Med Psychol (Leipz) 22:247–249
Hammer H (1956) Die Mitarbeit des Zahnarztes in forensischen Fragen. Vortrag, FDITagung, Kopenhagen, 19.8.1955. Zahnarztl Mitt 44:156–160
Helmer R (1998) Die Weichteilbedeckung des Gesichtes und Kopfes. In: Leopold D (Hrsg) Identifikation unbekannter Toter. Schmidt-Romhild, Lubeck, pp 469,483,496
Hennis I, Schienbein H, Scholl E (1981a) Die forensische Verwertbarkeit von menschlichen Bisspuren bei Stellungsanomalien der Zahne (II). Quintessenz 11:2141–2150
Hennis I, Schienbein H, Scholl E (1981b) Die forensische Verwertbarkeit von menschlichen Bisspuren bei Stellungsanomalien der Zahne (III). Quintessenz 12: 2349–2360
Hennis I, Schienbein H, Scholl E (1981c) Menschliche Bissspuren bei Stellungsanomalien der Zahne und ihre forensische Verwendbarkeit. Teil 2. Kriminalistik 35(4):176–180
Houtrow T (1963) Uber die gerichtlich-medizinische Wurdigung von Bisverletzungen durch Mensch und Tier. Dtsch Z Gesamte Gerichtl Med 16:89
Humble BH (1933) Identification by means of teeth. Br Dent J 54:528–536
Keiser-Nielsen S (1947) Retsodontologisk casuistik. Identfikation paa grundlag af et bidspor. Tandlaegebladet 51(2):41–52
Kerr NW (1977) Apple bite mark identification of a suspect. Int J Forensic Dent 4(13):20–23
Langer AK (1861) Zur Anatomie und Physiologie der Haut. Sitzungsber, vol 19. Wiss D K Akademie, Dresden, p 179
Ligthelm AJ, van Niekerk PJ (1995) Comparative review of bitemark cases from Pretoria, South Africa. J Forensic Odontostomatol 12(2):23–29
Lundevall J (1989) Courtesy of Universitetsforlaget, Oslo. *Rettsmedisin*. Forensic Med
Luntz LL, Luntz P (1973) A case in forensic odontology: a bite-mark in a multiple homicide. Oral Surg Oral Med Oral Pathol 36:2–78
MacFarlane TW, MacDonald DG, Sutherland DA (1974) Statistical problems in dental identification. J Forensic Sci 14:247–252
Marshall W, Potter J, Harvey W (1974) Bite marks in apples – forensic aspects. Criminol 9:21–34
Martin O (1959) Suche, Sicherung, Untersuchung und Auswertung von Spuren in Sittlichkeitsstrafsachen. Kriminalistik 13:330–335
Mehl A, Gloger W, Kunzelmann KH, Hickel R (1996) Entwicklung eines neuen optischen Oberflachenmesgerates zur prazisen dreidimensionalen Zahnvermessung. Dtsch Zahnarztl Z 51:23
Mehl A, Gloger W, Kunzelmann KH, Hickel R (1997) A new optical 3D-device for the detection of wear. J Dent Res 76:1799
Melchior (1929) Mitarbeit des Zahnarztes bei der Identifizierung von Leichen. Med. Dissertation, Berlin
Mills PB (1976) An unusual case of bite mark identification. Int J Forensic Dent 11:38–39
Mittleman RE, Stuver WC, Souvron R (1980) Obtaining saliva samples from bitemark evidence. FBI Law Enforc Bull 49:16–19
Mollaret P (1969) Infektionen nach Katzen- und Rattenbis. Munch Med Woschenschr 111:13
Nehrkorn K, Sturm F (1974) Uber den Aussagewert der Identifikation menschlicher Bisspuren an Weichgeweben. Med. disseration, Dresden
Pilz W, Zerndt B (1963) Eine Analyse menschlicher Zahnschartenspuren. Arch Kriminol 132:61–76
Pilz W, Reimann W, Krause DH (1980) Biß und Bißspur. In: Gerichtliche Medizin für Stomatologen. JA Barth, Leipzig, pp 150–174, 183–186
Prokop O (1966) Forensische Medizin, 2nd edn. Volk und Gesundheit, Berlin, p 458
Rotzscher K (1972) Die forensische Stomatologie – eine forensische Wissenschaft. IV. Die Bedeutung der Bisspur als Beweismittel. Dtsch Stomatol 22Jg(H.5): 390–398
Rotzscher K, Reimann W (1975) Die forensische Stomatologie. In: Prokop O, Gohler W (eds) Forensische Medizin, 3rd edn. Volk und Gesundheit, Berlin, pp S545–S564
Ruddick RF (1974) A technique for recording bite marks for forensic studies. Med Biol Illus 24:128–129

Saar H (1952) Untersuchungen uber das Verhalten nichtverletzender Bisse. Kriminalistik 6:32
Selle G (1966) Zahnarztliche Moglichkeiten zur Identifizierung von Bisspuren. Dtsch Stomatol 16(561):566
Simon A, Adam J, Jordan H (1971) Zur Beurteilung und Identifizierung von Bisverletzungen der menschlichen Haut – zugleich ein Beitrag ihres Beweiswertes im Ermittlungs- und Gerichtsverfahren. Kriminalistik Forens Wiss 6:161
Sobel MN, Perper JA (1985) Self-inflicted bite mark on the breast of a suicide victim. Am J Forensic Med Pathol 6(4):336–339
Sognnaes RF (1977) The case for better bite and bite mark preservations. Int J Forensic Dent 4(13):17–19
Solheim T (1980) Unusual dental forensic cases in Norway. Am J Forensic Med Pathol 1:197–203
Solheim T, Leidal TI (1976) Scanning electron microscopy in the investigation of bite marks in foodstuffs. Forensic Sci 6:205–215
Sorup A (1926) Odontoskopie. Ein Beitrag zur zahnarztlichen Kriminalistik. Dtsch Monatschr Zahnheilkd 21:777–784
Stimson PG (1980) Maintaining chain of evidence from beginning of case. In: Siegel R, Sperber N (eds) Forensic odontology workbook, ASFO II, New York, p 1
Stimson PG, Mertz CA (1997) Chapter 7: Bite mark techniques and terminology. In: Stimson PG, Mertz (eds) Forensic dentistry. pp 137–159
Strauch N (1927) Über Anfressen von Leichen durch Hauskatzen. Dtsch Z Gesamte Gerichtl Med 10:457–469
Strom F (1963) Investigation of bite-marks. J Dent Res 42:312–316
Sweet DJ (1995) Chapter 5. Bitemark evidence. Human bitemarks: examination, recovery and analysis. In: Bowers CM, Bell GL (eds) Manual of forensic odontology, 3rd edn. ASFO, AAFS, P.O. Box 669, Colorado Springs, pp 148–169
Thompson IOC, Phillips VM (1994) A bitemark case with a twist. J Forensic Odontostomatol 12(2):37–40
Trube-Becker E (1973) Bisspuren bei Kindsmishandlung. Beitr Gerichtl Med 31:115
Tsokos M, Schulz F (1999) Indoor postmortem animal interference by carnivores and rodents: report of two cases and review of the literature. Int J Legal Med 112:115–119
Ulrich K (1963) Uber die Haufigkeit und Vielgestaltigkeit der Verletzungen durch Menschenbisse und ihre Brauchbarkeit bei der Aufklarung von Verbrechen. Med. dissertation, Leipzig
Wood RE, Miller PA, Blenkinsop PB (1994) Image editing and computer assisted bitemark analysis: a case report. J Forensic Odontostomatol 12(2):30–36
Zerndt B (1964) Zur forensischen Beurteilung von Bisverletzungen. Arch Kriminol 133:1
Zerndt B, Simon A (1962) Uber den Nachweis von Epidermisresten an Kleidern bei Bisverletzungen. Arch Kriminol 129:27–33

Lip Marks

24

Klaus Rötzscher and Wolfgang Pilz

Similar to the skin (ridges) and the palatal mucosa (rugae and plicae), the lips have a surface shaped by characteristic sulci (Rackowitz 1968). Because these features remain unchanged throughout life, lip marks (cheiloscopy) may identify a person as well as fingerprints (dactyloscopy) (Rackowitz 1968; Suzuki and Tsuchihashi 1970; Pilz et al. 1980; Whittaker and MacDonald 1993) (Fig. 24.1). Labyt-Leroy, Laborier, and Georget presented a comparative study in 1999; see also Figs. 24.2, 24.3, 24.4 and 24.5.

Lip reliefs in model types can be classified as (modified from Suzuki 1970; Tsuchihashi and Suzuki 1970):

1. Type I: vertical furrows over the entire lip
2. Type Ia: partial vertical furrows
3. Type II: branched furrows
4. Type III: crossed furrows
5. Type IV: net-drawing
6. Type V: other patterns

A complete copy of the upper and lower lips (on letters or mirror) allows not only individual identification (after Rackowitz 1968; Fig. 24.3) but also an approximate determination of age. A fine classification and a percentile age distribution of lip pattern types was worked out by Rackowitz (1968).

Pathological changes in the lip redness (*benigne tumores*) are not stable features, but may be significant (in addition to the lip pattern) in identifying a person, e.g., in a comparison with a photograph (Labyt-Leroy et al. 1999). Lip relief types (Rackowitz 1968) (see Fig. 24.3) are:

(a) Vertical grooves (I)
(b) Vertical furrows net fine (II_1)
(c) Vertical furrows net coarse (II_2)
(d) Net without wrinkles, fine (III_1)
(e) Net without wrinkles, coarse (III^1)
(f) Net with many folds (III_2)
(g) Net with a few wrinkles (III^2)
(h) Dedifferentiated with horizontal folding (IV_1)
(i) Dedifferentiated with irregular folding (IV^1)
(j) Dedifferentiated with furrows and folds poverty (IV_2)

Lip print marks can be conveniently photographed.

K. Rötzscher, Dr. med. Dr. med. dent. (✉)
German Academy of Forensic Odontostomatology (AKFOS),
Wimphelingstraße 7, 67346 Speyer, Germany
e-mail: roetzscher.klaus.dr@t-online.de

W. Pilz, Univ.-Prof. (em) Dr. med. dent.
Department of Preservative and Pediatric Stomatology, Academy Carl Gustav Carus,
Dresden, Germany

K. Rötzscher (ed.), *Forensic and Legal Dentistry*,
DOI 10.1007/978-3-319-01330-5_24,

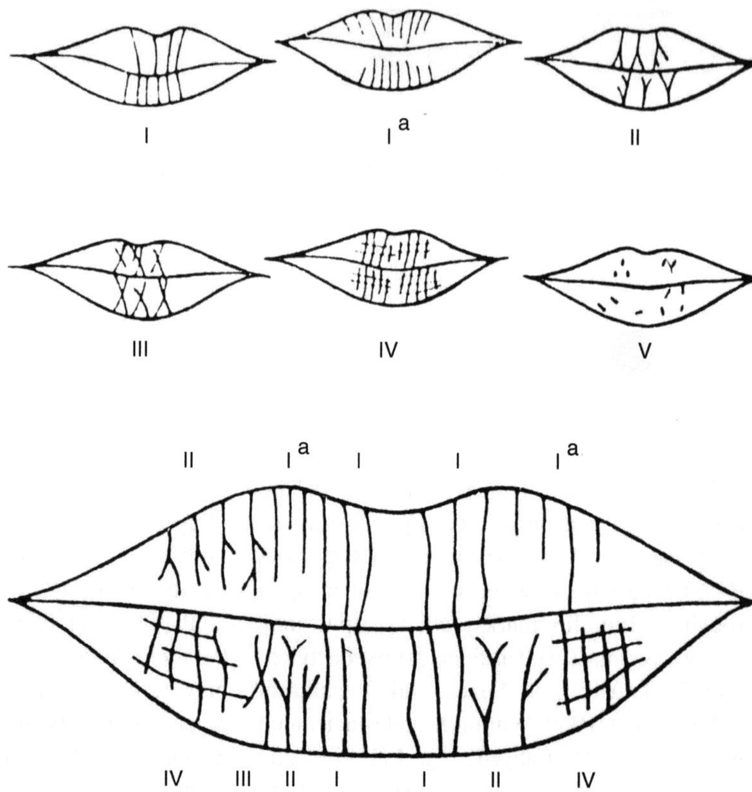

Fig. 24.1 Types of lip reliefs (Suzuki 1970; Suzuki and Tsuchihashi 1970)

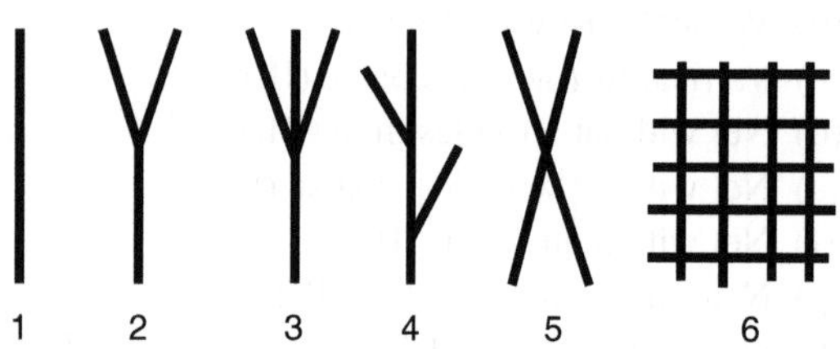

Fig. 24.2 Comparative studies by Georget and Laborier (1999)

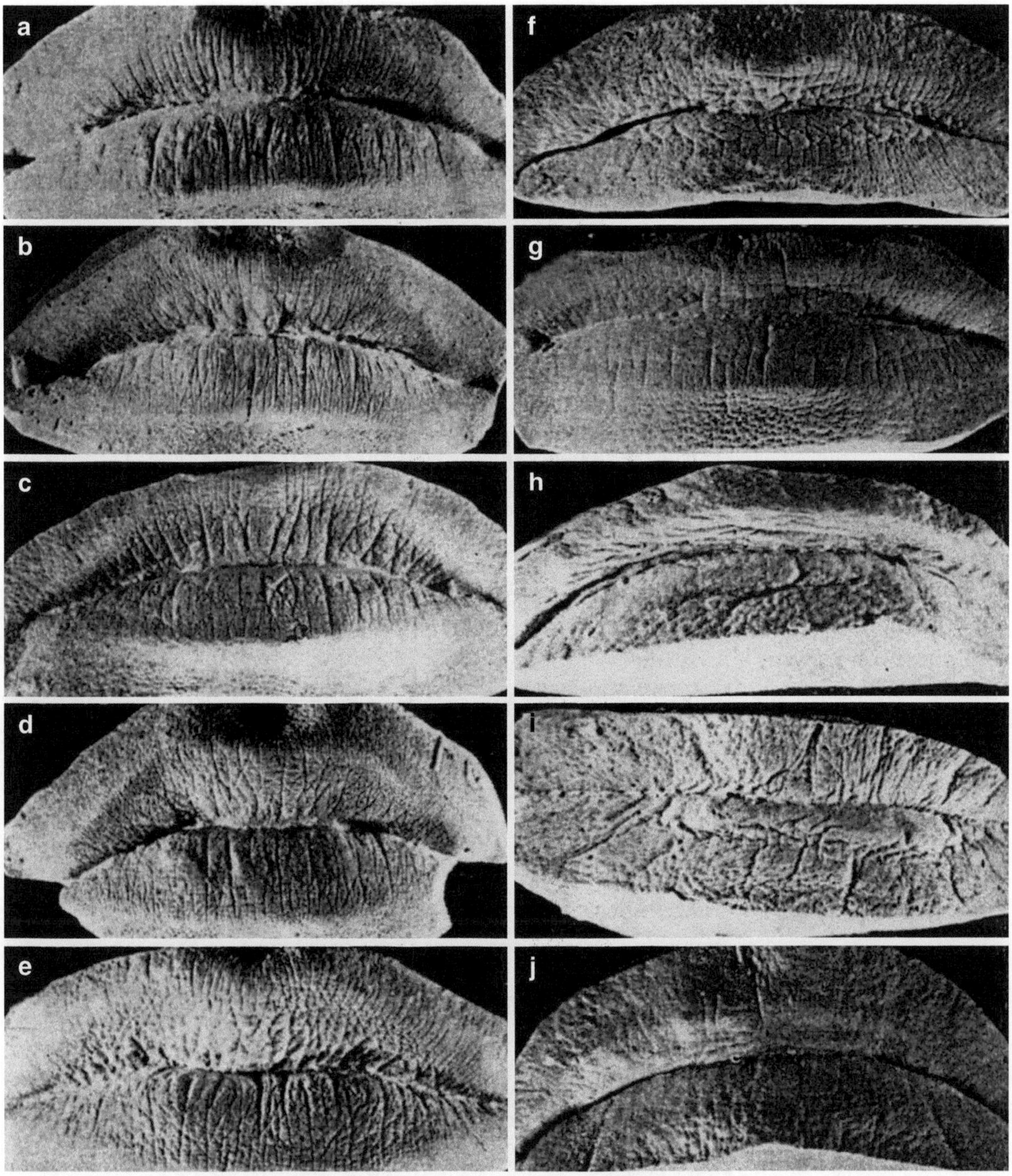

Fig. 24.3 Lip relief types (Rackowitz 1968)

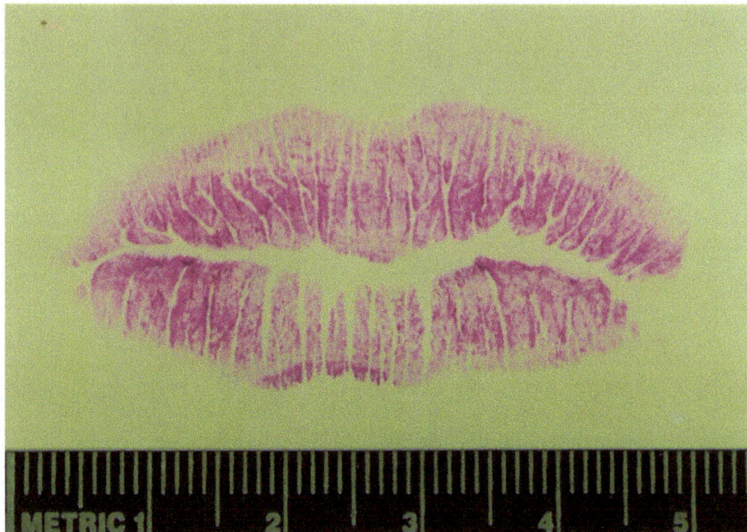

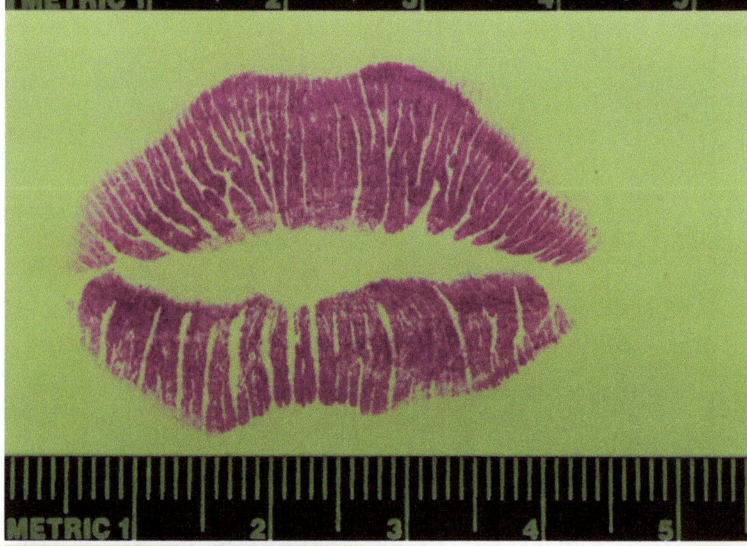

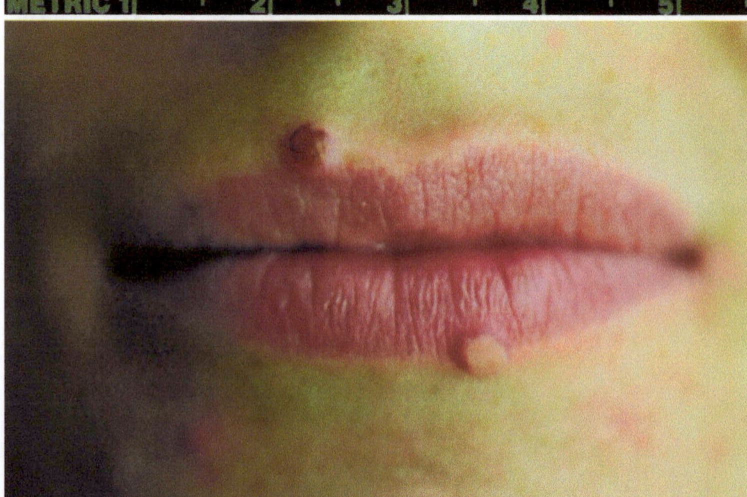

Figs. 24.4 and 24.5 One person can have different reliefs depending on the intensity of the print (Courtesy of Ch. Georget, AFIO 1999)

References

Pilz W, Reimann W, Krause DH (1980) Biß und Bißspur. In: Gerichtliche Medizin für Stomatologen. JA Barth, Leipzig, pp 150–174, 183–186

Rackowitz M (1968) Das Oberflächenrelief des menschlichen Lippenrots. Med. Dissertation, Dresden

Suzuki K (1970) Forensic odontology and criminal investigation. Acta Crim Jpn 36(3):88–102

Suzuki K, Tsuchihashi Y (1970) New attempt of personal identification by means of lip print. J Forensic Med 17:52

Whittaker DK, MacDonald DG (1993) Lippenabdrücke. In: Whittaker DK, MacDonald DG (eds) Atlas der forensischen Zahnmedizin. Deutscher Ärzte-Verlag, Köln, S. 55

Index

K. Rötzscher (ed.), *Forensic and Legal Dentistry*,
DOI 10.1007/978-3-319-01330-5, © Springer International Publishing Switzerland 2014

MIX
Papier aus verantwortungsvollen Quellen
Paper from responsible sources
FSC® C105338

If you have any concerns about our products,
you can contact us on
ProductSafety@springernature.com

In case Publisher is established outside the EU,
the EU authorized representative is:
Springer Nature Customer Service Center GmbH
Europaplatz 3, 69115 Heidelberg, Germany

Printed by Libri Plureos GmbH
in Hamburg, Germany